HUMAN INTESTINAL FLORA

HUMAN INTESTINAL FLORA

B. S. DRASAR

Bacterial Metabolism Research Laboratory,
Central Public Health Laboratories, London, England
and
Medical Research Council Gastroenterology Unit,
Central Middlesex Hospital, London, England

and

M. J. HILL

Bacterial Metabolism Research Laboratory,
Central Public Health Laboratories, London, England

1974

ACADEMIC PRESS

LONDON   NEW YORK   SAN FRANCISCO
A Subsidiary of Harcourt Brace Jovanovich, Publishers

ACADEMIC PRESS INC. (LONDON) LTD.
24/28 Oval Road,
London NW1

United States Edition published by
ACADEMIC PRESS INC.
111 Fifth Avenue
New York, New York 10003

Library of Congress Catalog Card Number: 73-18997
ISBN: 0—12—221750—0

Printed in Great Britain by
The Whitefriars Press Ltd,
London and Tonbridge

PREFACE

Because our relationship with our intestinal flora is stable and symbiotic it is usually ignored. Disease may result from the disturbance of this relationship. Thus the displacement of *Escherichia coli,* a benign organism, by *Salmonella typhi* or *Shigella sonnei* results in severe disease. A change in the balance of the large intestinal flora as a result of antiobiotic action often results in diarrhoea; a change in the distribution of the flora down the gut results in steatorrhoea and folate deficiency. There is a growing interest in the nature and the causes of these changes, and for these and a host of other reasons the gut flora and its biochemical activities are no longer simply the academic interest of some bacteriologists and biochemists but also occupy the minds of many pharmacologists and gastroenterologists.

Research can be divided into two parts, these being (a) problem identification followed by (b) problem solving. The subject of this book is young and fast growing, but is still largely concerned with problem identification. In this work we have attempted to provide a integrated picture of the intestinal flora and its activities in health and disease. The book is divided into three sections. In section I the flora is described in health and disease; we outline the shortcomings in our knowledge as well as the results of the remarkable progress that has been made in the last 15 years. In section II some of the biochemical activities have been outlined. This is an enormous subject and our choice had been restricted to a few topics, shamelessly chosen for their interest to the authors and assumed by them to be important; others may wish other topics had been examined. In section III we bring the flora and their metabolism together in the discussion of a few disease states, again dominated by our research interests. By choosing the topics in this way we can better portray the concepts and rationale behind the experiments and hope that these might be of use to other specialists in their own chosen field.

We would like to thank Professors R. E. O. Williams and R. T. Williams who awakened our initial interest in the subject and were a constant source of encouragement. Our colleagues Vivienne Aries, Gabrielle Hawksworth, Susan Peach, John Crowther and Paul Goddard were enthusiastic workers responsible for many of the results described in this book. Much of the clinical work was done with the help and support of the MRC Gastroenterology Unit at Central Middlesex Hospital; our collaborative experiments with that department has been a major source of our data and of our constant intellectual renewal and for this we are especially grateful to Doctors Margot Shiner, E. N. Rowlands, Hugh Wiggins and John Cummings. Finally we must thank our wives for their forbearance while this book was being written, that they are still with us is a great tribute to their patience and fortitude in our hour of need.

London   B. S. DRASAR
July, 1974   M. J. HILL

CONTENTS

PREFACE v

SECTION I

Composition of the Gut Flora

Introduction

Limitations of the Data

I	Limitations to study of micro-organisms in the environment .	3
	A Collection of specimens	4
	B The isolation of intestinal bacteria	5
II	Limitations of the study of pure isolated strains of micro-organisms	7
III	Limitations to the study of physiological aspects of environment	8
IV & V	The study of washed cell suspensions or purified enzymes . .	8

Chapter 1

Factors Controlling and Influencing the Gut Flora

I	Host physiology	9
	A Intestinal secretions	10
	B The intestinal mucosa	11
	C Immune mechanisms	12
	D Intestinal motility	14
II	Environmental factors	15
	A Bacterial contamination	15
	B Diet	18
	C Antibacterial drugs	20
III	Bacterial interactions	22
	A Stability of the flora	22
	B The exclusion of implants	22
	C Bacterial interactions	23

Chapter 2

The Intestinal Bacteria

I   Taxonomic relationship 26
II   The bacterial species isolated from the intestine 28
III The biochemical characteristics of some intestinal bacteria . . 28

Chapter 3

The Distribution of Bacterial Flora in the Intestine

I   The mouth 36
II   The stomach 38
III The small intestinal flora in people resident in Europe and
North America 38
IV The small intestinal flora in tropical residents 40
V   The large intestine and faeces 43

Chapter 4

Changes in the Bacterial Flora Associated with Alterations in the Intestine due to Disease or Surgery

I   Alteration in gastric function 44
    A   Pernicious anaemia and gastric achlorhydria 44
    B   Surgical procedures for gastric and duodenal ulcer . . . 46
    C   Colonic transplant 47
II   Conditions producing small intestinal stasis 47
    A   Small intestinal diverticulosis 47
    B   Other conditions 47
    C   Conditions allowing direct access from the colon to the
       upper intestine 47
    D   Ileostomy 50

SECTION II

The Metabolic Activities of Gut Bacteria

Introduction

Gut Bacteria, Importance in the Environment

Chapter 5

Bacterial Glycosidases

I   Introduction 54
II   Metabolism of glucuronides 54

III   Metabolism of glucosides 57
IV   Metabolism of disaccharides   65
V   Gut bacteria and the enterohepatic circulation of foreign
      compounds 68

Chapter 6

Metabolism of Nitrogen Compounds

I   Metabolism of primary amino groups 72
      A   Deamination   72
      B   N-esterification   78
II   Metabolism of secondary amino groups 79
      A   N-dealkylation 79
      B   N-nitrosation   80
III   Metabolism of tertiary and quaternary amines 83
IV   Hydrolysis and reduction of diazo compounds   85
V   Reduction of a nitro group, nitrate or nitrite   88
VI   Degradation of amino acids 90
      A   Amino acid decarboxylases 91
      B   Miscellaneous other reactions 94
VII   Production of phenols and phenol acids from tyrosine   . . . 96
VIII Metabolism of 3,4-dihydroxyphenylalanine (dopa) 98
IX   Metabolism of tryptophan   100

Chapter 7

Bile Acid Degradation

I   Cholanoylglycine hydrolase 104
II   Hydroxy-steroid-oxido-reductases   109
      A   7α-hydroxycholanoyl dehydrogenase   111
      B   12α-hydroxycholanoyl dehydrogenase   114
      C   3α-hydroxycholanoyl dehydrogenase   115
      D   Summary of properties of the hydroxysteroid dehydro-
           genases 116
III   Hydroxycholanoyl dehydroxylases 116
IV   Bile acid degradation in the human intestine   122

Chapter 8

Cholesterol Metabolism

I   Reduction of cholesterol to coprostanol 125
II   Cholesterol side chain cleavage   132

Chapter 9

Nuclear Dehydrogenation of Steroids

I Introduction of a double bond conjugated to an oxo group . 135
II Nuclear dehydration reactions 136
III Removal of the C-10-methyl substituents 138
IV Introduction of a nuclear bond conjugated to other double bonds 141

Chapter 10

The Metabolism of the Major Non-steroidal Biliary Components

I Introduction 144
II Bile pigment metabolism 145
III Metabolism of phospholipids 146

Chapter 11

Metabolism of Antibiotic Compounds

I Chloramphenicol metabolism 150
II Metabolism of sulphonamide antibiotics 153
III Metabolism of the penicillins 154
IV Inactivation by bacteria of streptomycin and other amino-glycosides 155

Chapter 12

Other Metabolic Reactions

I Hydrolysis of sulphate esters 159
II Ester and amide hydrolysis 161
III Aromatization reactions 162
IV Reduction of double bonds 163
V Dehydroxylation reactions 164
VI Decarboxylation reactions 166
VII Metabolism of intestinal mucin 167

SECTION III

The Significance of Gut Bacteria

Introduction

Some Problems in relation to the Intestinal Flora

Chapter 13

Malabsorption

I   Post pathogen malabsorption 173
II   The blind loop syndrome 174
    A   Alterations in the bacterial flora of the small intestine in the blind loop 175
    B   The mechanism of B_{12} malabsorption in the blind loop syndrome 175
    C   Steatorrhoea in the blind loop syndrome 175
    D   Other defects in the blind loop syndrome 175
III   Malabsorption and malnutrition in the tropics 178
    A   The tropical intestine 178
    B   Tropical sprue 179
IV   Whipples disease 181
V   The influence of malabsorption not caused by bacteria on the intestinal flora 181

Chapter 14

Acute Diarrhoeal Disease

I   Protective function of the flora 184
II   The agents of diarrhoeal disease 184
III   Diarrhoeas thought to be infective 189
    A   Weanling diarrhoea 189
    B   Travellers' diarrhoea 190
IV   Alterations in the flora 190
V   General considerations 191

Chapter 15

Role of Bacteria in the Aetiology of Cancer

I   Bacterial production of carcinogens 193
    A   From steroids 193
    B   Production of phenols and their possible significance . . 197
    C   Bacterial metabolism of tryptophan and its reactions to cancer 198
    D   Bacterial production of N-nitrosamines 201
    E   Miscellaneous bacterial reactions yielding carcinogens . . 201

II   Production of nitrosamines by bacteria, and its relation to
       human cancer 201
       A   The fate of ingested nitrate 204
III   Bacteria, steroids and cancer of the colon 212
       A   Epidemiological considerations 212
       B   Hypotheses 214
       C   Conclusions 220
IV   Bacteria, steroids and cancer of the breast 222

Chapter 16

Gut Bacteria and Hepatic Disease

I   Hyperammonemia 226
II   Production of toxic amines and phenols 229
III   Steatorrhoea and gallstones associated with hepatic disease . . 230

Chapter 17

The Significance of Gut Bacteria in Normal People

I   Ageing and survival 233
II   Nutrition and digestion 234
       A   Vitamins 234
       B   Intestinal structure and function 235
III   Body defence mechanism 235
       A   Humoral defence systems 236
       B   Cellular defence systems 236
IV   Ulcerative colitis 237

REFERENCES 239

SUBJECT INDEX 259

SECTION I

Composition of the Gut Flora

Limitations of the Data

The study of the ecology of a microbial environment such as the intestine may be examined at various levels, the ultimate aim of the study being to explain, in terms of the biochemical properties of purified enzymes, the biochemical modifications of the environment and the microbial interactions. In the intestine complexity is maximal, not only are the ecological interactions very varied but also variation in host physiology, and alimentation can cause short or long term environmental variations. Chemical microbiologists have considered five levels of research for the examination of microbial ecology (Woods, 1953) and a re-definition of these categories to accommodate the problem of the intestinal flora seems useful.

(i) *The study of micro-organisms in the natural environment.* This is the most complex level of experimentation. Studies at this level are usually limited to the enumeration of the bacteria present and measurement of the resultants of complex metabolic processes.

(ii) *The studies of isolated strains of micro-organisms in the laboratory.* Studies are usually directed to determining the identity and metabolic ability of the bacteria in an attempt to suggest which organisms are responsible for reactions found to occur in the intestine.

(iii) *The study of physiological aspects of the environment.* Animal experiments may be regarded as attempts to elucidate the human intestinal environment; for example, physiological mechanisms only postulated in man may be demonstrated in animals.

(iv) *The study of cell suspensions* enables the conditions under which reactions and transformations occur to be more closely defined.

(v) *The study of purified enzymes,* in theory at least, enables the mechanisms of the biochemical reactions and hence of the bacteria-bacteria and host-bacteria interactions occurring in the intestine to be explained.

I. Limitations to study of micro-organisms in the natural environment

Studies on the human intestine are complicated by the problems of obtaining specimens from locations other than the mouth or anus. The number of bacteria isolated is dependent on the sensitivity of the cultural methods used and the types of bacteria reported upon and the methods used for their identification. The analytical studies in this group are subject to all of these difficulties, in attempting to present an integrated picture of the intestinal flora we first consider the technical difficulties that may have influenced the results.

A. COLLECTION OF SPECIMENS

Several workers have obtained specimens from patients undergoing abdominal surgical operations without antibiotic pre-treatment and various methods of sampling the intestine have been used. In one method buffered saline, introduced and aspirated with a needle and syringe, is used to wash out a length of intestine between clamps (Cregan and Hayward, 1953; Anderson and Langford, 1958; Bishop and Allcock, 1960; Bornside and Cohen, 1965). In another the intestine was opened and the contents sampled (Hewetson, 1904; Barber and Franklin, 1946; Bach-Neilson, 1965). Excised appendices have also been examined (Hewetson, 1904; Seeliger and Werner, 1963).

The results obtained from washings are difficult to quantitate because it is never possible to recover all the wash fluid, and it is impossible to estimate how efficient the washing process may be. However, Anderson and Langford (1958) reported that their results with washings were similar to those obtained from intubation specimens and the animal experiments of Gorbach et al (1967a) seem to confirm this. However, specimens can be obtained at operation only from fasting anaesthetized subjects who are usually abnormal, but the section of the intestine sampled can be accurately and easily defined, and this is the major advantage of the method.

1. *Intubation techniques*

Specimens of intestinal juice can be obtained through a peroral or nasal tube. Intubation techniques can be used to obtain samples from non-anaesthetized subjects; repeated samples can be obtained from any particular locus and the period for which sampling can be continued is not limited, thus enabling studies to be performed before, during, and after meals. The technique has, however, several disadvantages apart from the discomfort to the subject; the tube may stimulate peristalis and gastric or biliary secretions and thus affect the state of the intestinal contents, organisms may be carried down from above by the tube and contaminate the specimen, and the part of the intestine sampled is difficult to determine.

Open-ended tubes have been used extensively (e.g. Hess, 1912; Kalser *et al.*, 1966) but in an attempt to overcome the risk of contamination from the mouth, special sampling capsules have been devised which open and close only when they are in the position to be sampled (Van der Reis, 1925; Henning *et al.*, 1959; Shiner, 1963). Kalser *et al.* (1966) compared the results from 10 patients sampled using both the Shiner capsule and an open-ended polyvinyl tube and found no significant difference; similar results have been reported by other workers (Gorbach *et al.*, 1967; Williams and Drasar, 1972). The location of the sampling point is greatly assisted by the use of radioopaque tubing and X-rays (Van der Ries, 1925; Kendall *et al.*, 1927). The rapid transit tube devised by Wiggins *et al.* (1967) enables multiple samples to be obtained with one intubation and small samples are brought to the surface, so avoiding the reactions that can occur in the column of intestinal contents trapped in less complex tubes.

Though intubation is not an ideal technique its advantages out-weigh its disadvantages and it is to be preferred to the other techniques available.

2. *Self-opening capsule*

A free capsule was devised by Hirtzmann and Reuter (1963). It could be swallowed by the subject and opened by remote control when in the intestine; it was subsequently collected from the faeces. Discomfort to the subject is minimal. The sample is, however, incubated for a long time during the passage of the capsule from the collecting point to the anus and bacterial multiplications must occur.

B. THE ISOLATION OF INTESTINAL BACTERIA

1. *Preservation of specimens*

Crowther (1971) studied the survival of bacteria in faeces stored in various ways. Whole faeces could be held at room temperature for up to 24 h without loss of even the most fastidious bacteria; for prolonged storage the preferred method was ten-fold dilution in 10% glycerol broth and storage at −25°C or below. Freezing at −78°C in solid carbon dioxide or at −196°C in liquid nitrogen was satisfactory. Intestinal aspirates, have a much lower total bacterial count than faeces, and it seems best to insist either on immediate cultivation or immediate dilution in glycerol broth and freezing (Drasar *et al.*, 1969).

2. *Cultivation of bacteria*

The techniques employed in medical bacteriology have usually been devised for the selective isolation of "pathogens", similarly chemical microbiologists have concentrated upon the isolation of bacteria with particular metabolic properties. The examination of the intestinal flora requires the isolation of bacteria in the same numbers and relative proportion as they occur in the specimen. There are three types of system employed.

(a) *Standard methods.* The dominant organisms in the large bowel are strictly anaerobic (Sanborn, 1931) and although conventional methods are adequate for their isolation recovery is not quantitative. The loss of anaerobes probably results from the oxidation of media components and from the prolonged exposure of bacteria to oxygen dissolved in aerobically inoculated media even when placed in an anaerobic atmosphere (Drasar, 1967; Smith and Holdeman, 1968). Recently attempts have been made to overcome the problems of aerobically prepared media by use of oxidation-reduction buffering systems (Moore, 1968; Collee *et al.*, 1971) and these have considerably extended the range of application of standard methods.

(b) *Pre-reduced roll tube methods.* The cellulolytic bacteria occurring in the bovine rumen cannot be isolated by standard techniques. In order to isolate these bacteria Hungate (1950) devised a technique by which media can be prepared, distributed, sterilized and inoculated under an atmosphere of oxygen-free gas. Various modifications of the basic technique have been described (Bryant and Burkey, 1953; Moore, 1966; Latham and Sharpe, 1971; Anaerobe Laboratory Manual, 1972). The viable counts obtained from faeces are equal to the direct microscopic count (Moore *et al.*, 1969).

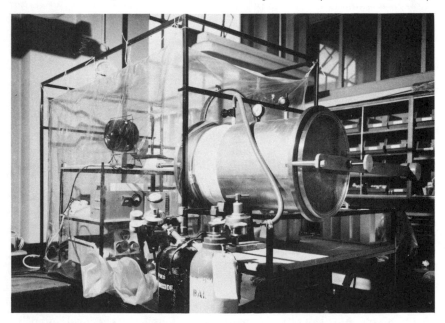

Fig. 1. An anaerobic cabinet

(c) *Cabinet methods* (Fig. 1). Anaerobic cabinets of various types have been devised to enable all standard bacteriological techniques to be carried out under an oxygen-free atmosphere. (Drasar, 1967; Lee *et al.*, 1968; Aranki *et al.*, 1969). The use of an anaerobic cabinet enables approximately 100 times more bacteria to be isolated from a specimen of faeces than can be isolated using the standard techniques.

The numbers of bacteria isolated from faeces using the anaerobic cabinet and pre-reduced media techniques approximates to the direct microscopic count, however, even using these advanced techniques the numbers of bacteria isolated from the duodenum and jejunum (maximally 10^4/ml falls far below the direct microscopic count (at least 10^5/ml). Until recently it was commonly stated that the majority of bacteria in faeces were dead, improved techniques disproved this statement thus we should perhaps hesitate before declaring the un-cultivable duodenal and jejunal flora, non-viable.

II. Limitations of the study of pure isolated strains of micro-organisms

The study of isolated strains of bacteria can yield important results that may help to explain the effect observed *in vivo*. Many of the studies described in Section II have utilized pure strains of bacteria or intestinal contents incubated *in vitro* to demonstrate a bacterial role in the metabolism of foreign compounds. It must be noted, however, that the metabolic activities of a bacterium may depend on the growth conditions with respect to (a) type of nutrients available, (b) E_h and pH of the growth medium, (c) external restraints on growth, such as immunological controls. This topic has been discussed at length with respect to growth in tissues versus growth *in vitro* (e.g. Smith, 1972) and is undoubtedly equally true of studies on gut organisms. Thus, demonstrations that bacteria are able to perform a metabolic step *in vitro*, is no guarantee that the same organisms will be able to perform the same reaction *in vivo;* it also gives no proof of the quantitative importance of bacteria on metabolizing a compound.

Many reactions known to be carried out by gut bacteria (e.g. reduction of cholesterol, hydrolysis of cyclamate) are readily carried out by mixed bacterial populations, such as cultures of caecal contents, but are difficult to demonstrate using pure cultures. The uncertainties of bacterial classification especially with respect to the numerically important non-sporing anaerobes complicates the problem of assigning biochemical activities to bacterial groups. It is hoped that the work at present in progress at the anaerobe laboratory (Anaerobe Laboratory Manual, 1972), will solve many of the taxonomic problems.

III. Limitations to the study of physiological aspects
of environment

Much of the evidence regarding host-flora interactions is based on work with germ-free (Gordon and Pesti, 1971) and antibiotic treated animals (Scheline, 1968). Although such evidence is suggestive it should be remembered that species differences (Williams, 1959) in metabolism do occur and that the multiple differences between germ-free and normal animals are interlinked and can seldom be ascribed to any component of the flora. Antibiotics can affect host metabolism directly without any action on the flora (e.g. Ling and Morin, 1971).

IV and V. The study of washed cell suspensions of purified enzymes

Studies of this sort are not directly applicable to the study of the metabolic activities of the gut flora *per se* and are of more interest in answering such questions (a) why does the flora metabolize a compound more or less efficiently *in vivo* than *in vitro*? (b) what are the conditions needed to maximize the rate of metabolism of a compound? (c) what are the conditions that determine which of a range of alternative products is formed?.

Such studies should also facilitate predicting with more precision the effect of lowering the gut pH, increasing the rate of passage of material through the gut, and suppression of a bacterial species not directly participating in a reaction etc.

CHAPTER 1

Factors Controlling and Influencing the Flora

From birth man is subject to bacterial contamination from his environment; some of these organisms are able to grow on body surfaces and may become part of the body flora. Whether a particular organism is able to colonize the body depends upon its ability to compete with established forms and its interaction with host physiology.

Physiological mechanisms, bacterial interactions and environmental influences, such as diet and antibiotics, all inter-relate in determining the nature and distribution of bacteria in the gut. Ageing and changes in habits may modify the physiological status with corresponding adjustment in the flora. Some changes, such as alteration in diet, may both directly influence the flora and produce physiological changes.

I. Host physiology

Although intestinal physiology and host defense mechanisms must play an important role in preventing the flora overrunning the host and determining the distribution of the flora within the intestine, the exact mechanisms are largely obscure.

Animal experiments suggest that the flora is growing at much below the maximum rate (Gibbons and Kapsimalis, 1967); how the host induces a low rate of bacterial multiplication is not known. Explanations of these observations have concentrated upon those characteristics of the flora analogous to continuous flow cultures, but the colon, unlike a fermenter, is not physiologically inert.

Variations in host physiology associated with ageing and, in animal studies, with folate deficiency may bring about changes in the flora (Haenel, 1963; Klipstein and Lipton, 1970). The mechanisms governing such changes are not known. Gastric acidity and small intestinal motility are important in determining the distribution of bacteria within the intestine, but the way that the colonic flora is regulated and invasion of the tissues prevented are less well understood.

A. Intestinal Secretions

1. *Gastric acid*

The germicidal activity of gastric acid has been realized for many years (Sternberg, 1896; Knott, 1923; Bartle and Harkins, 1925). The paucity of bacteria in the stomach of fasting subjects and the normal decline in the bacterial content of the stomach after a meal are related to the acidity, (Fig.1.1) (Drasar *et al.*, 1969). The achlorhydric stomach is usually heavily

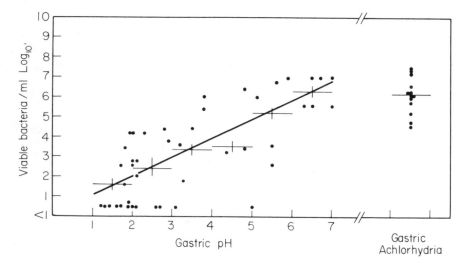

Fig.1.1. Influence of gastric pH on the total bacterial numbers in the stomach.

colonized with bacteria (Van der Reis, 1925; Knott, 1927) and a slight increase in the numbers of bacteria in the jejunum has also been reported (Knott, 1927; Davidson, 1928; Cregan *et al.*, 1953; Sherwood *et al.*, 1964; Drasar *et al.*, 1969). Animal studies suggest that gastric acid is important in controlling the passage of bacteria into the small intestine (Smith, 1965), and in man the acid is probably important in preventing the invasion of pathogenic bacteria (Giannella *et al.*, 1971).

2. *Enzymes, mucus and bile salts*

No anti-bacterial factors other than gastric acid have been definitely demonstrated to be active in the human stomach and intestine although some must be present. In contrast the stomach of the suckling rabbit contains a specific enzyme system which produces antibacterial factors, including decanoic acid, from ingested milk.

There is no evidence to suggest that intestinal bacteria are destroyed by the action of the succus entericus or pancreatic juice (Dack and Petran, 1934). Although the enzyme lysozyme, which can disrupt bacterial cell walls, is found in intestinal mucus (Goldsworthy and Florey, 1930) the significance of this observation is uncertain. Intestinal mucus seems to be involved principally in the mechanical cleansing of the small intestine associated with intestinal motility.

Bile salts disrupt the cells of *Streptococcus pneumoniae* (Neufeld, 1900), *Streptococcus faecalis* and other enterococci are resistant to bile salts (Weissenbach, 1918), similarly bile salts are incorporated in selective media used in the isolation of enterobacteria. These facts support the suggestion that bile has some selective action on the bacteria in the bowel, but there is little direct evidence of this and it should be noted that streptococci that will not grow on bile containing media occur in faeces in significant numbers. In the laboratory, bile salts are in general more inhibitory of Gram positive than Gram negative bacteria, but their bactericidal action is not striking (Leifson, 1935; Stacey and Webb, 1947; Floch *et al.*, 1970). Some Gram negative anaerobic bacteria, notably *Bacteroides fragilis*, are stimulated by whole bile (Beerens *et al.*, 1960; Barnes and Goldberg, 1968).

There is some indirect evidence for an effect of bile secretion on the gut flora. In studies of the faecal bacteria from people in various countries, it was noted that those living on a mixed "western" diet, who have relatively high concentration of bile salts and their degradation products in their faeces, also had relatively high counts of bacteroides (Hill *et al.*, 1971a). Whether this is a direct relation, or whether there is some other factor concerned is not known.

B. THE INTESTINAL MUCOSA

In some sense, the intestinal mucosa functions as a barrier preventing the flora leaving the lumen of the intestine. Although some small molecular weight bacterial products, and perhaps bacterial somatic antigens (Ravin *et al.*, 1960) may be absorbed, bacterial invasion of the mucosa seems to be a specialized property of pathogenic bacteria such as the *Shigella*.

Interest in the mucosa has centred principally on the existence of a specific mucosa dependent flora. The anterior regions of the stomach of rats and mice has a keratinized squamous epithelium and supports a dense palisade of bacteria (Dubos *et al.*, 1965; Savage, 1970). The human stomach has no such keratinized region and bacteria are not normally associated with the gastric mucosa (Nelson and Mata, 1970). A few organisms are demonstrably adherent to the small intestinal mucosa of both mice and man (Savage *et al.*, 1968; Plaut *et al.*, 1967), but there are no pallisaded masses of bacteria comparable to those found in the mouse stomach. Only in the large intestine is there evidence for colonization of the human intestinal mucosa (Nelson and Mata, 1970).

Adhesion of *Streptobacillus moniliformis* to the ileal epithelium of mice was demonstrated after the organisms were administered by stomach tube (Hampton and Rossario, 1965). Similarly, adhesion of bacterial cultures to pieces of human gastric mucosa excised at gastrectomy is easily demonstrated by a modification of the replica plate technique (Drasar, unpublished). As discussed later, these adherence phenomena may be important in the pathogenesis of intestinal infections (e.g. Takeuchi *et al.*, 1965; Labrec *et al.*, 1964).

C. IMMUNE MECHANISMS

The intestine is one of the major sites of immunological activity, but the role of this activity in controlling the indigenous bacteria is not well understood. The intestinal immune response has been studied in the context of infectious intestinal disease, and of oral immunization to these diseases. Infection with, or the oral administration vaccines derived from intestinal pathogens such as *Vibrio cholerae, Salmonella typhi* or *Shigella*, brings about an immune response (e.g. Davies, 1922; Dupont *et al.*, 1972; Freter, 1962; Freter *et al.*, 1965; Cvjetanovic *et al.*, 1970). Immunoglobulins, referred to as coproantibody, may be demonstrable in the faeces. The earlier work on oral immunization was reviewed by Thomson *et al.*, 1948).

1. *The origin of intestinal antibody*

Antibody may reach the intestinal lumen by transudation from the serum or by local synthesis. Orally administered antigen may stimulate systemic, as well as local antibody production.

Investigations of experimental cholera in the guinea pig demonstrated two distinct antibody responses. Coproantibody appeared before serum antibody and reached peak titres and declined before serum antibody (Burrows *et al.*, 1967; Burrows and Havens, 1948). Further studies on experimental cholera indicate that in germ-free animals transudation does not occur, all intestinal antibody being synthesized locally, but that in animals with an intestinal flora the low grade inflammation induced by the flora allows transudation (Freter and Fabara, 1972). These studies and others reviewed by Shearman *et al.*, (1972) clearly illustrate the importance of local antibody synthesis in the intestine. That serum antibody plays no crucial role in control of the flora is illustrated by the failure of Robinet (1962) to find any relation between serum antibody levels and intestinal *Escherichia coli*.

Immunofluorescent antibody studies have shown that IgA is the major immunoglobulin synthesized in the gut mucosa; IgG and IgM are also produced and interstitial IgM, probably of serum origin is also demonstrable. Within the intestine secretory IgA (an IgA dimer coupled to a glycoprotein "secretory piece") is probably most important. This immunoglobulin complex is highly resistant to intestinal enzymes and maintains its integrity in the gut (Tomasi and Bienenstock, 1968; Shearman *et al.*, 1972).

2. *Role of intestinal antibody in the control of the flora*

Patients with immunoglobulin deficiencies have more bacteria in their small intestines than do normal people. This increase, cannot be explained solely on the basis of the other intestinal abnormalities, such as achlorhydria, often encountered in these conditions (Hersh *et al.*, 1970; Parkin *et al.*, 1972; Brown *et al.*, 1972). These findings illustrate the importance of intestinal antibody in controlling the normal flora as well as preventing the establishment of pathogens, but the mechanism by which these important functions are performed wait to be elucidated.

Immune-lysis of bacteria requires the combined action of antibody and the complement system. In serum this action is usually performed by the action of IgM antibody and complement. Adinolfi *et al.*, (1966) reported that S IgA could activate the lysis of bacteria by complement and lysozyme. The most recent evidence suggests that the reaction of S IgA starts from C_3 and not the earlier complement components (Tomasi, 1972).

Opsonization of bacteria may result from the action of IgA antibody thus rendering them available for phagocytosis. Coating of bacteria with IgA may also prevent their adherence to the mucosa and prevent the growth of those bacteria that do adhere (Freter, 1969, 1970). IgA might be regarded as a biological anti-fouling paint.

The ability of antibody to interfere with bacterial growth (Stollermann and Ekstedt, 1957) may contribute to the low overall growth rate of the flora.

3. *The role of cellular immunity in the control of the flora*

When germ-free animals acquire a bacterial flora a marked cellular response occurs within the villi (Bauer *et al.*, 1963). A similar cellular response is seen within the normal human intestine. Many of these cells are lost into the intestine (Hobbs, 1971). The report that small intestinal juice can stimulate phagocytosis (Girard and Kalbermatten, 1970) and the known opsonizing properties of IgA antibody suggests that cells migrating into the intestine probably ingest bacteria. Thus some cellular control of the flora is feasible.

D. INTESTINAL MOTILITY

The cleansing action of the movement of intestinal contents down the intestine is probably the most important determinant of the distribution of bacteria within the intestine (Donaldson, 1968; Gorbach, 1967). The normal peristaltic flow is fastest in the jejunum and upper ileum and slows in the distal ileum, and there is normally a degree of stagnation proximal to the ileo-caecal valve. This doubtless accounts for the higher bacterial population normally found in the terminal ileum.

Animal experiments have demonstrated that bacteria introduced into the small intestine are cleared mechanically in a way analogous to that of an inert marker (e.g. Dack and Petran, 1934, Dixon, 1960; Dixon and Paully, 1962). The particles cleared from the intestine are probably wrapped in intestinal mucus (Florey, 1933).

Disorders that impair the normal peristalsis of the gut commonly lead to a greatly increased bacterial population in the ileum; these include strictures due to Crohn's disease or tuberculous adhesions, scleroderma (Salen et al., 1966) and diabetic neuropathy (e.g. Gorbach, 1971). Patients with single or multiple diverticula, or with blind loops of gut following surgical operations, especially Poly-gastrectomy, also commonly show heavy bacterial colonization of the jejunum or ileum as well as of the stagnant pouch itself. The actual bacterial count observed in the intestinal canal naturally depends on the relation of the sampling point to the stagnant area; Drasar and Shiner (1969) recorded counts of 10^8-10^9 per ml of aspirate.

Although impaired motility undoubtedly contributes to alterations in the distribution of bacteria within the small intestine, the exact mechanism is not known since in animal experiments only gross alterations in propulsion consistently result in alterations in the flora (Sumner and Kent, 1970). Furthermore, germ-free animals appear to have lessened gut motility and it has been suggested that, in mice at least, the normal bacteria of the gut stimulate motility (Abrams et al., 1963).

The bacteria present in stagnant areas of small intestine are pre-dominantly the non-sporing anaerobic bacteroides and bifidobacteria, and enterobacteria (Drasar and Shiner, 1969; Krone et al., 1968; Gorbach and Tabaqchali, 1969). The flora is often referred to as "colonic" or "faecal" in type; this should not be taken to mean that the bacteria are derived by retrograde spread from the large intestine, since, bacteria of these varieties are present in saliva, and not uncommonly in small numbers in the jejunum and ileum. A similar flora develops above a complete obstruction (Bishop and Allcock, 1960), and in a patient whose only abnormality was a slowed rate of peristalsis (Vince, 1971).

II. Environmental factors

A. BACTERIAL CONTAMINATION

The foetus *in utero* is sterile (Donaldson, 1968). The foetus at birth is contaminated with the vaginal and faecal flora of the mother and other bacteria are added from the environment, from this mixture the normal flora is selected.

Patients in hospital commonly seem to acquire new strains of *Escherichia coli* (Cooke *et al.*, 1969) and these can sometimes be traced back to foods (Cooke *et al.*, 1970); the *E. coli* in foodstuffs are certainly sometimes derived from animals (Shooter *et al.*, 1970). Presumably the same is happening outside hospital, and *E. coli* cannot be the only organism spread this way, although it might be that patients in hospital are especially liable to be colonized by the bacteria they ingest. In experiments reported by Buck and Cooke (1969), volunteers who consumed 10^6 *Pseudomonas aeruginosa* or more, excreted the bacteria transiently in the faeces but did not become colonized; the pseudomonads were generally isolated from faeces within 24 hours of ingestion and were rarely found after more than 7 days.

People living under different conditions and in different parts of the world must be exposed to very different loads of bacteria in their diet and it is clear from the volunteer experiments reported by Shooter and his colleagues that some of these bacteria must pass beyond the stomach. There is some evidence that apparently healthy people in India (Gorbach *et al.*, 1969) and Guatemala (Nelson and Mata, 1970) have more bacteria in the small intestine than people living in temperate countries; this might be related to a greater exposure. However, recent studies suggest that nutritional status may also be important (Gorbach *et al.*, 1970).

Analogous observations have been made by Dubos and his colleagues in their studies of mice from a "specific pathogen free" colony; preserved under conditions of stringent hygiene, these animals had a much simpler gut flora than when exposed to more normal animal house conditions (Dubos and Schaedler, 1962) and they also gained weight faster and utilized food more efficiently.

Animals that indulge in coprophagy are dependent on this habit for the maintenance of a normal gut flora (Gustafson and Fitzgerald, 1960). In man, who is not habitually coprophagic, the upper intestinal flora is probably only influenced by faeces in patients with a gastro-colic fistula.

Bacterial contamination is important in establishing the flora but during adult life functions only as a means of acquiring fresh strains of bacteria.

TABLE 1.1

Comparison of the numbers of selected bacteria groups isolated from people on various diets

Diet	Country of origin	Log$_{10}$ bacteria/gram of faeces (Mean)					
		Entero-bacteriaceae	Bacteroides	Enterococci (faecal streptococci)	Lactobacilli	Gram+ non-sporing anaerobes	Clostridia
Mixed western diet 3000-3200 calories/day 85-100 g protein/day 50-70 g animal protein/day	U.S.A. England Scotland Uganda	7.4 7.9 7.6 7.4	9.7 9.8 9.8 9.8	5.9 5.8 5.3 5.3	6.5 6.5 7.7 5.3	10 9.8 9.9 9.5	5.4 5.7 5.6 4.7
High carbohydrate diets (a) Rice 1700-2000 calories/day 45-50 g protein/day 0-5 g animal protein/day	India	7.9	9.2	7.3	7.6	9.6	5.7
2000-2500 calories/day 60-80 g protein/day 10-30 g animal protein/day	Japan	9.4	9.4	8.1	7.4	9.7	5.6
(b) Matoke 1500-2000 calories/day 50 g protein/day 0.5 g animal protein/day	Uganda	8.0	8.2	7.0	7.2	9.3	5.1
Vegan diet 2000-3500 calories/day 80-100 g protein/day	England	7.0	9.7	4.8	7.4	9.6	5.4
Liquid formulae diet 1800 calories/day 35 g aminoacids/day	England	8.2	10.2	4.0	4.3	9.9	3.1

TABLE 1.2

Prominence of some bacterial species in faecal specimens

Bacterial groups	Bacterial species	Percentage of bacterial groups studied identified as species designated	
		Mixed Western diet: England, Scotland and U.S.A.	High Carbohydrate diet: Uganda, India and Japan
Enterobacteriaceae	*Escherichia coli*	92	81
Bacteroides	*Bacteroides fragilis*	92	98
Enterococci	*Streptococcus faecalis*	65	38
	Streptococcus faecium	30	45
Gram-positive non-sporing anaerobes	*Bifidobacterium adolescentis*	35	28
	Eubacterium aerofaciens	16	34
Clostridia	*Clostridium (perfringens) welchii*	39	41
	Clostridium parapatrificum	35	7

B. Diet

The nature of a meal affects the rate of gastric emptying (Hunt, 1959) and indirectly affects the distribution of bacteria within the small intestine. Diet has more usually been considered to be of major significance in determining the nature of the flora of the large intestine. It used to be considered that the predominant groups of intestinal bacteria were determined by the chemical nature of the diet consumed (Rettger and Cheplin, 1921; Dugeon, 1926). There is evidence that diet may affect the constitution of the intestinal flora in animals (Porter and Rettger, 1940; Smith, 1965; Dubos, 1965), but the work on the faecal flora of man has produced equivocal results (Sanborn, 1931a, b; Torry and Monteau, 1931; Haenal et al., 1957).

Studies of people on different diets in various countries (Hill et al., 1971a) have demonstrated some differences in relative numbers of various groups of bacteria which may well reflect the effect of diet, although there were also other substantial differences between the populations. These inter-group variations reflected both the counts of the various bacterial groups present in the faeces (Table 1.1) and the relative proportions of the various bacterial species comprizing these groups (Table 1.2), (Drasar et al., 1972). The most striking differences were that people living in Britain or the U.S.A. on a mixed "western" type of diet had more bacteriodes and fewer enterococci and other aerobic bacteria than people living on the native, largely vegetarian diet in Uganda or South India; Japanese living on a vegetarian diet showed similar though less well-marked trends. It was postulated that the differences might be attributable to the low fat content of the diet in Uganda, India and Japan. The significance of these findings with respect to intestinal cancer is discussed later.

One particular bacterial species has been found virtually confined to the vegetarian populations, namely, *Sarcina ventriculi*; in some vegetarians the faecal count reached 10^8 per gram (Crowther, 1971b). Filamentous fungi are also more common in the faeces of the vegetarian peoples than those from Britain and the U.S.A.

Faecal samples from a number of people living on a strict "vegan" diet in London had bacterial counts very similar to those of people living on mixed diets (Aries et al., 1971).

Although differences are demonstrable between groups of people living on different diets, attempts to change the composition of the flora by variations in diet have, in general, been unsuccessful. A change to a vegetarian diet produces no change in the predominant faecal flora (Moore et al., 1969). One study on the faeces of astronauts (Gall, 1965) showed changes in the flora on a synthetic diet; however, a further study demonstrated no such effect (Corardo et al., 1966). On the other hand, cellulose (Haenel *et al.*, 1964) and lactulose (Haenel *et al.*, 1958) apparently produced slight changes. In one long-term study in which one subject was fed successively for periods of some weeks on high protein, high carbohydrate and high fat diets, the high protein diet did not affect the faecal flora whereas the high carbohydrate diet increased the relative numbers of the bifidobacteria, and the high fat diet favoured the bacteroides (Hoffman, 1964).

Winitz *et al.* (1970) fed volunteers with a no-residue diet composed of amino-acids, vitamins and glucose or sucrose and found, with the glucose-based diet, a substantial reduction in both numbers and variety of bacteria, counts as low as 10^3 per gram of faeces being observed. With sucrose replacing glucose the changes were less marked. The effect was attributed to "starvation" of the bacteria. A similar study reported by

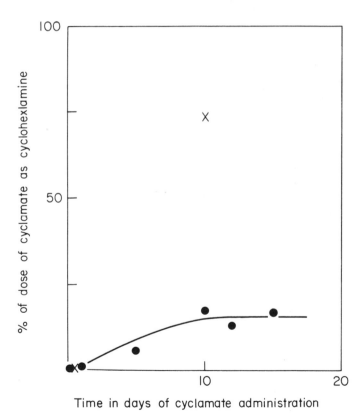

Fig. 1.2. The induction of cylamate metabolism in the intestinal flora of a human subject as judged by urinary excretion of cyclohexylamine and faecal metabolism. ●: Urinary excretion; X: metabolism by faecal homogenate.

Finegold *et al.* (1972) showed that extremely oxygen sensitive anaerobes disappeared from the faeces if a completely absorbable diet was consumed, but that no other consistent change occurred.

Our studies in volunteers maintained on similar diets for shorts periods, and in a few patients treated with these diets for long periods, have not confirmed the findings of Winitz *et al.* The total number of anaerobes remained constant at pre-diet levels, but some fluctuation was observed in the number of aerobes; enterococci and lactobacilli apparently disappeared in some patients (unpublished studies by Drasar, Crowther *et al.*).

It is noteworthy that in these experiments the volume of faeces was greatly reduced, though the concentration of bacteria was not substantially altered. This would be consistent with the idea that the colon bacteria are normally living on gut secretions and the products of shed cells from the mucosa, rather than on unabsorbed residues of the diet.

Although changes in the bacterial species and genera comprizing the flora are difficult to demonstrate, changes in the metabolic properties of the flora due to changes in dietary compounds do occur. During studies on the metabolism of cyclamate by man it was observed that administration of cyclamate was followed by the excretion of cyclohexylamine resulting from the breakdown of the cyclamate by the gut flora. Before exposure to cyclamate the flora was not able to perform this reaction (Fig. 1.2.) (Drasar *et al.*, 1972b).

Thus, important changes in the bacterial flora may be induced by compounds in the diet. The major nutrients are well absorbed and, probably, only gross variations in diet alter the amount of these substances reaching the colon. The difficulty in changing the flora with respect to the bacterial species and genera isolated may reflect the procedures used in bacterial identification. These have been developed to distinguish bacterial groups in the laboratory, not biological types in an ecological situation. Thus many of the substrates whose utilization is important in bacterial identification may be without significance in the bio-economics of bacterial growth in the intestine.

Additional support for this idea is provided by studies on bile salt degradation by bacteria. Thus, bacteria isolated from persons living on a high fat diet and therefore having a higher concentration of bile salts in the faeces, were more active in the degradation of bile salts than were bacteria isolated from people on a low fat diet, although the same groups of bacteria were tested (Hill *et al.*, 1971).

C. Antibacterial Drugs

The reaction of the intestinal flora to the administration of antibacterial substances or a mixture of substances depends both on the specificity of the compound and the resistance of the bacteria comprising the flora. Interest in the effects of antibiotics on the intestinal flora has centred around the use of antibiotics to stimulate the growth of farm animals (Stokestad, 1954) and the use of antibiotics in the pre-operative preparation of the bowel.

Studies on the effect of antibiotics on the flora have been limited by the inadequacy of bacteriological techniques. The studies of Finegold and his colleagues (1965) contain the most complete data. Rather than recapitulate their whole data here a few points must suffice. Several antibiotics suppress the aerobic flora, the enterobacteria, streptococci and lactobacilli. Bacteriodes are resistant to neomycin, kanamycin and similar agents, and although when first studied a combination of neomycin and tetracycline would suppress the whole flora (Finegold *et al.*, 1965) this treatment is now less effective (Finegold, 1970). Lincomycin seems to be the drug most active against bacteroides.

The use of antibiotics as part of the pre-operative preparation for colonic surgery is surrounded by controversy. Controlled trials of neomycin and kanamycin prophylaxis have demonstrated no benefit (Everett *et al.*, 1969; Gaylor *et al.*, 1960). Combinations of kanamycin or neomycin with polymixin or bacitracin have been strongly advocated by Cohn (1965, 1970) but the absence of any controlled trial renders evaluation impossible. In mice the administration of streptomycin greatly increases susceptibility to oral challenge with salmonellae due to suppression of the protective function of the flora (Miller and Bohnhoff, 1962; Bohnhoff and Miller, 1962; Bohnhoff *et al.*, 1964; Meynell, 1963). Presumably the prolongation of intestinal carriage of salmonellae in patients given neomycin (Association for Study of Infectious Diseases, 1970) is the clinical counterpart of the mouse experiments.

Some years ago there were numerous reports of patients developing acute staphylococcal enterocolitis following treatment with broad spectrum antibiotics, particularly tetracycline (e.g. Altemeier *et al.*, 1963; Azer and Drapanes, 1968). It is not clear whether the lack of recent reports indicates a decline in frequency, nor, if there has been a decline, whether this is attributable to a change in the prevalent staphylococci, a decline in the use of the relevant antibiotics, or a change to greater resistance in the normal flora of the gut as hinted by Finegold (1970).

Any antibiotic treatment is liable to alter the balance of antibiotic-sensitive or resistant organisms in the gut. This has been well studied in relation to the use of antibiotics in feeding-stuffs for animals and there is evidence that most of the strains of antibiotic resistant Type 29 *Salmonella typhimurium* causing human infections in a recent epidemic resulted from the selection of R-factor carrying strains in intensively reared calves (Anderson, 1968).

The effects of a given antibiotic treatment on the bacterial populations of the intestinal tract are dependent upon a number of variables including the dose of the agent, frequency, duration and route of administration, and the previous antibiotic experience of the flora. The reaction of individuals is often idiosyncratic, and while some general principle may be delineated the subject requires further research. It should, however, be stressed that the over-use of antibiotics has undoubtedly reduced their value in therapy, indeed the outbreak of typhoid in Mexico caused by R-factor carrying chloramphenicol resistant *Salmonella typhi* probably results from misuse of this antibiotic (Anderson and Smith, 1972).

III. Bacterial interactions

A. STABILITY OF THE FLORA

Except when successful invasion by an external pathogen occurs, the gut flora is probably a stable, self-regulating system.

The gastric and small intestine flora are, because of their transient nature, subject to considerable variation (Drasar *et al.,* 1969). The flora of the large intestine has been little studied but numbers of the dominant anaerobes in faeces show little variation in repeat samples (Moore *et al.,* 1969). The minor components of the faecal flora are subject to considerable numerical variation (Zubrzycki and Spaulding, 1962; Keityi and Barna, 1964), but, despite this, Gorbach *et al.* (1967) noted that the variation between multiple samples from an individual was much less than between samples from different individuals. Variation in the dominant serotypes of *E. coli* has been extensively studied. Sears *et al.,* (1957) demonstrated the presence of "resident" and "transient" strains in successive samples from an individual and some of the "resident" strains were present for considerable lengths of time. Cooke *et al.* (1969) demonstrated that the number of different serotypes present was even greater than had been previously realized, the number of serotypes isolated from an individual being related to the number of samples examined. These workers did not, however, conduct long-term investigation that might reveal the existence of the "resident" types.

B. THE EXCLUSION OF IMPLANTS

There is a natural resistance to the alteration of the gut flora by the introduction of bacteria even if they are of species commonly encountered in the intestine. The role of the flora in excluding pathogenic bacteria has important consequences in the context of acute intestinal disease (Chapter 14).

The speculations of Metchnikoff (1903, 1907) on the noxious influence of intestinal putrefaction and the longevity of Caucasians consuming a diet rich in fermented milk products were followed by numerous attempts to alter the intestinal flora. The many attempts to convert a "putrefactive flora" to a "lactic flora" by the administration of lactobacilli were reviewed by Rettger *et al.* (1935) and Rettger and Cheplin (1921). More recently the use of *Lactobacillus acidophilus* in the treatment of hepatic coma has revived interest in bacterial implantation (Macbeth *et al.*, 1965; Fenton *et al.*, 1966). Attempts to implant lactobacilli in the intestine have in general proved unsuccessful although if very large amounts of bacteria are administered they can be detected in the faeces. These findings are paralleled by those of Buck and Cooke (1969) using *Pseudomonas aeruginosa* and as mentioned previously even *Salmonella* can only be reliably implanted if the flora is depressed with antibiotics (Meynell, 1963).

The resistance of the flora to change is understandable; the bacteria comprising the flora are adapted to growth in the intestine whereas freshly introduced strains require time to adapt. The importance of the mode of growth of administered bacteria was strikingly illustrated by the studies of Ozawa and Freter (1964) who showed that *Escherichia coli* grown in continuous culture, and thus adapted to a low rate of multiplication, was more successful in colonizing the mouse intestine than inocula prepared on plates.

C. BACTERIAL INTERACTIONS

The large intestine can be considered as a continuous culture fermenter, indeed attempts have been made to explain the whole of host-flora interactions in these terms (Boni, 1967). Although faecal output is variable in health it can seldom exceed one third of the colonic volume. Thus at least 3 days elapse before replacement of the whole colonic contents. As has been demonstrated in animal experiments (Gibbons and Kapsemalis, 1967) the multiplication rate of the intestinal bacteria is very low. The bacteria in the colon must be adapted for this low growth rate, and for the maximal utilization of substrates. As has been demonstrated such adaptation of itself confers considerable advantages on bacteria (Ozawa and Freter, 1964) and the ability to undergo such adaptation is undoubtedly selective.

Interactions between the bacteria must play an important part in determining both the total numbers and the relative frequency of the various species. If any confined environment, such as the large intestine, space and nutrients are limited and the bacteria that are able to transform nutrients into bacterial cells fastest under the prevailing conditions will occur in the greatest numbers. Bacteria able to utilize available nutrients that are not used by other bacteria, will also possess an ecological advantage. The presence of the bacteria themselves thus changes the environment. Direct measurements have shown that the Eh of the gut contents in germ-free animals is much higher than in re-contaminated animals, (Worstmann *et al.*, 1965) or than in the normal state. Administration of antibiotics that supress coliforms leads to a reduction in the bacteroides count and a rise in the Eh (Meynell, 1963). Facultatively anaerobic bacteria such as enterobacteria and streptococci use oxygen and this tends to produce anaerobic conditions under which anaerobic bacteria can grow. During ruminal conversion of carbohydrates to acetic, propionic and butyric acids, carbon dioxide and methane, the cell yield is greater than by other theoretically possible pathways for carbohydrate fermentation. Pure fermentations such as the homo- and heterolactic fermentations, the acetic-butyric types, or formic-acetic types are replaced by types more efficient in the production of new cells (Hungate, 1966).

Experimental studies have also demonstrated that bacteroides and coliform bacteria produce, during growth, volatile fatty acids that can inhibit or, in rare cases stimulate, the growth of other bacteria (Meynell, 1963; Hentges, 1969), and such acid production appears to be responsible for the normal resistance of the mouse to salmonellae or shigellae given by mouth (Meynell, 1963; Bohnhoff *et al.,* 1964).

It has also been suggested that exhaustion of some nutrient, such as available carbon sources, may be a limiting factor for some bacteria but later evidence does not support this idea (Hentges, 1970).

Many of the coliform bacteria found in the gut liberate "colicines" that are able to kill other related bacteria and it is assumed that this must happen in the intestine. Studies by Branche *et al.* (1963) on five healthy individuals over a period of six months indicated that resident serotypes of *Escherichia coli* produced colicine far more consistently than did transient serotypes, and that a greater variety of serotypes was present in the subjects whose strains produced relatively little colicine.

CHAPTER 2

The Intestinal Bacteria

Most types of bacteria have at some time been isolated from the intestine. Those that have been isolated more frequently fall into three classes: (1) organisms present in small numbers, probably contaminants from other regions of the body, e.g. staphylococci, or from the environment, e.g. *Bacillus* spp.; (2) organisms normally present in small numbers and apparently part of the resident flora e.g. enterobacteria, and (3) organisms almost always present in large numbers, e.g. bacteroides. Organisms belonging to groups (1) and (2) are easily cultivated and thus have been much more extensively studied than organisms belonging to group (3) which, due to difficulties of isolation, have often been overlooked, notwithstanding their numerical dominance. Recent studies (Anaerobe Laboratory Manual, 1972) have to some extent improved the situation but our knowledge of the anaerobic components of the flora is still far from complete.

Bacteria usually identified by means of their culture in specific media, and morphological characteristics as determined by specific stains, most importantly Gram's stain. Sugar reactions, the ability to dissimilate various sugars, alcohols etc, have long been a stable part of schemes for bacterial identification. In an attempt to find a more scientific, biochemical basis for distinction of species and genera, Kluyver and van Niel (1936) directed attention to the importance of studying the end products of fermentation rather than simple consideration of the production of acid. Wide-scale application of such studies was delayed because of technical difficulties but the advent of gas liquid chromatography has much simplified these procedures. End product analysis has been most fruitful in the study of strict anaerobes.

The specificity of bacterial antigens, the sensitivity of bacteria to bacteriocins and 'phages, the chemical composition of the bacterial cell wall and the chemical composition and structure of bacterial DNA are all important in bacterial classification but they will not be described here.

The purpose of this section is to describe briefly the bacterial groups known to occur in the intestine and to recapitulate such information derived from taxonomic studies which may be of significance when considering host-intestinal flora metabolic interactions. It is not intended to be taxonomically definitive nor serve as a guide for the identification of the organism discussed. For aid in the identification of the bacteria and information as to their classification and nomenclature the reader is referred to Bergey's Manual of Determinative Bacteriology (Breed *et al.,* 1957), Index Bergeyana (Buchanan *et al.,* 1966) and The Principles of Bacteriology and Immunity (Wilson and Miles, 1964). Information on anaerobic bacteria is most readily available in the Pathogenic Anaerobic Bacteria (Smith and Holdeman, 1968), and the Anaerobe Laboratory Manual (Anaerobe Laboratory, 1972).

I. Taxonomic relationship

Family Pseudomonadaceae

Genus *Pseudomonas.* Gram-negative, non-sporing, oxidative, strictly aerobic rods very seldom occur in large numbers in any part of the intestine, usually less than 50 per gram of faeces, enrichment media are necessary to ensure isolation. The interest in these organisms centres around the possibility that the intestine may be the source of the *Pseudomonas aeruginosa* causing infections in deprived hosts.

Family Enterobacteriaceae.

Gram-negative, non-sporing, fermentative, facultatively anaerobic rods, when motile having peritrichous flagella. Due to the prominence of pathogenic and potentially pathogenic bacteria in this group it has been the subject of especially extensive studies (Edwards and Ewing, 1972; Kauffman, 1969). *Escherichia coli* is usually the predominant organism revealed by the aerobic cultivation of faecal specimens. *Klebsiella aerogenes* and *Proteus mirabilis* also commonly occur. These bacteria are widely distributed and often occur in food and may be isolated from the mouth and small intestine. Organisms belonging to this group are often identified on the basis of colonial appearance on selective media and referred to as "coliforms".

Family Bacteroidaceae

Genus *Bacteroides.* Gram-negative, non-sporing anaerobic rods. *Bacteroidis fragilis* is the most numerous bacterial species in the intestine, the very similar *Bacteroides oralis* is common in the mouth. Bacteroides is probably the most important genus of intestinal bacteria.

Genus *Fusobacterium* (Sphaerophorus). Following the practice of the Anaerobe Laboratory Manual (1972) these genera are combined: Gram-negative, non-sporing, pleomorphic, rods often with pointed ends producing butyric acid from glucose.

Family Micrococcaceae

Genus *Staphylococcus.* Gram-positive, fermentative, facultatively anaerobic cocci occurring in clusters producing catalase, occur in the mouth and intestine as contaminants from skin and environment. *Staphylococcus aureus* is of particular significance in the causation of staphylococcal entero-colitis after antibiotic treatment.

Genus *Sarcina*. Gram-positive, fermentative, cocci occurring in cubical packets. The genus should probably be restricted to anaerobic organisms. *Sarcina ventriculi* occurs in the faeces of persons on a vegetarian diet (Crowther; 1971b).

Genus *Peptococcus*. Gram-positive, anaerobic cocci occurring in irregular masses, ferment a wide variety of organic compounds including purines and amino-acids. *Peptococci* are found in the mouth, intestinal tract and faeces but their distribution has not been systematically studied. These organisms may be difficult to distinguish from the peptostreptococci.

Family Neisseriaceae

Genus *Neisseria*. Gram-negative, facultatively anaerobic cocci usually occurring in pairs. Usually present in the mouth and in smaller numbers in the intestine and faeces. *Neisseria catarrhalis* is typical of the indigenous neisseria.

Genus *Veillonella*. Gram-negative, strictly anaerobic cocci occurring in masses, some produce catalase. Occur constantly in the mouth, intestine and faeces but are not a dominant part of the flora. *Veillonella parvula* and *Veillonella alcalescens* are common species.

Family Lactobacillaceae

Genus *Streptococcus*. Gram-positive, facultatively anaerobic cocci occurring in chains; do not produce catalase. Common in the mouth and intestinal tract, *Streptococcus salivarius*, *Streptococcus sanguis* and *Streptococcus viridans* (mitior) are most common in the mouth while *Streptococcus faecalis* and *Streptococcus faecium* are more common in the lower reaches. However, any or all of these species may be isolated from any intestinal location.

Genus *Lactobacillus*. Gram-positive, facultatively anaerobic, non-sporing rods occurring in chains, do not produce catalase. Stricly anaerobic strains do occur and care should be taken to distinguish these from bifidobacteria. Interest has centred on *Lactobacillus acidophilus*; this and other species can usually be isolated from the mouth and intestinal tract.

Genus *Bifidobacterium*. Gram-positive, strictly anaerobic, fermentative rods, often Y shaped or clubbed at the ends. Numerically one of the most important groups in the intestine, numbers 10^{10}-10^{11} per gram of faeces but may also occur in the mouth and small intestine. *Bifidobacterium bifidum* and *Bifidobacterium adoloscentis* are important species.

Genus *Peptostreptococcus*. Gram-positive, strictly anaerobic cocci occurring in chains. May occur in the mouth, intestine and faeces in large numbers.

Family Propionobacteriaceae

Genus *Propionobacterium*. Gram-positive, non-sporing rods producing propionic acid as the major end-product of fermentation. *Propiono-bacterium acnes* is a skin organism but propionobacteria have been isolated from faeces.

Genus *Eubacterium* (Ramibacterium and Catanabacterium). Gram-positive, non-sporing rods producing a mixture of acids as the end product of fermentation. Following the suggestion of Smith and Holdeman (1968) these genera have been transferred from the Lactobacillaceae and following the Anaerobe Laboratory Manual (1972) the genera are combined. *Eubacterium aerofaciens* may be a major component of the faecal flora.

Family *Corynebacteriaceae*

Genus *Corynebacterium*. Gram-positive, non-sporing, facultatively anaerobic irregular rods producing catalase. Diptheroids seem to be part of the normal flora of the mouth and intestine (Vince, 1971). Little is known about them. *Corynebacterium pseudo diptheriticium* is an example of this group.

Family Bacillaceae

Genus *Bacillus*. Gram-positive, spore-forming aerobic and facultatively anaerobic rods. They are often isolated from faeces usually on high-salt media used in the search for *Staphylococcus aureas*. These isolations probably represent spore survival as the vegetative organisms are usually sensitive to the lysozyme of the intestinal mucus.

Genus *Clostridium*. Gram-positive, spore-forming, strictly anaerobic rods. *Clostridium perfringens*, *Clostridium sporogenes*, *Clostridium bifermentans*, and other clostridia can usually be isolated from the faeces; they do not occur in very large numbers.

II. The bacterial species isolated from the intestine

While it is obviously not possible nor perhaps desirable to provide a complete list of all the bacterial species that have been isolated from the intestine, some list must be provided before the complexity of the flora can be appreciated. The species present in the intestine are listed in Table 2.1; this table is based on the data on Rosebury (1961), Eggerth and Gagnon (1933), Eggerth (1935), Anaerobe Laboratory Manual (1972) and Drasar *et al.* (1973).

III. The biochemical characteristics of some intestinal bacteria

Many of the substances used in bacterial identification are not available in the intestine so biochemical data derived from identification procedures may be irrelevant when considering the bio-economics of the intestinal flora. However, the biochemical tests used in bacterial identification

TABLE 2.1

The bacterial groups represented in the healthy intestine. The species listed reflect the interests of various investigators and is not an exhaustive survey

Families and Genera represented	Prominent species	Other species isolated from the intestine
Pseudomonadaceae		
Pseudomonas		*Pseudomonas aeruginosa* (pyocyanea) *Pseudomonas* (Alkaligenes) *faecalis*
Enterobacteriaceae	*Escherichia coli*	
Klebsiella		*Klebsiella* (Aerobacter) *pneumoniae*
Enterobacter		*Enterobacter* (Aerobacter) *aerogenes*
Proteus		*Proteus mirabilis*
Bacteroidaceae		
Bacteroides	*Bacteroides fragilis*	*B. capillosus*　*B. oralis* *B. clostridiformis*　*B. putredinis* *B. coagulans*　*B. ruminicola*
Fusobacterium		*Fusobacterium mortiferum* *Fusobacterium necrogenes* *Fusobacterium fusiforme* *Fusobacterium girans*
Neisseriaceae		
Neisseria		*Neisseria catarrhalis*
Veillonella		*Veillonella parvula* *Veillonella alcalescens*
Micrococcaceae		
Staphylococcus		*Staphylococcus albus*
Acidaminococcus		*Peptococcus asaccharolyticus*
Sarcina		*Sarcina ventriculi*
Peptococcus		*Acidaminococcus fermantans* *Streptococcus salivarius*
Lactobacilliaceae		
Streptococcus	*Streptococcus faecalis*	*Streptococcus sangius* *Streptococcus viridans* (mitior) *Streptococcus faecium*

TABLE 2.1 (cont.)

Families and Genera represented	Prominent species	Other species isolated from the intestine
Lactobacilliaceae		
Lactobacillus	Lactobacillus acidophilus	Lactobacillus brevis Lactobacillus casei
		Lactobacillus catenaforme
		Lactobacillus fermentum
		Lactobacillus leichmanii
		Lactobacillus plantarum
Leptotrichia		Leptotrichia buccalis
Bifidobacterium	Bifidobacterium adolecentis	Bifidobacterium (Actinomyces lactobacillus) bifidum (bifidus)
	Bifidobacterium longum	Bifidobacterium breve
		Bifidobacterium cornutum
		Bifidobacterium eriksonii
		Bifidobacterium infantis
Ruminococcus	Ruminococcus bromii	
Peptostreptococcus		Peptostreptococcus intermedius
		Peptostreptococcus productus
Propionbacteriaceae		
Propionobacterium		Propionobacterium (Corynebacterium) acnes
		Propionobacterium granulosum
Eubacterium	Eubacterium (Bacteroides) aerofaciens (biforme)	Eu. contortum., Eu. cylinderoides., Eu. lentum, Eu. limpsum., Eu. rectale., Eu. tortuosum., Eu. ventriosum
Corynebacteriaceae		
Corynebacterium		Corynebacterium pseudo-diphtheriticum (hofmanni)
		Corynebacterium xerosis Corynebacterium ulcerans

Bacillaceae		
Bacillus		*Bacillus cereus., Bacillus subtilis*
Clostridium	*Clostridium perfringens* (welchii)	*Clostridium cadaveris., Cl. innocum., Cl. malenominatum., Cl. ramosum Cl. sordelli.,*
	Clostridium paraputri-ficum	*Cl. tertium., Cl. bifermentans., Cl. sporogenes., Cl. indolis., Cl.oroticum Cl. splenoides., Cl. felsineum., Cl. difficile*

TABLE 2.2

Metabolic characteristics of bacterial genera found in the intestine

	Metabolism					Substrate utilization									
		End products				Carbohydrates						Protein		Lipid	
						Monosaccharides									
	Metabolic type	Volatile fatty Acids	Substituted fatty acids	Alcohols	Amines	Pentose	Hexose	Other	Disaccharides	Trisaccharides	Polysaccharides	Amino-acid fermentation	Protein hydrolysis	Lipase	Lecithinase
Pseudomonadaceae															
Pseudomonas	Oxidative					−	+	−	−	−	−	+	+	±	−
Enterobacteriaceae															
Escherichia	Fermentative	+	+	+	+	+	+	+	+	+	±	±	−	−	−
Klebsiella	Fermentative	+	+	+	+	+	+	+	+	+	+	+	−	−	−
Proteus	Fermentative	+	+	+	+	+	+	+	+	+	+	±	+	+	−
Bacteroidaceae															
Bacteroides	Fermentative anaerobe	+	+	±	+	+	+	+	+	+	+	±	±	−	−
Fusobacterium	Fermentative anaerobe	+	+	−	+	−	+	±	±	−	−	+	±	+	−

Family / Genus	Metabolism													
Micrococcaceae														
Staphylococcus	Fermentative	+	+	+	+	+	+	+	±	−	+	+	+	+
Sarcina	Fermentative anaerobe	+	+	+	+	+	+	+	+	+	−	+	−	−
Peptococcus	Fermentative anaerobe	+	+	−	±	−	+	−	−	+	−	+	−	−
Neisseriaceae														
Neisseria	Oxidative	+	+	−	±	−	−	−	−	−	−	−	−	−
Veillonella	Fermentative anaerobe	+	−	−	−	−	−	−	−	+	−	±	−	−
Lactobacillaceae														
Streptococcus	Fermentative	−	+	±	+	+	+	±	+	±	±	+	±	−
Lactobacillus	Fermentative	±	+	±	+	+	+	+	±	−	±	−	−	−
Bifidobacterium	Fermentative anaerobe	+	+	+	+	+	+	+	+	+	+	−	−	−
Peptostreptococcus	Fermentative anaerobe	+	+	±	±	±	±	±	±	+	+	±	±	−
Corynebacteriaceae														
Corynebacterium	Fermentative	−	+	+	+	±	±	−	±	−	+	−	−	−
Propionbacteriaceae														
Propionbacteria	Fermentative anaerobe	+	+	±	±	±	+	−	±	±	±	±	−	−
Eubacteria	Fermentative anaerobe	+	+	±	±	±	±	−	+	±	±	±	−	−
Bacillaceae														
Bacillus	Oxidative/fermentative	+	+	±	±	±	±	+	+	+	+	+	−	−
Clostridium	Fermentative anaerobe	+	+	±	+	±	±	±	±	+	±	±	±	±

+: Most strains of most species positive; ±: Some strains of species positive; −: Strains of any species seldom positive

TABLE 2.3

Metabolic reactions of some important intestinal bacteria

SPECIES	End products of metabolism							Substrates utilized														
	Volatile fatty acids				substituted fatty acids		Alcohol	Carbohydrates											Protein		Lipids	
								Mono-saccharides					Disacc-harides			Trisacc-harides		Poly-sacc-harides				
								Pentose		Hexose												
	Acetic acid	Propionic acid	Butyric acid	Others	Lactic acid	Succinic acid	Ethanol	Arabinose	Xylose	Fructose	Glucose	Mannose	Lactose	Maltose	Sucrose	Melezitose	Raffinose	Starch	Meat digestion	Gelatine digestion	Lipase	Lecithinase
Escherichia coli	+	−	−	−	+	+	+	v	+	+	+	+	+	+	v	v	v	−	−	−	−	−
Bacteroides fragilis	+	+	+	+	−	+	−	v	+	+	+	+	+	+	+	v	v	+	−	v	−	−
Streptococcus faecalis	±	−	−	−	+	−	−	v		+	+	−	+	+	+	v	v	+	−	v	−	−
Ruminococcus bromii	+	−	−	+	−	−	+	−	−	+	+	−	−	−	−	−	+	+	−	−	−	−
Bifidobacterium adolescentis	+	−	−	−	+	±	±	+	+	+	+	+	+	+	+	−	−	−	−	−	−	−
Eubacterium aerofaciens	+	−	−	+	+	±	+	−	−	+	+	+	+	+	+	v	−	−	−	−	−	−
Clostridium perfringens	+	±	+	−	±	±	−	−	−	+	+	+	+	+	+	−	−	+	+	+	−	+

+: fermented; −: not fermented; v: variable

provide information about the ability of bacteria to metabolize carbohydrate, proteins and fats and some general picture of the range of metabolic types among the flora is useful (Table 2.2). The characteristic reactions of some of the major species of intestinal bacteria are listed in Table 2.3.

CHAPTER 3

The Distribution of Bacterial Flora in the Intestine

The bacteria demonstrable in specimens of intestinal contents are in part dependent upon methods used for their collection and cultivation. Although advances have been made both in the method of obtaining and of cultivating specimens, our knowledge of the intestinal flora is as yet far from adequate, and the classification of the anaerobic bacteria in particular is still unsatisfactory (Anaerobe Laboratory 1972). Furthermore, although current methods seem to permit the cultivation of virtually all the bacteria present in large numbers in faeces, bacteria in other locations may still remain uncultivated. Thus bacteria can often be seen in Gram stained preparations of material from the jejunum or stomach in numbers that are very seldom approached by the viable counts. It may be that these organisms are the dead residue of salivary and food-borne bacteria; however, the similar assumption that most of the organisms in faeces were dead was disproved when improvements were made in culture methods and the same may yet prove to be true for stomach contents.

I. The mouth

The mouth has a complex structure and its flora probably reflects the differing micro-environments of its various regions (Farmer and Lawton, 1966). Bacteria cultivated from saliva are probably a mixture of those washed from tooth surfaces, gingival crevice and soft tissue surfaces; together with those added from the environment in food and on objects introduced into the mouth (Gibbons *et al.,* 1963, 1964).

To review the complex subject of oral microbiology is beyond the scope of the present work, however, the saliva is among the main sources of bacteria entering the intestine. The bacteria cultivated from saliva in the largest numbers in the various surveys (Table 3.1) were streptococci, veillonella and fusobacteria; other organisms such as spirochaetes and anaerobic vibrios are also reported to occur in large numbers. Neisseria appear to be an important group, though seldom counted (Richardson and

TABLE 3.1

Occurrence of selected bacterial groups in saliva of normal people

Number of subjects	Enterobacteriaceae	Bacteroides	Streptococcus	Lactobacillus	Gram$^+$ non-sporing anaerobes	References
			Log$_{10}$ bacteria/ml saliva. Mean (Range)			
14	N	4.7(3.0-5.3)	7.3(6.0-7.8)	4.5(3.0-5.4)	3.4(3.0-4.3)	Richardson and Jones (1958)
132	D(N-4)	2(N-5)	6(5-7)	2(N-3)	2(N-4)	Drasar, et al. (1969)

N = Not detected; D = Less than 100 bacteria

Jones, 1958). Staphylococci. lactobacilli, corynebacteria and bacteroides (other than fusobacteria) are reported to be usually present, as are Gram positive anaerobic rods and filamentous forms, possibly bifidobacteria, included under the names *Actinomyces, Leptotrichia* and anaerobic lactobacilli (Bisset and Davies, 1960; Rosebury, 1962; Burnett, and Scherp, 1962; Farmer and Lawton, 1965). Yeasts, mainly *Candida albicans,* occur in between 29% and 60% of salivary samples (Handleman and Mills, 1965). Enterobacteria seldom occur in saliva and usually only transiently; although in some individuals they are constantly present.

II. The stomach

Acid stomach contents are usually sterile (Sternberg, 1896; Knott, 1923; Wichels, 1924; Dick, 1941; Drasar *et al.,* 1969). The germicidal action of gastric juice is considered to be due mainly to free hydrochloric acid. The stomach sampled at operation has been found to contain numbers of salivary organisms (Barber and Franklin, 1946; Bach-Nielson and Amdrup, 1965), probably because anaesthesia and premedication depresses gastric secretion. Immediately after a test meal a count of around 10^5 bacteria per ml of gastric juice can be recorded, the bacteria including streptococci, enterobacteria, bacteroides and bifidobacteria derived from the mouth and from the meal (Drasar *et al.,* 1969). As the pH falls the bacterial count declines, and relatively few bacteria are grown after a pH of about 3 has been attained.

III. The small intestinal flora in people resident in Europe and North America

Samples of intestinal contents obtained from the proximal small intestine of fasting subjects contain few bacteria, indeed most investigators have reported on samples from which they were unable to isolate bacteria. The count of viable bacteria seldom exceeds 10^4 per ml of intestinal contents (Table 3.2). For a period after a meal an increased number of bacteria can be isolated from jejunal samples (Gorbach *et al.,* 1967a; Drasar *et al.,* 1969; Hamilton *et al.,* 1970). It is of note that Dellipiani and Girdwood (1964), who also examined their subjects after a meal, obtained higher counts than some other investigators. The evidence suggests that the upper small intestine contains at least in part transient bacterial flora.

The bacteria found in samples from the proximal small intestine are sometimes referred to as "contaminants from the mouth", it would probably be better to refer to them as "transients from the mouth" since it is a normal phenomenon for some mouth bacteria to be conveyed to the small intestine.

TABLE 3.2

Occurrence of selected bacterial groups in the small intestine of normal people

| | Number of subjects | $\log_{10}$ bacteria/ml intestinal contents. Mean (Range) | | | | | References |
		Entero-bacteriaceae	Bacteroides	Streptococcus	Lactobacillus	Gram+ non-sporing anaerobes	
Jejunum	6	N	N	3.5(N-5.5)	N	N	Dellipiani and Girdwood, (1964)
	20	D	D	2.4(N-3.9)	2.4(N-3.9)	D	Gorbach, et al. (1967)
	22	D(N-3)	D(N-3.1)	D(N-6)	D	D(N-3.2)	Drasar, Shiner and McLeod, (1969)
	12	D(N-3)	N	4.2(N-8.9)	2.2(N-6)	D(N-5)	Hamilton, et al. (1970)
Ileum Distal	6	D(N-6)	N	N	D(N-3.7)	D	Dellipiani and Girdwood, (1964)
Ileum Terminal	12	5.4(3.5-6.3)	5.5(3.1-8.8)	2.5(2-6.3)	3.5(3-4)	2.5(2-3)	Gorbach, et al. (1967)
Ileum	7	3.3(N-6)	5.7(3.4-8)	3.4(3.1-4.1)	D(N-8)	5.7(4.1-8)	Drasar, et al. (1969)
	6	5.6(N-8.5)	5.2(N-8)	4.9(N-9)	4.2(N-8)	4(N-8)	Hamilton, et al. (1970)

N = Not detected; D = Less than 100 bacteria

Recent investigations have confirmed older reports on the prominence of Gram positive organisms (Hewtson, 1904; Van der Reis, 1925; Kendall *et al.*, 1927; Cregan and Hayward, 1953; Martini *et al.*, 1957). Streptococci, usually of the viridans group and lactobacilli are the bacteria most often isolated but enterobacteria and bacteroides also occur fairly frequently though in small numbers (French, 1961; Bornside and Cohn, 1961; Legler and Zeitler, 1962).

The lower small intestine, the distal and terminal ileum, appears to contain a richer and more permanent flora than the upper (Table 3.2). Although lactobacilli and streptococci are still prominent, bacteroides and enterobacteria occur more constantly (Cregan and Hayward, 1953; Nichols and Glenn, 1940; Bornside and Cohn, 1965; Kalser *et al.*, 1966). Most specimens contain bacteria. Thus of 155 specimens from the ileum examined by Henning *et al.* (1959) only seven were reported as sterile while 124 contained considerable numbers of bacteria. In the distal ileum bacterial counts in the region of 10^5-10^7 per ml are not uncommon. (Drasar *et al.*, 1969; Gorbach *et al.*, 1967). The flora of the lower ileum is qualitatively similar to that of faeces.

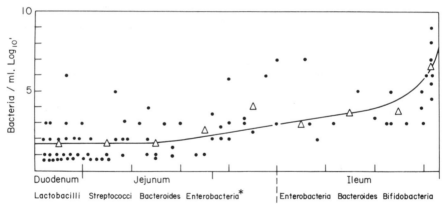

Fig. 3.1. The distribution of viable bacteria in the small intestine.

The overall distribution of bacteria in the small intestine is probably best represented by Fig. 3.1. Thus, although the distribution of bacteria along the intestine varies throughout the day, the bacteria in the small intestine being replenished after each meal, the concentration of bacteria is probably always lowest in proximal intestine and greatest at the terminal ileum.

IV. The small intestinal flora in tropical residents

The account of the flora presented here is based on studies performed in Western Europe and North America. Studies in India and Guatemala

TABLE 3.3

Occurrence of selected bacterial groups in the small intestine of normal people resident in the tropics

	Entero-bacteriaceae	Bacteroides	Streptococcus	Lactobacillus	Gram$^+$ non-sporing anaerobes	References
Jejunum	5(N-5)	6(N-6)	4.3(N-5)	4(N-4)	5(N-5)	Nelson and Mata (1970)
	3.5(N-5)	D(N-6)	5.5(N-8)	2.5(N-3)	D(D-6)	Bhat, et al. (1972)
Ileum	4(N-6)	D(N-3)	D(N-4)	D(N-4)	D(N-5)	Gorbach, et al. (1969)
	6(N-8)	5(N-7)	5(N-7)	4(N-6.5)	5(N-7)	Bhat, et al. (1972)

Header note: Log$_{10}$ bacteria/ml intestinal contents. Mean (Range)

N = Not detected; D = Less than 100 bacteria

TABLE 3.4

Occurrence of selected bacterial groups in the large intestine of normal people

Number of subjects	Entero-bacteriaceae	Bacteroides	Streptococcus	Lactobacillus	Gram$^+$ non-sporing anaerobes	References
	Log$_{10}$ bacteria/ml intestinal contents. Mean (Range).					
11 (Appendix)	6.9(6.7-9)	7.1(4-9.3)	7.0(5-9.7)	6.4(4-9)	5.6(4-8.6)	Seeliger and Werner, (1962)
3 (Caecum)	6.2(5.6-7.4)	7.9(6.4-9.1)	2.6(N-3.6)	D(N-2.8)	5.2(2.3-7.6)	Gorbach, et al. (1967)

N = Not detected; D = Less than 100 bacteria

TABLE 3.5

Occurrence of selected bacterial groups in faeces

Entero-bacteriaceae	Bacteroides	Streptococcus	Lactobacillus	Gram$^+$ non-sporing anaerobes	References
Log$_{10}$ bacteria/gram faeces. Mean (Range)					
7.6(7-7.8)	8.4(6-9)	7.(5-9.7)	6.4(4-9)	6.6(4-8.6)	Seeliger and Werner, (1962)
7.1(6.5-7.6)	10(9.5-10.5)	4(3.2-4.5)	4.5(4-5)	D	Zubrzychi and Spaulding, (1962)
8.4	8	7.4	7.5	8.1	Ketyi and Barna, (1964)
7(5-8)	8.8(8-9.5)	5(5-5)	3.6(3-4)	6.6(5-8)	Gorbach, et al. (1967)
6(4-9)	10.5(10-11.5)	5(2-8)	4(2-7)	10.5(9-11)	Drasar, et al. (1969)
6.6(N-10.1)	9.8(8-11.4)	4.9(N-9.4)	3.5(N-10)	5.6(N-10.8)	Finegold, et al. (1970)

N = Not detected; D = Less than 100 bacteria

suggest that a richer and more permanent flora is found in the small intestine of normal people living in these areas (Table 3.3). However, the nutritional status of the people studied may also be important (Gorbach *et al.*, 1970).

These studies provide important pointers for future research. Should their conclusion be maintained, the implications with respect to intestinal physiology would be very important. Some implications are discussed in Chapter 13.

V. The large intestine and faeces

Many studies on the intestinal flora have been primarily with the bacterial content of faeces. Such studies on faeces are relevant to the discussion on the significance of the intestinal flora, in so far as the findings reflect the bacterial flora of the colon.

Few studies have been made of the flora of the large intestine; it seems, however, to be qualitatively similar to that of faeces (Table 3.4). Estimates of total bacterial numbers vary, some investigators (Moore *et al.*, 1969) have suggested higher counts than those in faeces.

The bacteria isolated from faeces are predominantly non-sporing anaerobes (Table 3.5). Bacteroides are present in very large numbers and many investigators have found them to be the predominant organisms. However, bifidobacteria are also found in large numbers and Haenel (1961) considered these to be the dominant microbes. Enterobacteria and streptococci are constantly present and lactobacilli are usually isolated; these latter groups constitute a proportion of the total population isolated dependent upon the investigator. Bacteria of other groups are reported irregularly in small numbers.

The faecal flora is much more complex than was realized. Of the 230 strains of faecal bacteria from two people examined by Moore *et al.* (1969), 46% represented a single species, *Bacteroides fragilis;* however, at least 36 other species were also represented. Many of the bacterial groups known to be present in faeces in large numbers for example, Peptostreptococci have seldom been enumerated.

CHAPTER 4

Changes in the Bacterial Flora Associated with Alterations in the Intestine due to Disease or Surgery

The bacterial flora of the intestine is controlled by the anatomy and physiology of the intestinal tract. Surgical operations for intestinal conditions, intestinal disease and the effects of ageing alter the physiology of the intestinal tract. The effect of intestinal changes on the flora are little understood but some data is available.

I. Alteration in gastric function

A. PERNICIOUS ANAEMIA AND GASTRIC ACHLORHYDRIA

The stomach. The achlorhydric stomach, whether associated with pernicious anaemia or resulting from ageing, is usually heavily colonized with bacteria, (van der Reis, 1925; Knott, 1927). Enterobacteria, a faecal type of flora (Wichels, 1924; Engel, 1929) or salivary streptococci, an oral type of flora may be present (Dick, 1941; Cregan *et al.*, 1953; Drasar *et al.*, 1969).

The small intestine (Table 4.1). Gastric achlorhydria results in an increase in the number of bacteria entering the small intestine. A slight increase has been reported in the number of bacteria present and in the frequency with which enterobacteria are isolated (Knott, 1927; Davidson, 1928; Cregan *et al.*, 1953; Sherwood *et al.*, 1964; Drasar *et al.*, 1969).

Faeces. Enterobacteria, clostridia and streptococci are reported to be present in increased numbers in the faeces of subjects suffering from pernicious anaemia and gastric achlorhydria (Moench, Kahn and Torry, 1925; Davidson, 1928; Legler and Zeitler, 1964). But similar changes have been reported to occur in older people (Haenel, 1963), and those suffering from gastro-intestinal disorders and various diseases (Legler and Zeitler, 1964). These changes are probably non-specific.

TABLE 4.1

Occurrence of selected bacterial groups in the jejunum of patients with achlorhydria associated with Pernicious Anaemia or Gastric Surgery

Log_{10} bacteria/ml intestinal contents. Mean (Range)

Condition	No. of patients studied	Entero-bacteriaceae	Bacteroides	Streptococcus	Lactobacillus	Gram⁺ ve non-sporing anaerobes (e.g. Bifidobacteria, Eubacteria)	References
Pernicious anaemia	10	1.5(1-4)	2(1-4)	1.4(1-4)	1.5(1-4)	1.2(1-3)	Drasar et al. (1969)
	5	N	N	5(1-6.3)	1.2(1-2.7)	N	Dellipiani and Girdwood (1964)
Billroth I Gastrectomy	8	4.7(1.7-8.2)	1.7(1.7-3)	5.2(1.7-7)	2.2(1.7-6)	3.5(1.7-7.5)	Parkin et al. (1972)
	5	N	N	1.8(1-4)	1.8(1-4)	1.4(1-3)	Drasar and Shiner (1969)
Vagotomy and Pyleroplasty	14	2(1-6)	2.7(1-6)	2(1-6)	N	2.2(1-6)	Drasar (unpublished results)
Billroth II (Polya) Gastrectomy	18	4.7(1-8)	N	4(1-5)	N	N	Goldstein et al. (1961)
	43	2.1(1-9)	3.3(1-9)	1.7(1-9)	1.6(1-7)	1(1-2)	Drasar and Shiner (1969)
Gastro-enterostomy	6	4.1(1-6.9)	N	N	N	N	Dellipiani and Girdwood (1964)
	3	4.6(3-7)	5.6(4-7)	2.6(1-6)	N	N	Drasar and Shiner (1969)

N = Not detected

B. Surgical Procedures for Gastric and Duodenal Ulcer (Table 4.1)

Attempts to explain post-gastrectomy and post-vagotomy symptoms have produced several studies on the intestinal flora following gastric surgery. Further impetus was provided by studies on the Blind Loop Syndrome (Chapter 13). Operations that result in a by-passed or blind loop of small intestine provide a region of stasis that may become colonized. Polya (Billroth 2) gastrectomy provides a blind afferent loop of duodeneum; a similar blind loop results from the Roux en Y (Poth's modification of the Billroth 2) gastrectomy, while gastroenterostomy produces a by-passed loop of duodenum. Billroth 1 gastrectomy and vagotomy and pyloroplasty do not give rise to such areas of stasis (Fig. 4.1).

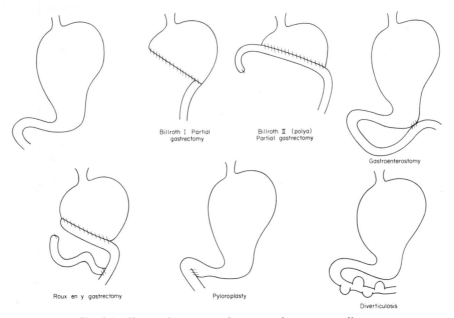

Fig. 4.1. Changes in anatomy due to gastric surgery or disease.

All patients who undergo operations producing a potential area for colonization do not become colonized, however, typically faecal bacteria such as enterobacteria and enterococci are often demonstrable in duodenal and jejunal aspirates in large numbers (10^8 per ml of intestinal fluid) (Bishop, 1965; Duncan *et al.*, 1954; Goldstein *et al.*, 1961; Stammers and Williams, 1963; Shiner *et al.*, 1963; Tabaqchali and Booth, 1966) Some patients develop a mixed bile salt resistant flora including enterobacteria, enterococci and bacteroides (Drasar and Shiner, 1969). The flora of patients who undergo Billroth 1 gastrectomy or vagotomy and pyloroplasty do not undergo colonization and their flora is comparable to that of other achlorhydric subjects.

C. COLONIC TRANSPLANT

The colon may be used as a replacement for the oesophagus. Patients who have had their colons mobilized and inserted in place of the oesophagus were studied by Mallinson and Drasar (1971). The colon retains the rich bacterial population that it harbours in its more usual location.

II. Conditions producing small intestinal statis

A. SMALL INTESTINAL DIVERTICULOSIS

Diverticuli of the small bowel are found in many older people; these may provide areas of stagnation that can be colonized by bacteria. The process of colonization is assisted by the frequency of achlorhydria in people with diverticulosis. The flora is similar to that found in other "colonized" locations being bile resistant; enterobacteria and bacteroides are often isolated (Table 4.2).

B. OTHER CONDITIONS (TABLE 4.2)

Colonization of the small intestine has also been reported in various other conditions. Patients with Crohn's disease having strictures of the small intestine are often colonized (Drasar and Shiner, 1969; Krone *et al.*, 1968; Prizoht *et al.*, 1970). Intestinal obstruction (Bishop and Allcock, 1960), Diabetic diarrhoea (Goldstein *et al.*, 1970), Scleroderma (Salen *et al.*, 1966), X irradiation of the abdomen (Gorbach and Tabaqchali, 1969), and cirrhosis of the liver (Martini *et al.*, 1957) have all been associated with an abnormal small intestinal flora in some patients.

C. CONDITIONS ALLOWING DIRECT ACCESS FROM THE COLON TO THE UPPER INTESTINE

Gastro-colic and jejunocolic fistulae allow the reflux of colonic contents into the small intestine and produce profound disturbance of the small intestinal flora (Table 4.2). Fistulae and stricture of other types presumably give rise to blind loops of small intestine that become colonized.

Massive resection of the small intestine may alter the small intestinal flora. A very short small intestine may be associated with an abnormal intestinal flora (Krone *et al.*, 1968).

TABLE 4.2

Occurrence of selected bacterial groups in the jejunum of patients with small intestinal abnormalities

Condition	No. of patients studied	Log$_{10}$ bacteria/ml intestinal contents. Mean (Range)					References
		Entero-bacteriaceae	Bacteroides	Streptococcus	Lactobacillus	Gram$^+$ve non-sporing anaerobes (e.g. Bifidobacteria, Eubacteria)	
Duodenal and jejunal diverticulosis	4	4.6(1-8.7)	N	N	N	N	Dellipiani and Girdwood (1964)
	4	8.2(8-8.5)	4.5(1-8.5)	6(4-7)	4.2(2-6)	5(3-7)	Gorbach and Tabaqchali (1969)
	15	2.3(1-6(	3.3(1-8)	1.5(1-4)	1.5(1-4)	1.5(1-6)	Drasar and Shiner (1969)
Ileal strictures	2	4(1-8)	N	6(5-7)	2(1-4)	4.5(4-5)	Gorbach and Tabaqchali (1969)
Gastrocolic fistulae	4	3.3(2-5)	4.8(3-8)	2.2(1-6)	2.5(1-5)	3.75(1-7)	Drasar and Shiner (1969)
Regional enteritis (Crohn's disease)	6	2(1-6)	3.3(1-7)	1.5(1-3)	N	1.5(1-3)	Drasar and Shiner (1969)
Hypogamma-globulinaemia	5	4.9(1.7-7.1)	4(1.7-7)	6(3-7)	2(1.7-3.5)	6(3.2-7.2)	Parkin et al. (1972)

N = Not detected

TABLE 4.3

Occurrence of selected bacterial groups in Ileostomy effluent

Condition	No. of patients studied	Log_{10} bacteria/ml intestinal contents. Mean (Range)					References
		Entero-bacteriaceae	Bacteroides	Streptococcus	Lactobacillus	Gram⁺ve non-sporing anaerobes (e.g. Bifidobacteria, Eubacteria)	
Ileostomy	13	7.0	7.7*	6.7	5.8	6.7	Gorbach et al. (1967)
	6	7.7(5.3-8.8)	1(1-3)	8.1(4-8.8)	3.6(1-7.3)	3(1-7.3)	Finegold et al. (1970)
	10	5.6(3-7)	7.3(6-10)	4.7(1-8)	5.1(1-9)	5.6(3-8)	Drasar and Shiner (1969)
Transverse colostomy	2	3.7(3-4.5)	7.5(8-6.9)	6.1(5.2-6.6)	4(0-8)	7.7(6.9-8.5)	Finegold et al. (1970)

* = Total Anaerobes

D. ILEOSTOMY

Removal of the colon and construction of an ileostomy is an important
surgical procedure. The ileostomy represents a new ecological situation and
is rapidly colonized (Gorbach *et al.*, 1967).

Bacterial counts on ileostomy fluid, reported by Gorbach *et al.*, (1967)
and Finegold *et al.*, (1970) were much higher than those on aspirates from
the normal ileum, but rather lower than those from faeces; aerobic bacteria
were observed in large numbers but anaerobes were much less numerous
than in faeces (Table 4.3).

SECTION II

The Metabolic Activities of Gut Bacteria

Gut Bacteria, Importance in the Environment

The metabolic activity of the gut bacteria is potentially equal to that of the liver. Thus the contribution of the gut bacterial flora to the metabolism of any compound administered orally or any substance secreted into the intestine may be considerable and has been mentioned in a number of articles (Williams *et al.*, 1965; Smith, 1966; Williams *et al.*, 1971) and reviews (Scheline, 1968a). In view of the increasing interest in the role of environmental factors in the aetiology of human disease, it is pertinent to recognize that the gut bacteria are an important factor in our environment. Although the literature abounds with reports of the enzymic activity of intestinal microbes, the studies have often concerned only single strains of aerobic organisms acting on obscure substrates.

In this section we describe the metabolism of some endogenous compounds (e.g. biliary components, intestinal mucin etc.) of common dietary components (e.g. amine acids, glycosides) and food additives (e.g. food colours, preservatives etc.) and of commonly used drugs (e.g. antibiotics, cathartics etc.). These components have been arranged in this section under the broad headings of glycosides, nitrogen compounds, biliary components (three chapters), antibiotics and miscellaneous. This is not an exhaustive review, but an attempt has been made to illustrate the range of metabolic activities and to assess the importance and relevance of these reactions to the well-being of the human host whether in health or disease.

CHAPTER 5

Bacterial Glycosidases

I. Introduction

Glycosides entering the gut are from three principal sources, (a) the diet, (b) therapeutic glycosides, and (c) the glucuronides produced by the liver and secreted in the bile.

Glycosides are widely distributed in the plant world and are synthesized by plants as a means of detoxifying potentially harmful metabolites which are then secreted as flower pigments. They are also present in seed coats and appear to act as a protection against bacterial attack (when the aglycone is bactericidal) or against ingestion by animals (when the glycoside or aglycone is toxic). Because of their widespread occurrence in the plant world, glycosides are present in the normal diet.

Since many glycosides are pharmacologically active (giving them a protective function in the plant) they can be used in controlled treament therapeutically. Thus the anthraquinone cathartics, senna and cascara sagrada, are glycosides as are the Lanatoside cardioactive agents. In many cases the glycosides owe their pharmacological effect to gut bacteria since they release the active aglycone. In addition, a number of antibiotics are administered as their glycosides. As part of the normal detoxification process many compounds are metabolized in the liver to their glucuronides, which are then secreted via the bile into the gut lumen. Although this is the major source of glucuronides, the liver does not produce significant amounts of the other glycosides.

The principle glycosidases produced by the gut bacteria are β-glucuronidase, β-galactosidase and β-glucosidase.

II. Metabolism of glucuronides

In 1932 Quick demonstrated that, when p-hydroxybenzoic acid diglucuronide was administered orally to man, p-hydroxybenzoic acid and p-hydroxyhippuric acid but no glucuronide was excreted in the urine. He concluded that the conjugate was hydrolysed in the gut, presumably by the gut bacteria, and then to some extent reconjugated with glycine. As part of their study of benzene metabolism Gorton and Williams (1949) showed that orally administered phenyl glucuronide was excreted as a mixture of the sulphate and the glucuronide by rabbits, they concluded that the conjugate was hydolysed in the gut then reconjugated as the sulphate or glucuronide either in the gut mucosal wall or in the liver before being excreted in the urine. When phenyl glucuronide was administered to the rabbits by injection it was excreted unchanged in the urine.

β-glucuronidase from *Esch. coli* was isolated and characterized by Buehler *et al.* (1951). They showed that enzyme was inducible and was produced optimally in shaken cultures grown for eight days at 25°C in broth at pH 7.3. The enzyme had a pH optimum of 6.2 when sodium phenolphthalein glucuronide was used as substrate and a broad optimum of pH 4.5-7.0 with sodium estriol glucuronide. Marsh *et al.* (1952) investigated the β-glucuronidase activity in the intestinal tract of a number of laboratory animals; they showed that the enzyme was at maximal activity in the colon and caecum of all animals studied (sheep, cattle, rats, rabbits, pigs, cats and fowls) and was of low activity in the small intestine and stomach. The activity of the enzyme was higher in the rat small intestine than in that of the rabbit.

In a survey of gut bacterial speices and genera, Hawksworth *et al.*, (1971) showed that *Esch. coli* produced much more β-glucuronidase per strain than did the other genera tested (Fig. 5.1). They used *p*-nitrophenyl glucuronide and phenolphthalein glucuronide as substrates; the two substrates gave essentially similar results. From the mean activity per 10^9 organism of the various species, and from data on the normal intestinal flora of various laboratory animals, the amount of bacterial enzyme at

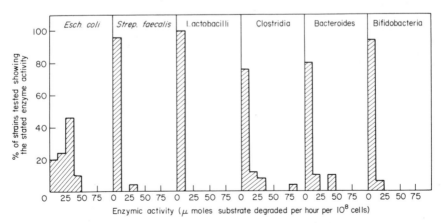

Fig. 5.1. Histograms of β-glucuronidase activity of rat intestinal bacteria. Fifty strains of each of the six genera were tested and the histograms are plotted as % frequency against activity.

various points in the intestinal tract may be calculated (Tables 5.1 and5.2).

It is evident from Table 5.1 that although *Esch. coli* produces the highest activity of enzyme/cell, they are greatly outnumbered by the *Lactobacillus* spp., *Bacteroides* spp. and *Bifidobacterium* spp. with the result that they contribute only 3% of the total bacterial enzyme in the rat upper small intestine and only 0.2% of the total in the lower small intestine.

The amount of β-glucuronidase in the upper small intestine of the rat and mouse is very much greater than that in the guinea pig, rabbit and man (Table 5.2) and in all animals the enzyme activity is much higher in the colon and caecum than in the small intestine. These calculated results are, therefore, in agreement with those of Marsh *et al.* (1952). The agreement is qualitative; the results are not comparable because Marsh *et al.* performed their assays of total enzyme activity under conditions optimal for the

TABLE 5.1

Estimated bacterial β-glucuronidase activity in the small intestine of the rat

Bacteria	Mean enzyne activity[+] per 10^8 cells	Estimated activity in the proximal small intestine		Estimated activity in the distal small intestine	
		No. of bacteria per gram contents	Total* activity	No. of bacteria per gram contents	Total* activity
Esch. coli.	24.7	3.2×10^4	7.9	1.3×10^4	3.2
Strep. faecalis	2.9	5.0×10^4	1.5	1.0×10^5	2.9
Lactobacilli	1.6	5.0×10^6	80.0	6.3×10^6	101.0
Clostridia	11.3	1.0×10^3	0.1	2.0×10^3	0.2
Bacteroides	6.0	2.0×10^6	120.0	7.9×10^6	474.0
Bifidobacteria	1.9	5.0×10^6	95.0	4.0×10^7	760.0

* activity = n moles substrate degraded/hr/gram. + activity = μ moles substrate degraded/hr.

TABLE 5.2

Estimated β-glucuronidase activity in the small intestine of man and four laboratory animal species

Animal species	Estimated β-glucuronidase activity	
	Proximal small intestine	Distal small intestine
Man	0.02	0.9
Rabbit	2.4	45.4
Guinea-pig	2.7	139.0
Rat	304.0	1341.0
Mouse	1200.0	5015.0

mammalian enzyme and different from those used by Hawksworth *et al.* The higher enzyme activity in the small intestine of the rat and mouse suggest that β-glucuronides would be much more readily hydrolysed in the small intestine of these animals; this is of importance in the enterohepatic circulation of foreign compounds (Section V), and affects the retention of such compounds within the body.

Most of the glucuronides entering the intestine are the result of conjugation reactions in the liver followed by biliary excretion. Foreign compounds ingested and entering the gut will be absorbed from the intestine by passive diffusion if they are lipid soluble; such compounds are potentially toxic to the body but are metabolized in the liver to yield non-toxic products which must then be excreted. With many compounds this is achieved by conjugation with glucuronic acid to yield a water soluble product which is then excreted in the bile. Since it is hydrophilic it will not be passively absorbed from the gut and may be passed in the faeces.

In addition to the hepatic glucuronides, a number of therapeutic agents may be administered orally as the glucuronide. This is especially so when the active agent is lipid soluble and is being used to treat the large bowel contents. Thus in infant diarrhoea chloramphenicol is often given as the glucuronide which then passes virtually quantitatively into the large bowel, where it is hydrolysed by the gut bacteria to release the active antibiotic. This method of administration may also be used when slow release of a pharmacologically active compound into the circulation is required. For example, when using prednisolone as an anti-inflammatory agent, an oral dose of the steroid would be rapidly absorbed from the small intestine giving an initially high blood concentration which would then fall as the steroid was excreted in the urine. The glucuronide is not absorbed from the small intestine and is slowly hydrolysed in the gut, so that although there is no initial high concentration in the blood, there is a continuous release of prednisolone over a prolonged period giving a lower but flatter blood level.

III. Metabolism of glucosides

The majority of plant glycosides are glucosides, where the sugar moiety may be α- or β-linked (in contrast to the glucuronides which are all β-linked); the β-glucosides are the more common. Adult mammals lack intestinal β-glucosidase (although the enzyme is present in the gut of infant animals) but this enzyme is produced by a wide range of intestinal organisms (Fig. 5.2). Using as substrates *o*-nitrophenyl-β-*D*-glucoside and aesculin (4,5-dihydroxycoumarin-β-*D*-glucoside) the most active enzyme producers were *Strep. faecalis* strains (Hawksworth *et al.*, 1971), but they are so outnumbered in the gut by the lactobacilli and the strict anaerobes that they contribute a negligible proportion of the total enzyme activity in

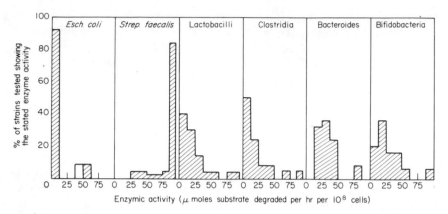

Fig. 5.2. Histograms of β-glucosidase activity of rat intestinal bacteria. Fifty strains of each of the six genera were tested and the histograms are plotted as % frequency against activity.

the small intestine (Table 5.3). The enzyme is constitutive, and in a strain of *Strep. faecalis* has an optimum pH between 6 and 7. In general, the conditions leading to optimal bacterial growth result in optimal enzyme production.

The intestinal bacteria are exposed to a wide range of glucosides, some of dietary origin and some administered for their therapeutic activity (e.g. the cardiac glucoside cathartics). There is also a range of glucoside compounds whose harmful effect is due to the aglycone released by bacterial action.

The cathartic agent cascara sagrada and senna are both mixtures of glycosides. Cascara sagrada contains six major components all related to emodin (1,3,8-trihydroxy-6-methyl-anthraquinone) β-linked to a glucose molecule (Fig. 5.3). Senna contains sennosides A and B, each containing a

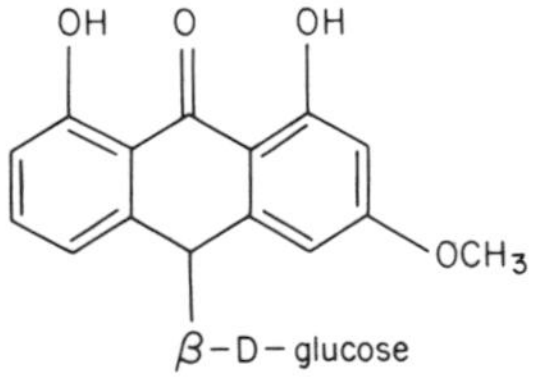

Fig. 5.3. One of the six major emodin glucosides present in cascara sagrada.

molecule of rheindianthrone linked to two molecules of glucose. The glycosides have no pharmacological action but, on hydrolysis they yield active aglycones. In experiments on colonic motility Hardcastle and Wilkins (1970) showed that the aglycone stimulated colonic peristalsis whereas the parent glycoside had no such action. If the aglycone is administered orally

TABLE 5.3

Estimated bacterial β-glucosidase activity in the small intestine of the rat

Bacteria	Mean enzyme activity[+] per 10^8 cells	Estimated activity in the proximal small intestine		Estimated activity in the distal small intestine	
		No. of bacteria per gram contents	Total activity*	No. of bacteria per gram contents	Total activity*
Esch. coli.	5.8	3.2×10^4	1.9	1.3×10^4	0.8
Strep. faecalis	192.7	5.0×10^4	96.4	1.0×10^5	192.7
Lactobacilli	26.0	5.0×10^6	1300.0	6.3×10^6	1638.0
Clostridia	22.1	1.0×10^3	0.2	2.0×10^3	0.4
Bacteriodes	35.1	2.0×10^6	702.0	7.9×10^6	2775.0
Bifidobacteria	29.3	5.0×10^6	1465.0	4.0×10^7	11,720.0

* activity = n moles substrate degraded/hr/gram; + activity = μ moles substrate degraded/hr.

it has little carthatic effect, indicating that it might be inactivated by stomach acid or in the small bowel; the glucoside group must therefore protect the aglycone against the inactivation. Fingl (1965) showed that faecal bacteria could perform this hydrolysis and Hawksworth *et al.* (1971) found that cascara sagrada was a suitable substrate for the β-glucosidase of a *Strep. faecalis* strain.

The role of gut bacteria in the action of cathartic glycosides is therefore clear. Their role in the action of the cardiac glycosides is not so apparent. The cardiac glycosides include the digitalis group, the straphanthosides and the squill toad venom group. A characteristic of the digitalis glycosides is their slow excretion which, in addition to causing problems of overdosing may also permit extensive metabolism. Lauterback and Repke (1960) demonstrated that Lanatoside A (Fig. 5.4) is hydrolysed by the rat faecal suspensions to release acetyl-digitoxin by removal of the terminal glucose residue, and then digitoxin by subsequent removal of the acetyl group. These reactions were also demonstrated with lanatoside C using a strain of *Strep. faecalis* (Hawksworth *et al.*, 1971). Similarly, *K*-straphanthoside (Fig. 5.5) is hydrolysed by rat faecal suspensions to release cymarin by the removal of two glucose molecules (Holtz, 1958; Engler *et al.*, 1958). Both oral and parenteral administration of *K*-straphanthoside caused cymarin to be excreted in the urine and faeces, and it was suggested that cymarin might be responsible for some of the side effects of straphanthoside administration (e.g. emesis, convulsions) since it is known to be an intensely toxic compound. Thevetin is one of the poisonous principles of the betel nut and contains a digitoxigenin aglycone (as does Lanatoside A,

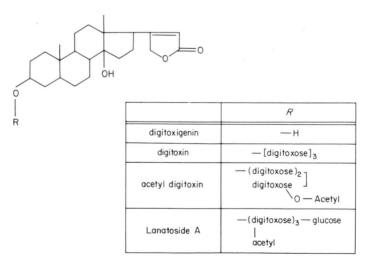

	R
digitoxigenin	— H
digitoxin	— [digitoxose]₃
acetyl digitoxin	— (digitoxose)₂ ⌉ digitoxose ⌋ ＼O — Acetyl
Lanatoside A	— (digitoxose)₃ — glucose | acetyl

Fig. 5.4. The structure of the Lanatoside A group of cardiac glycosides.

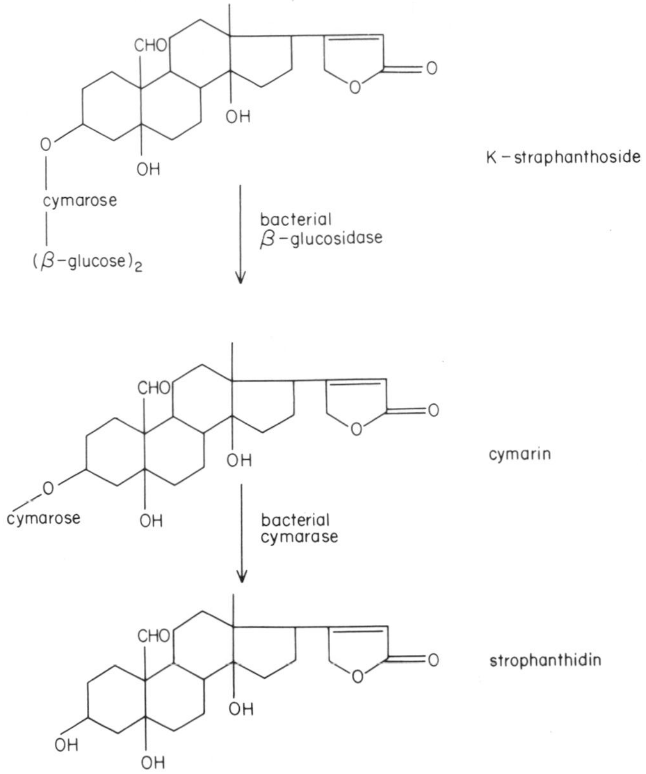

Fig. 5.5. The metabolism of *K*-straphanthoside.

see Fig. 5.4) linked to thevetose and two glucose molecules; again, it has been postulated that its action may be due to the aglycone released by gut bacterial action.

In addition to the harmless dietary glucosides and those with a therapeutic pharmacological effect, there are a number of glycosides which, if taken orally, have harmful effects. Amygdalin (Fig. 5.6) which is present in bitter almonds is practically non-toxic to mice when administered intraperitoneally with an LD^{50} greater than 5,000 mg/kg, but is extemely toxic when given orally (Williams, 1970b). It has been postulated that amygdalin is hydrolyzed in the gut by bacterial β-glucosidase to yield mandelonitrile, which is unstable and is readily hydrolysed to release cyanide, the postulated toxic agent. Amygdalin is readily hydrolysed *in vitro* by pure bacterial strains and, indeed, is one of the glucosides used in bacterial classification (together with salicin, aesculin etc.) (see Table 5.4). The cyanogenetic glucosides are ubiquitous in the plant kingdom and, in

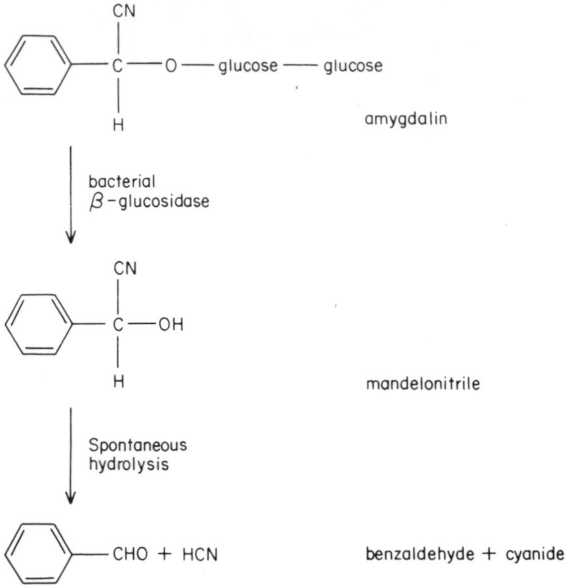

Fig. 5.6. The metabolism of amygdalin.

particular, are present in quite high amounts in certain plants used as human food-stuffs. The three major cyanogenetic glucosides are amygdalin, dhurrin (the glucoside of p-hydroxybenzaldehyde cyanohydrin) and linamarin (the glucoside of acetone cyanohydrin) linamarin is also known as phaseolunatin; the major food-stuffs habitually containing large amounts of cyanide include cassava, sweet potato, yams, butter beans and sorghum. In addition, many plants used as animal food-stuffs may also contain high levels of cyanogenetic glucoside. The poisoning of General Kitchener's transport animals in the Sudan by *Lotus arabicus* first led to the identification of linamarin (Dunstan and Henry, 1903). The poisonous properties of cassava were first recorded in 1605 by Clusius; before being consumed the cassava must be mashed and soaked to extract the cyanogenetic compounds, then boiled to hydrolyse any remaining glucoside and evaporate the HCN released. The lethal properties of oil of bitter almonds (due to the amygdalin content) has been well known for many centuries and it used to be commonly used in suicide or homicide. The toxicity of cyanogenetic plants has been reviewed by Montgomery (1969).

Perhaps the most widely publicized glucoside known to be hydrolysed by gut bacteria to yield a toxic aglycone is cycasin and the toxicity of this compound has been described by Mawdesley-Thomas (1971). During Captain Cook's exploration of the Pacific in 1770, his crew suffered severe

TABLE 5.4

Some glucosides used in bacterial taxonomy, and their hydrolysis by some organisms

	Baptisin	Aesculin	Amygdalin	Salicin	Coniferin	Arbutin	Saponin
Enterobacteria							
Proteus	–	+	+	–	+		–
Escherichia	–	+	+	–	+	+	–
Klebsiella	+	+	+	+	+		+
Salmonella	–	+		–			–
Shigella	–			–			–
Streptococci							
Strep. faecalis		+	+	+			
Strep. faecium		+	+	+			
Lactobacilli		+	+				
Staphylococci				+			
Clostridia		+	–	–			
Non-sporing anaerobes							
Bacteroides		+	–	–			
Fusobacteria		–	–	–			
Propionibacteria		+	–	+			
Bifidobacteria		+	+	+			
Eubacteria		+	–	–			

vomiting and gastrointestinal discomfort after eating raw cycad nuts (Hooker, 1896), and similar symptoms were reported after World War 2, when starving Japanese soldiers ate cycad nuts and suffered considerable discomfort as a result. Further interest was aroused following reports of the high incidence of neurological disorders amongst cycad eaters on Guam (Arnold *et al.*, 1953; Whiting, 1963), and amongst cattle fed cycads (Mason and Whiting, 1966; Hall and McGavin, 1928). Cycads are the principal starch source for people living in many areas of South East Asia, but only after long and careful preparation which involves the leaching out of toxic components. When this treated cycad flour was used in prolonged feeding experiments in rats no toxic effects were produced. However, if the whole untreated cycad was used, tumours were produced in the gut, liver and kidney (Laquer and Spatz, 1968). The toxic agent has now been shown to be cycasin, the glucoside methylazoxymethanol-β-D-glucoside (Fig. 5.7) via its aglycone methylazoxymethanol (MAM). The glucoside was first isolated by Cooper in 1941, and the structure was established by Nishida *et al.* (1955). Cycasin is not toxic when given parenterally but, when given orally, is extremely heptatoxic. Spatz (1964) fed guinea pigs on a tryptyphan-deficient diet containing cycad meal and induced liver tumours. Laqueur (1964) reported the carcinogenic effects of cycad meal, cycasin and MAM

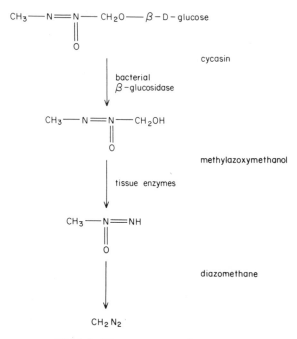

Fig. 5.7. The metabolism of cycasin.

in conventional rats but was unable to show any toxic effects with the first two in germ-free animals. It was later shown that the proximate carcinogen was MAM; cycasin is hydrolysed by the β-glucosidase of the gut bacteria to release the active aglycone (Laqueur *et al.*, 1967) which is thought to be further metabolized by the tissue enzymes to give the powerful methylating agent diazomethane (Williams, 1971b). In germ-free rats orally administered cycasin was excreted quantitatively unchanged, but in conventional rats only 18-35% of the dose was excreted (Spatz *et al.*, 1966) demonstrating the role of β-glucosidase of the gut bacterial flora (Spatz *et al.*, 1967; Dahlquist *et al.*, 1965). Spatz *et al.* (1967) showed that pure strains of streptococci and lactobacilli could hydrolyse cycasin to MAM *in vitro*.

IV. Metabolism of disaccharides

The ability of bacteria to metabolize disaccharides is well known and is used extensively in bacterial classification; such disaccharides are distributed extensively in the diet. The major disaccharides (e.g. sucrose, lactose and maltose) are hydrolysed by enzymes located in the enterocytic brush border and so do not reach the bacterially colonized regions. Consequently the bacterial enzymes are not utilized (due to lack of substrate) and the inducible enzymes (e.g. β-galactosidase in *Esch. coli*) are not produced. However, in certain disease states or syndromes the disaccharides are not hydrolysed by mucosal enzymes and are therefore not absorbed from the gut; under these conditions the bacterial enzymes become relevant and the result may be fermentative diarrhoea. The major enzymes of interest in this respect are lactase (β-galactosidase), sucrase (α-glucosidase) iso-maltase (β-glucosidase) and maltase (α-glucosidase). Although maltase and sucrase are both α-glucosidases, the mammalian enzymes are distinct and have different substrate specificities.

The most widely investigated disaccharidase deficiency, acquired lactase deficiency, is widespread throughout Africa, Asia and the indigenous peoples of Australia and America. The incidence is greater than 80% in Thailand (Flatz *et al.*, 1969), in Greeks living in London (McMichael *et al.*, 1966) in Chinese (Bolin *et al.*, 1968) in Bantu Africans (Cook and Kajubi, 1966; Jersky and Kinsley, 1967) as well as the indigenous people of New Guinea (Bolin *et al.*, 1968) and Australia (Elliott *et al.*, 1967). The term lactase deficiency is a misnomer since, of the populations investigated, only those of Anglo-Saxon or Scandinavian stock produce the intestinal enzyme (Table 5.5).

Lactose is present in the milk produced by most mammalian species and β-galactosidase is present in the intestinal mucosa of their off-spring during infancy. However, lactose and other β-galactosides are absent from

TABLE 5.5

The global incidence of lactose intolerance in adults

Population studied	% lactose intolerant
European	
Swiss	17
English	6
Danish	2-7
Swedish	3
Finnish	15
Greeks in London	90
American	
White	13
Indian	67
Negro	70
African	
Bantu	90
Ibo	98
Yoruba	98
Non-Bantu Ugandans	25
Australian	
European	0
Aboriginal	80
New Guinea	100
Asian	
Thais	100
Chinese	86
Asians in USA	100

non-milk products, so that after the weaning period the enzyme is no longer utilized and is lost in all animal species tested, and in humans except for N. W. Europeans and their descendants. There is still considerable controversy concerning the reasons for this anomaly and a number of reviews have been written on the subject (e.g. Bayless, 1971; Neale, 1972; McCracken, 1970). Simoon (1969, 1970) has hypothesized that lactose tolerance is a characteristic of populations who have traditionally consumed milk or milk products whilst those who do not are now lactose intolerent. It is possible that people in the non-milk drinking areas have never had the capacity to produce lactase in adulthood and that the non-milk diet is a natural result of this; alternatively the people living on non-milk diets gradually lose the enzyme (Bolin and Davis, 1969).

In lactose intolerant people a loading dose of lactose will not be absorbed and will then be metabolized in the caecum and colon to fatty acids, ethanol, CO_2 and H_2 giving rise to abdominal discomfort, flatulence and diarrhoea. Infants with disaccharidase deficiency often pass watery stools with a pH of less than 5.5 and containing much less lactic acid (Weijers *et al.*, 1960) but although these are also the symptoms of extreme lactase deficiency in adults, flatulence and abdominal pain are more commonly experienced.

The so-called fermentative diarrhoea is largely the result of osmotic effects; 1 molecule of lactose is metabolized to at least 4 molecules of acid and consequently, the water retained within the stool is increased considerably. It is possible, also that the acid produced may reduce the colonic pH sufficiently to produce an irritant effect. Lactase, or β-galactosidase, is widely distributed amongst the gut bacteria (Table 5.6), and is an inducible enzyme in *Esch. coli* but constitutive in *Strep. faecalis*. The bacterial enzyme is relatively non-specific, and can utilize *o*-nitrophenyl galactoside, lactose or lactulose as substrate.

TABLE 5.6

Production of β-galactosidase by gut bacteria

Bacteria tested	Mean activity (μ moles substrate degraded/hr/10^8 cells)
Esch. coli	42.4 ± 3.2*
Strep. faecalis	53.8 ± 6.0
Lactobacilli	90.6 ± 10.7
Clostridia	13.7 ± 2.7
Bacteroides	50.0 ± 4.9
Bifidobacteria	39.1 ± 4.7

* Standard error of mean

Because β-galactosidase is located in the small intestinal mucosal cells, lactose intolerance is a common secondary symptom associated with a range of small intestinal disorders, such as gastro-enteritis (Burke and Anderson, 1966), and may be an acquired feature of such disorders as Crohn's disease, ulcerative colitis, blind loop syndrome and tropical sprue. In protein malnutrition the activity of a range of small intestinal enzymes is reduced, so that lactose intolerance is often associated with kwashiorker. This is discussed more extensively later in this book.

The symptoms of fermentative diarrhoea are utilized in the lactulose treatment of hepatic coma. Although the β-galactosidase of the intestinal bacteria is relatively non-specific, the mucosal enzyme is unable to hydrolyse lactulose (fructose β1-4 galactoside) with the result that the sugar is available for bacterial fermentation. This is discussed extensively in

Chapter 15 which discusses the role of gut bacteria in cirrhosis and hepatic coma.

Deficiency in the other disaccharidases (e.g. sucrase, iso-maltase) is much rarer (Neale, 1971), presumably because these sugars are so widespread in the diet. Most patients suffering from acid diarrhoea not associated with lactose have their symptoms relieved by taking a diet free of sucrose. This is often associated with starch malabsorption, but not always so (Burgess *et al.*, 1964); when this is so, rice starch (which contains fewer α1-6 linkages) is often better tolerated. As with lactose intolerance, sucrase deficiency permits sucrose or starch substrate to reach the bacterially colonized area where it is hydrolysed to short chain fatty acids, CO_2 and H_2. The mean activity of the α-glucosidase of a range of bacterial species is shown in Table 5.7.

TABLE 5.7

Production of α-glucosidase by gut bacteria

Bacteria tested	Mean activity (μ moles substrate degraded/hr/10^8 cells)
Esch. coli	5.9 ± 0.5*
Strep. faecalis	14.0 ± 1.1
Lactobacilli	26.6 ± 3.5
Clostridia	30.1 ± 6.4
Bacteroides	9.8 ± 2.0
Bifidobacteria	20.7 ± 3.0

* Standard error of mean

A number of other disaccharides, polysaccharides and glycosides are present in small amounts in the diet and are hydrolysed by gut bacteria (Table 5.8). On occasions these reactions are of significance in bacterial classification but are not clinically important since the amount of substrate present in food would be insufficient to give significant quantities of acid.

V. Gut bacteria and the enterohepatic circulation of foreign compounds

The biological activity of foreign compounds in the body is limited by the rate at which they are metabolized and excreted. The metabolism undergone by such compounds is usually such as to increase the ease of elimination. One route of elimination is via the formation of hydrophilic metabolites which are then secreted in the bile and excreted in the intestine. This route is of major importance in the elimination of hydrophobic compounds, but is subject to interference by the gut bacteria.

TABLE 5.8

Disaccharides and glycosides normally present (sometimes in small amounts) in the diet and hydrolyzed by gut bacteria

Compound	Nature of glycoside
Trehalose	Disaccharide
Raffinose	Trisaccharide
Dextran/laevan	Polyglucose
Pectins	Polygalactose
	Polyarabinose
	Polygalacturonic acids
Pentosans	Poly D-xylose
	Polymers of xylose and glucuronic acid
Hexosans	Polymannose
	Polygalactose

The role of the bacteria in the absorption of foreign compounds and their subsequent metabolism is best illustrated by the use of some examples.

The dye Red 10G (Fig. 5.8) is used by the food industry as a food colouring agent and is sufficiently hydrophilic to be non-absorbed from the gut; it is therefore excreted in the faeces. Prontosil rubrum (Fig. 5.8) is another hydrophilic dye which is hydrolysed to yield the metabolite sulphanilamide, which is absorbed from the gut and subsequently eliminated in the urine. Stilboestrol is sufficiently lipophilic to be absorbed from the gut; it enters the portal blood system and is transported to the liver where it is conjugated with glucuronic acid and secreted in the bile. The glucuronide is relatively hydrophilic and is poorly absorbed, but it is hydrolysed by the gut bacteria to release the parent stilboestrol which is

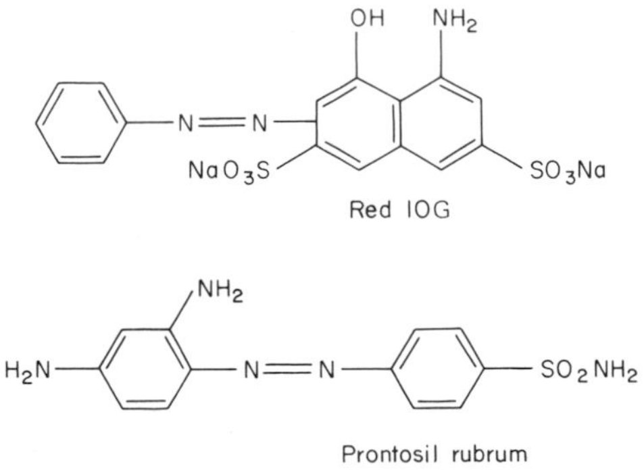

Fig. 5.8. The structure of Red 10G and prontosil rubrum.

then readily absorbed and returned to the liver for reconjugation. This enterohepatic circulation of stilboestrol is illustrated in Fig. 5.9, and results in a reduction in the efficiency of elimination of a compound.

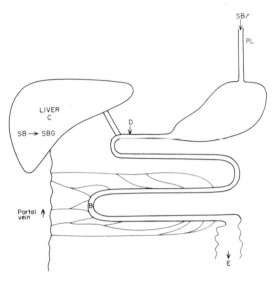

Fig. 5.9. The enterohepatic circulation of stilboestrol. Stilboestrol (SB) is orally administered (A), travels to the small intestine where it is absorbed, enters the portal blood and is carried to the liver C. There it is conjugated to give the glucuronide (SBG) and secreted in the bile (D) to enter the small intestine. That which is deconjugated by the bacteria is absorbed and returns to the liver for another cycle; undeconjugated material is excreted in the faeces E.

The factors determining the proportion of a compound excreted in the bile and the implication of such secretions have been reviewed by Smith (1966). The ease of hydrolysis of glucuronides by gut bacteria will vary depending on the nature of the aglycone; some glucuronides are poor substrates for the bacterial enzyme whilst others are readily hydrolysed. In view of the high activity of bacterial β-glucuronidase in the gut it is inevitable that many compounds secreted in the bile as conjugates will be eliminated very inefficiently. The proportion of compound retained in the body from each cycle will vary from person to person due to differences in the hydrolytic activity of the gut flora, and for the same reason there will be gross differences between animal species (see Table 5.2). Thus, rats, which have a relatively high bacterial β-glucuronidase activity in the small intestine, are likely to hydrolyse and recycle a higher proprtion of a compound than do rabbits; an example of this is stilboestrol which is rapidly eliminated by the rabbit but only slowly by the rat. As a consequence of the variation between persons in the degree of enterohepatic circulation of a compound there is a variation in the extent of cumulative effects of drugs. A result of the variation between species is the difficulty of safety testing of drugs, since an animal which extensively recycles a compound is more likely to modify its pharmacological effect (with either beneficial or harmful results).

Phenolphthalein is the active constituent of many purgatives and is said to stimulate the small intestinal motility. It is readily absorbed from the gut and is conjugated in the liver with glucuronic acid prior to secretion in the bile. During its transit through the small intestine it is hydrolysed to release the active compound which stimulates the gut motility and is reabsorbed for another cycle. Thus a single dose of purgative which undergoes enterohepatic circulation has as much effect as many doses of a similar compound which is not recycled. Phenolphthalein is only slowly eliminated by humans because, although they have little intestinal β-glucuronidase compared with other animals (Table 5.2), the glucuronide is an extremely good substrate for the bacterial enzyme (indeed it is the standard substrate used in the assay of β-glucuronidase). In a similar way chloramphenicol, an antibiotic which is chiefly used in the treatment of typhoid, is recycled efficiently and is therefore in contact with the target organism for a relatively prolonged period of time.

With both phenolphthalein and chloramphenicol the enterohepatic cycle prolongs the time available for the compound to act, and in both these cases this effect is harnessed therapeutically. However, in some cases it can cause difficulties in treatment. Morphine is extensively recycled and this can result in overdose and the problem of drug accumulation (Woods, 1954). Similarly, cumulative effects are important in treatment with the cardiac glycosides, especially the digitalis group (Okita et al., 1954). A further problem is the fact that compounds which are extensively recycled are more likely to induce bacterial degradative enzymes and this is thought to be responsible for some of the side-effects of treatment with cardiac glycosides and with chloramphenicol. The degradation of chloramphenicol to minor metabolites is discussed in Chapter 11.

CHAPTER 6

Metabolism of Nitrogen Compounds

I. Metabolism of primary amino groups

The two principle reactions of primary amino groups are deamination and N-esterification. These will be discussed in turn.

A. DEAMINATION

Gut bacteria are able to release ammonia from amino acids and amines and it was thought that this might be a significant source of intestinal ammonia. Sabbaj *et al.* (1970) showed that, although the ability to deaminate amino acids is widespread amongst the gut bacteria, ammonia from this source makes only a minor contribution to the total intestinal pool (the major source being urea hydrolysis). Table 6.1 summarizes the data in the literature on the ability of gut bacteria to deaminate amino acids.

Bacteria are able to deaminate by four direct pathways (Fig. 6.1) and an additional indirect route, the Stickland reaction. The four direct pathways are (i) oxidation, with the formation of an aldehyde and ammonia; (ii) reduction, with the production of a saturated fatty acid from an amino acid; (iii) hydrolysis, with the production of an alcohol or an α-hydroxy acid from an amine or amino acid respectively, and (iv) removal of the elements of ammonia yielding an unsaturated product.

Oxidative deamination is the major pathway used by mammalian cells but is of relatively minor importance in bacteria. According to Gale (1952), this mechanism for the deamination of amino acids is restricted to a few organisms (e.g. *Esch. coli*) acting on a restricted range of amino acids such as glycine, alanine and glutamic acid. Hawksworth (1973) showed that the oxidative deamination of putrescine and cadaverine (Fig. 6.2) was performed by a high proportion of strains of *Esch. coli*, bacteroides, bifidobacteria and clostridia (Table 6.2). This reaction is a step in the formation of the cyclic secondary amines piperidine and pyrrolidine from lysine and arginine respectively; these are produced by the gut flora in the large intestine and are discussed later. Similarly tryptophan is deaminated to indolepyruvic acid.

TABLE 6.1

Deamination of amino acids by intestinal bacteria

Organism tested	Arginine	Alanine	Aspartic acid	Cysteine	Glutamic acid	Glycine	Histidine	Leucine	Iso-leucine	Nor-leucine	Lysine	Methionine	Ornithine	Proline	Hydroxyproline	Serine	Threonine	Tyrosine	Phenylalanine	Tryptophan	Valine	Non-valine
Enterobacteria																						
Escherichia	O		R/D	R	O	O	D	O	O	O	-	O				R/H	R	O	-	R	O	O
Proteus	O		R/D	R	O	O	O	O	O	O	O	O				R	R	O	O	O	O	O
Klebsiella			+								-								-	-		
Salmonella		+					D				-								-	-		
Shigella							D				-								+	-		
Streptococci (unspec.)																						
Strep. faecalis			+													+		+				
Strep. faecium																-		-		-		
Lactobacillus spp.			R																			
Bacillus spp.	O				O	O																
Vibrio			+	R																		
Staphylococci	+	+	+		+	+	+							+		+	+			+		
Non-sporing anaerobes																						
Gram +ve								+						+	+	+		-		+		
Gram -ve																		-		-		
Clostridia spp.																						
Cl. welchii	S	S	S	S	S	S/D	S	O/S	S			S	S	S	S	S/R	R	S	S	S		
Cl. botulinum	S	S	S	S	S	S	S	S	S			S	S	S	S	S/O		S	S	S		
Cl. sporogenes	R/S	O/S	O/S	O/S	O/S	R/S	O/S	O/S	O/S			O/S	S/R/O	R/S	R/S	S/O		S/R/O	S/O	S/R/O	S/O	
Cl. tetanomorphum	S	S	S	S	S	S	S	S	S			S	S	S	S	S		S	S	S	S/R/O	
Cl. tetani	S	S	S	S	S	S	S	S	S			S	S	S	S	S		S	S	S	S/O	

D = removal of elements of ammonia; H = hydrolytic deamination; O = oxidative deamination; R = reductive deamination; S = Stickland; + = deamination by unspecified mechanism; — = claimed not to deaminate.

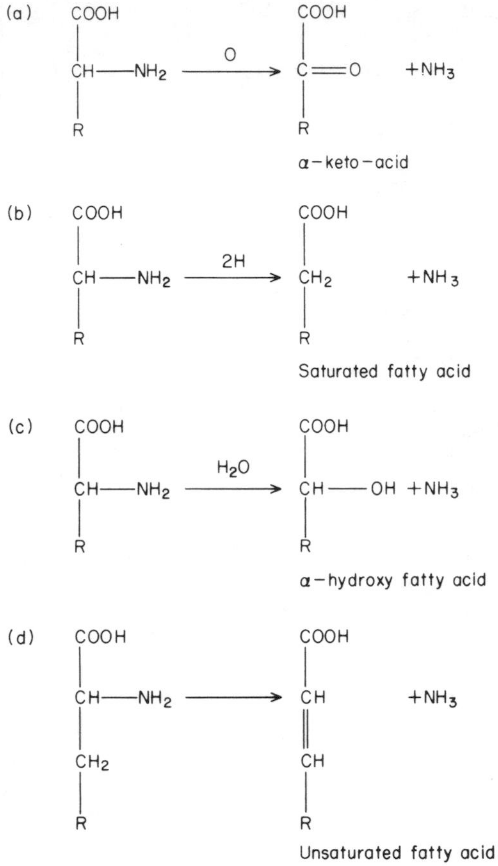

(a)
$$CH-NH_2 \xrightarrow{O} C=O \quad +NH_3$$

with COOH above each, R below each; α−keto−acid

(b)
$$CH-NH_2 \xrightarrow{2H} CH_2 \quad +NH_3$$

with COOH above each, R below each; Saturated fatty acid

(c)
$$CH-NH_2 \xrightarrow{H_2O} CH-OH \quad +NH_3$$

with COOH above each, R below each; α−hydroxy fatty acid

(d)
$$CH-NH_2 \longrightarrow CH \quad +NH_3$$

with COOH above; CH₂ and R below on left; CH below CH (double bond) and R below on right; Unsaturated fatty acid

Fig. 6.1. Major pathways of deamination of primary amines and amino acids by bacteria; (a) oxidative; (b) reductive; (c) hydrolytic; and (d) removal of the elements of ammonia.

Reductive deamination producing a saturated fatty acid from an amino acid is probably the most widely reported mechanism of microbial deamination. Aspartic acid is deaminated to succinic acid by a number of anaerobic organisms and *Mycobacterium phlei*; similarly tyramine is deaminated to p-hydroxyphenylpropionic acid (phloretic acid) and tryptophan to indoleproprionic acid by a range of gut bacterial species. L-3, 4-dihydroxyphenylalanine (L-dopa) is reductively deaminated to 3,4-dihydroxyphenylacetic acid by gut bacteria. Cohen *et al.* (1946) demonstrated the production of ethanol from ethanolamine by reductive deamination.

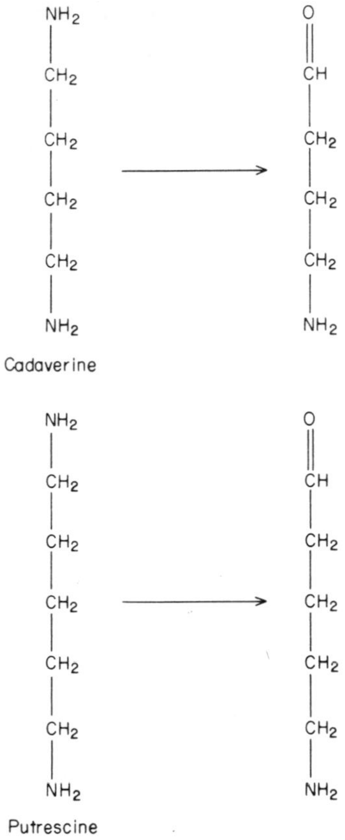

Fig. 6.2. The oxidative deamination of cadaverine and putrescine.

TABLE 6.2

The deamination of putrescine and cadaverine by gut bacteria

| Organism | % able to deaminate | |
	Putrescine	Cadaverine
Esch. coli	0	0
Strep. faecalis	0	0
Bacteroides spp.	75	38
Bifidobacteria	63	25
Clostridia	50	63

Hydrolysis is exemplified by the deamination of aspartic acid to yield malic acid by *Pseudomonas fluorescens*. One of the metabolites of tyrosine, p-hydroxyphenyllactic acid, may also be a product of hydrolytic deamination.

An example of the fourth type of deamination, removal of the elements of ammonia leaving an unsaturated product, is the "aspartase" produced by *Esch. coli* and a range of other facultative anaerobic bacteria. These organisms deaminate aspartic acid to yield fumaric acid, which is rapidly reduced to succinic acid unless enzyme inhibitors such as toluene are added to the reaction mixture. It is probable that many apparent examples of reductive deamination are in fact the result of such two stage reaction (as in a similar way, apparent examples of hydrolytic deamination are the result of oxidative deamination followed by reduction of the product).

In addition to these examples of direct deamination, there is a further type of deamination, a complex reaction involving two amino acids resulting in the mutal elimination of ammonia. This is the mixed amino acid fermentation, or Stickland reaction. Stickland demonstrated that, using reducible dyes as H-donators and acceptors, some amino acids are deaminated by strains of clostridia in the presence of H-donators and others are deaminated in the presence of H-acceptors. Thus, during the course of the reaction some amino acids can act as H-acceptors and others as H-donors; if an amino acid from each group is added to a suspension of the organisms then deamination of both occurs with the H-donor amino acid undergoing oxidative deamination to a keto acid and the H-acceptor undergoing reductive deamination to the corresponding saturated fatty acid (Fig. 6.3). This mixed amino acid fermentation is the pathway used in the putrefactive digestion of meat, the foul stench thought to be due to the products of such a reaction involving the sulphur amino acids, tryptophan etc.

A special case of the deamination of primary amines is the hydrolysis of urea to CO_2 and ammonia. This reaction is carried out by a wide range of organisms, amongst those identified by Sabbaj *et al.* (1970) were *Klebsiella Enterobacter* species, *Proteus mirabilis, P. vulgaris, Esch. coli,* Citrobacter, *Pseudomonas aeruginosa, Staph. aureus, Bacteroides fragilis, Staph. epidermidis,* and *Clostridium perfringens.* In a parallel study by Brown *et al.*

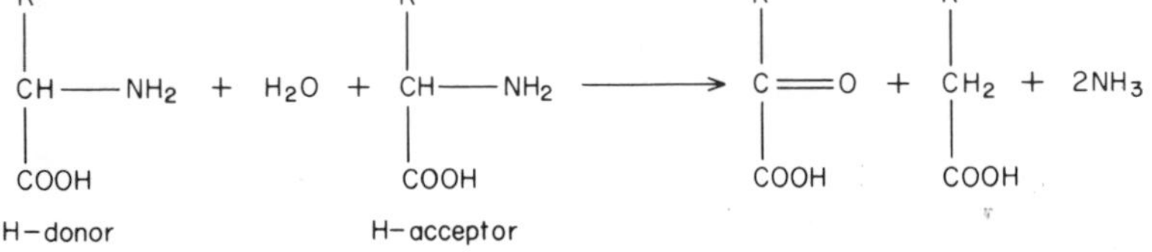

Fig. 6.3. Amino acid deamination via the STICKLAND reaction.

(1971) the urease-positive species included *Klebsiella* spp, *Clostridium sordelii, Bact. fragilis, Bifidobacterium* spp., anaerobic lactobacilli and *Eubacterium* spp. (Table 6.3); similar results were obtained by Donaldson (1964).

TABLE 6.3

Hydrolysis of urea by human intestinal bacteria

Organisms tested	Number of strains tested	% producing urease	Comments
Enterobacteria	220	2	All +ve strains were Klebsiellas
Strep. faecalis	118	0	—
Clostridia	100	5	All +ve strains were *Cl. sordelii*
Non-sporing anaerobes	161	11	+ve strains included Bacteroides, Bifidobacteria, Eubacteria, and Lactobacilli

Approximately 40% of the urea synthesized by the liver is hydrolysed to ammonia by gastrointestinal urease, and virtually all of the enzyme is bacterial. The metabolism of urea and its relevance to hepatic encephalopathy has been reviewed by Summerskill (1969). There is some evidence that the hydrolysis is carried out by bacteria which are closely associated with the gut mucosa cells (Wolpert *et al.*, 1971). It is necessary to posulate this since there is evidence that, despite the obvious effectiveness of the gut flora in the urea hydrolysis, the gut mucosa is relatively impermeable to the urea molecule; Wolpert *et al.* obtained evidence that, after cleansing the gut of luminal bacteria ureolysis was much more efficient if the urea was delivered to the colon by the circulation than when perfused through the lumen even though larger amounts were delivered by the latter route. Urease is the major source of intestinal ammonia with deamination of amino acids providing only a small proportion of the total (Sabbaj *et al.*, 1970).

In uraemia the blood urea level increases considerably although the proportion metabolized remains at about 40% (Walser and Bodenlos, 1959) and this is due to an increase in the proportion of bacteria able to hydrolyse urea (Brown *et al.*, 1971) as shown in Fig. 6.4, with no increase in the mean activity per strain. It was known that the urease of *Proteus* spp was constitutive and non-inducible; the evidence of Brown *et al.* implies that this is also true of the urease produced by the strictly anaerobic organisms. The increased ammonia release in uraemia results in urea nitrogen being converted to protein nitrogen (Richards *et al.*, 1967) and

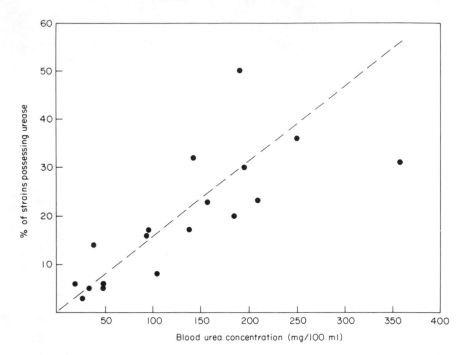

Fig. 6.4. Relation between the blood urea concentration and the proportion of faecal anaerobic bacteria possessing urease.

thus works to the advantage of the patient, since it means that the intake of dietary nitrogen can be curtailed without necessarily upsetting the nitrogen balance of the patient.

Whereas microbial ureolysis is of benefit to the uraemic patient, it is a major hazard to the cirrhotic or to the patient who has undergone systemoportal anastamosis (Ridwell, 1955). Portal ammonia is detoxified by the liver via the formation of urea or by incorporation into protein material. In cirrhosis the liver is unable to deal with the ammonia load and the systemic blood level, normally very low, rises resulting in ammonia intoxication. This is discussed more fully later.

B. N-ESTERIFICATION

The N-esterification of primary amino groups is the basis of the resistance of bacteria to the antibiotic effect of the sulphonamides and a number of amino glycosides; this is discussed more extensively in Chapter 11.

Urbach (1949), investigating the urinary excretion of N-acetyl histamine following the oral administration of the free amine, concluded that the intestinal flora was responsible for the reaction and demonstrated that strains of *Esch. coli* and *Aerobacter aerogenes* were able to perform the reation. The N-acetyl histamine in human urine seems to be largely the result of the metabolism of histidine by the gut bacteria.

The reverse reaction, the hydrolysis of an N-ester linkage, is exemplified in chloramphenicol metabolism (fig. 6.5) where the dichloroacetyl group is removed by *Esch. coli* (Smith and Worrall, 1950).

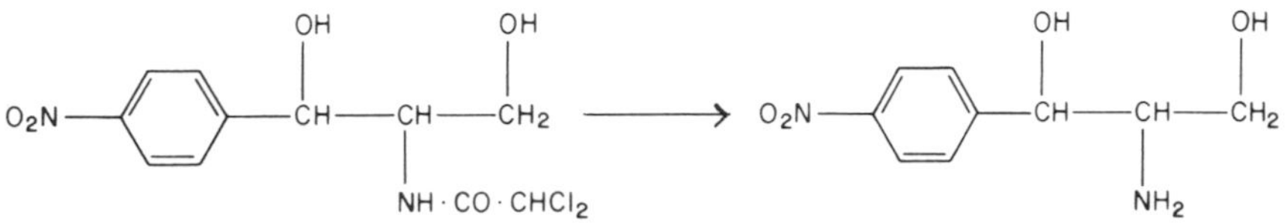

Fig. 6.5. Hydrolysis of the amide linkage in chloramphenicol by *Esch. coli.*

II. Metabolism of secondary amino groups

The two principle reactions of secondary amino groups are N-dealkylation to give a primary amine, and N-nitrosation.

A. N-DEALKYLATION

The N-dealkylation by gut bacteria has been examined mainly in the study of choline metabolism (which will be discussed in the next section), but there is a growing number of examples of secondary amines of clinical importance which undergo N-dealkylation. Thus methylamphetamine (Fig. 6.6) is demethylated to yield amphetamine by a range of species of intestinal bacteria (Table 6.4). Similarly imipramine is demthylated to yield desmethylimpramine (Fig. 6.6) by the gut bacterial flora (Minder *et al.*, 1971); this is of interest because it is the product of this reaction which is thought to be the proximate psychotropic agent rather than the drug itself (Parke, 1969).

There are a number of examples of cyclic secondary amines being hydrolysed to primary amines. It was shown as early as 1910 that gut bacteria could open the pyrrolidine ring of proline (Ackerman, 1910) and in a similar manner the heterocyclic rings of the purine and pyrimidine molecule are opened by N-dealkylation reactions. Thanhauser and Dorfmuller (1918) showed that adenosine, guanosine and inosine were converted to ammonia *in vitro*. Lethco and Webb (1966) demonstrated the formation of 5-sulphoanthranilic acid from the dye indigo carmine. Windmueller (1965) found that orotic acid was extensively catabolized by the gastrointestinal microflora of rats to ethanol, CO_2 and ammonia.

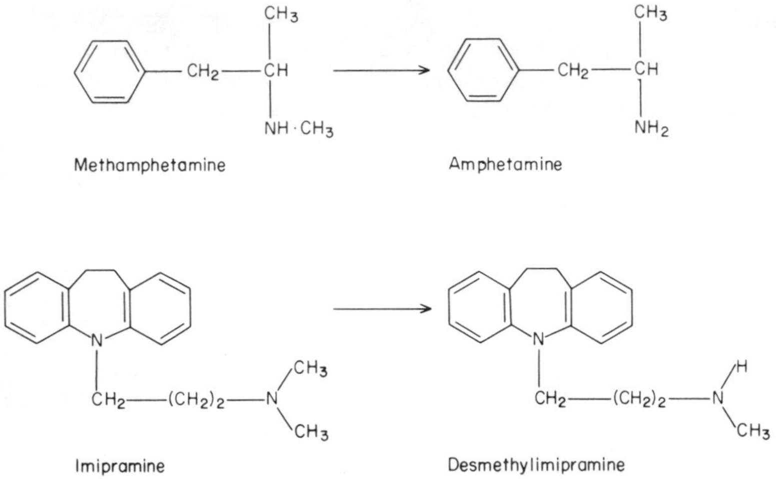

Fig. 6.6. The N-demethylation of methamphetamine and imipramine.

TABLE 6.4

N-demethylation of methylamphetamine by gut bacteria

| Organisms tested | N-demethylation of methylamphetamine | |
	Number of strains tested	%
Esch. coli	15	7
Strep. faecalis	15	67
Lactobacilli	8	75
Clostridia	23	35
Bacteroides	14	7
Bifidobacteria	6	0

Germ-free animals excreted 30% of an oral dose unchanged in the faeces. Conventional rats did not excrete any after the first five days, which were presumably necessary for adaptation by the gut flora. There seems little doubt, therefore, that the gut flora are responsible for the ring opening and destruction of orotic acid; at some stage in that destruction an N-dealkylation must have occurred.

B. *N*-NITROSATION

Nitrosamines are the product of an acid-catalysed reaction between secondary amines and nitrous acid (Fig. 6.7). In 1968 Sander demonstrated that certain strains of enterobacteria were able to N-nitrosate diphenyl-

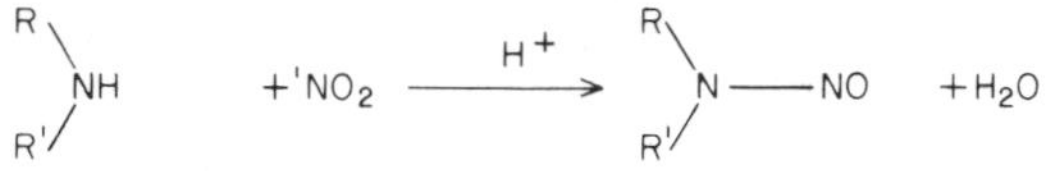

Fig. 6.7. The reaction between a secondary amine and nitrous acid to give an N-nitrosamine.

amine at neutral pH values using nitrate as the source of the nitrous group. This work was confirmed and extended by Hawksworth and Hill (1971a, b) and by Hill and Hawksworth (1973). The reaction involving nitrate is only performed by nitrate-reducing bacteria, but a proportion of the strains which do not produce nitrate are able to nitrosate secondary amines using nitrite as the nitrosating agent. These include enterococci, clostridia, bacteroides and bifidobacteria (Table 6.5). The ease of nitrosation is dependent to some extent on the basicity of the parent secondary amine (Table 6.6) varying from 68% for diphenylamine to less than 0.01% for dimethylamine. The reaction could be brought about by an enzymic reaction, or it could be merely due to the bacteria producing the reactants and the conditions necessary for the reaction. We have only been able to demonstrate the nitrosation of secondary amines by growing cultures of

TABLE 6.5

The N-nitrosation of secondary amines by gut bacteria

Organisms	N-nitrosation of diphenylamine	
	Number of strains tested	%[+]ve
Esch. coli	37	27
Strep. faecalis	10	40
Clostridia	21	10
Bacteroides	17	12
Bifidobacteria	22	18

TABLE 6.6

The nitrosation of various secondary amines related to their basicity

Secondary amine tested	% nitrosation	pK_6
Diphenylamine	68.0	13.1
Piperidine	0.4[+]	3.3
Pyrrolidine	0.4[+]	—
Dimethylamine	0.01	3.3
Diethylamine	0.01	2.9

[+] Assayed by GLC; remainder assayed by polarography

bacteria, and have not been able to isolate any enzymes from resting cultures; this would be in favour of the non-enzymic mechanism. Furthermore, growing cultures generate acid conditions during growth – the very conditions that would be expected to favour chemical nitrosation. However, addition of nitrite and secondary amines to the supernatant of an overnight broth culture results in negligible nitrosation, indicating that the acid generated is not sufficient alone to account for the nitrosation. Not all strains of *Esch. coli* produce nitrosamines to the same extent even though they all presumably produce the same conditions with respect to E_h and pH.

There are three secondary amines normally excreted in urine, dimethylamine is the most abundant, 20 mg being excreted per day (Asatoor and Simenhoff, 1965); most of this is derived from lecithin or choline (Fig. 6.8) and studies on germ-free and conventional pigs indicate that at least 50% of the dimethylamine is the result of gut bacterial action (Hawksworth, 1973). Piperidine and Pyrrolidine are excreted at the rate of 0.8 and 0.4 mg/day respectively and are the result of bacterial action on lysine and argine respectively (Fig. 6.9). There will also be a range of dietary secondary

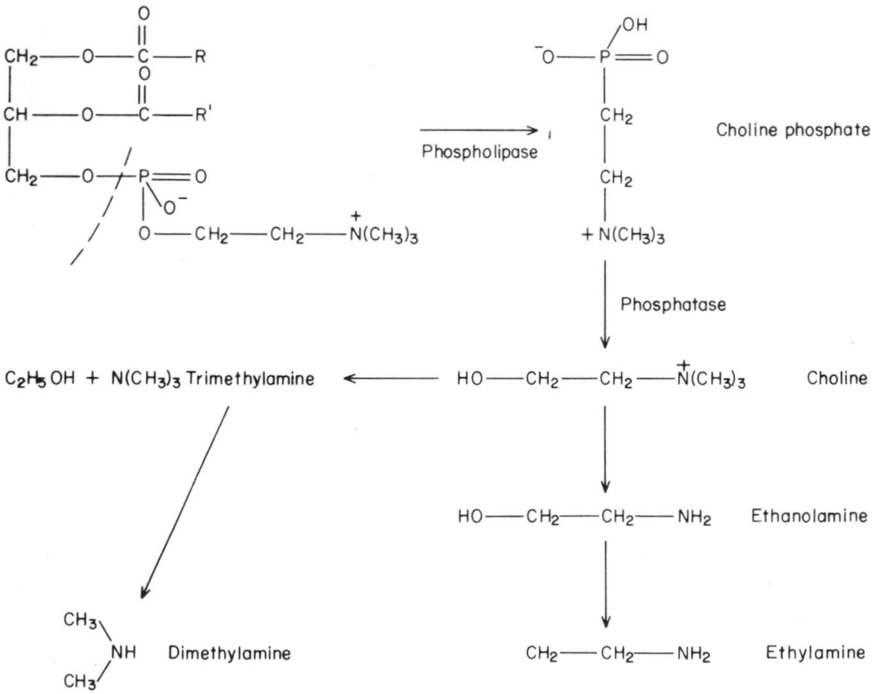

Fig. 6.8. The degradation of lecithin to yield dimethylamine.

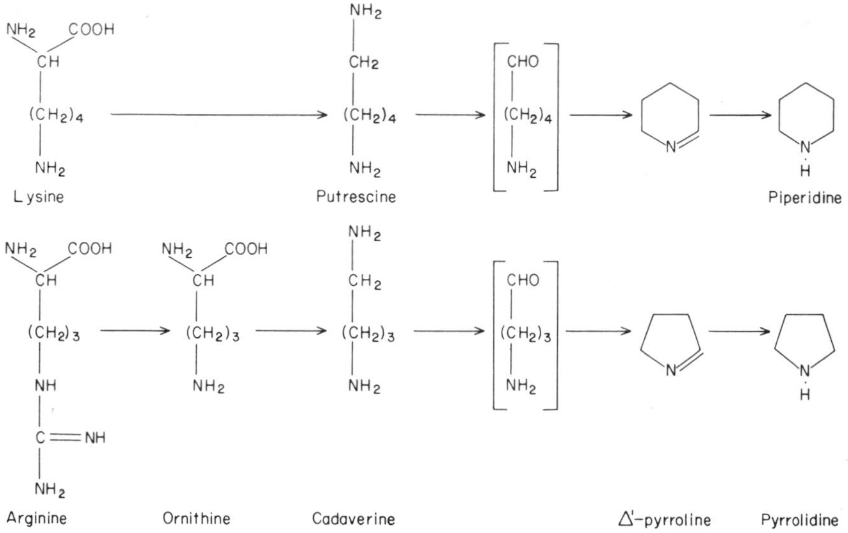

Lysine — Putrescine — Piperidine

Arginine — Ornithine — Cadaverine — Δ'-pyrroline — Pyrrolidine

Fig. 6.9. The formation of piperidine and pyrrolidine from lysine and arginine respectively.

amines excreted in the urine but these will, of course, be of variable amounts depending on the diet in the 24 hours prior to collection of the urine. Nitrate is rapidly excreted in the urine (Hawksworth and Hill, 1971b; Hill and Hawksworth, 1973) and so a person whose bladder is infected with a nitrosating strain will produce nitrosamines in his bladder if his nitrate intake is sufficient. This is discussed more extensively later.

III. Metabolism of tertiary and quaternary amines

The principle bacterial metabolic reaction with tertiary and quanternary amines is N-dealkylation and this has been extensively studied with respect to choline metabolism. Cohen *et al.* (1946) demonstrated that choline was metabolized by strains of *Bacillus* spp. and *Clostridium* spp. to trimethyl-amine which was further demethylated to dimethylamine, methylamine then ammonia. This metabolic sequence was also shown to be carried out by the gut bacterial flora by Michel (1962) and by Asatoor and Simenhoff (1965). Using isolated pure strains of human intestinal bacteria the N-dealkylation of choline was shown to be carried out by clostridia, bacteroides and bifidobacteria (Table 6.7); the pH optimum of the N-dealkylation by a strain of *Cl. bifermentans* was 5.5-6.5 (Hawksworth and Hill, 1971a).

TABLE 6.7

The N-dealkylation of choline by gut bacteria to release dimethylamine

Organisms tested	N-dealkylation of choline	
	Number tested	% producing dimethylamine
Esch. coli	9	11
Strep. faecalis	12	0
Bacteroides fragilis	11	27
+ Bifidobacteria		
Clostridia	19	53

Choline is released in the gut by bacterial action on lecithin and is metabolized in the gut to dimethylamine which is excreted in the urine. Asatoor and Simenhoff (1965) demonstrated that neomycin treatment of humans reduced the urinary dimthylamine level; further, the urinary dimethylamine concentration is much lower in germ-free than in conven-

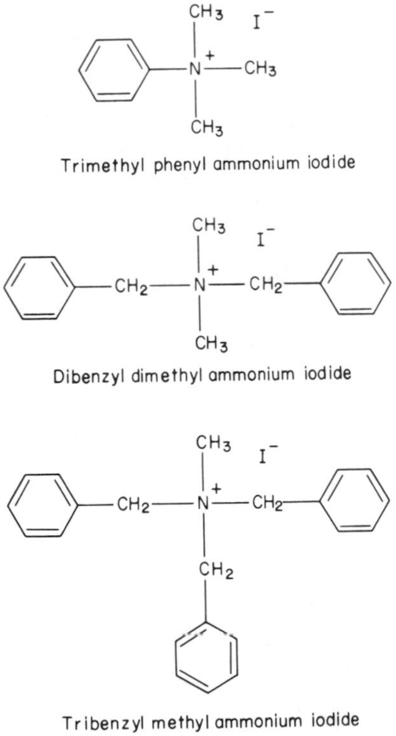

Trimethyl phenyl ammonium iodide

Dibenzyl dimethyl ammonium iodide

Tribenzyl methyl ammonium iodide

Fig. 6.10. Quaternary ammonium compounds which are N-dealkylated by gut bacteria.

tional pigs. Thus it is likely that at least half of the urinary dimethylamine is of bacterial origin.

In addition to choline, a number of other quaternary ammonium compounds are dealkylated by gut bacteria and some of these are illustrated in Fig. 6.10. Strains producing dimethylamine from choline also do so from acetyltrimethylammonium bromide.

IV. Hydrolysis and reduction of diazo compounds

The reduction of diazo compounds by gut bacteria first received general notice when it was observed that the anti-bacterial action of prontosil rubrum was due to the bacterial metabolite sulphanilamide (Fig. 6.11);

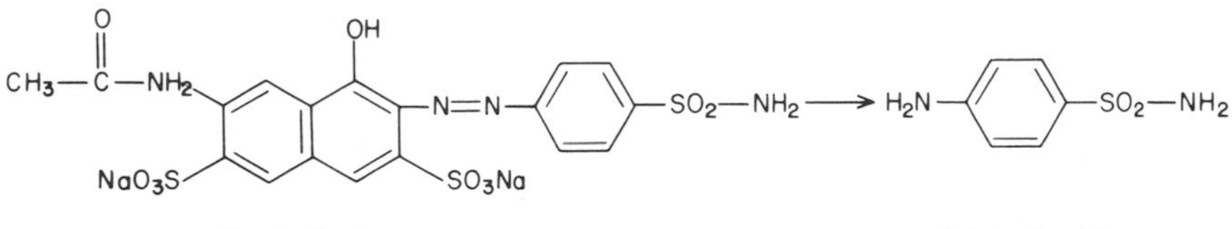

Fig. 6.11. Hydrolysis of prontosil rubrum to yield sulphanilamide.

similarly sulphanilamide is released from neoprontosil and sulphapyridine from salazopyrine by bacterial action. In all three cases the parent diazo compound had no anti-bacterial activity; the therapeutic aspects of this reaction are discussed more fully in Chapter 11.

We have studied the latter reaction, the reduction of the diazo linkage of salazopyrine by pure cultures of human gut bacteria. Overnight cultures were harvested by centrifugation, suspended in peptone water to give a suspension containing 10^{10} organisms/ml and incubated with salazopyrine at $37°$ C; the reduction was followed spectrophotometrically. During the course of the reaction the proportion of viable organisms in the suspension fell due to the release of sulphapyridine. The optimal pH of the reaction was 7 with *Strep. faecalis*, but 5 with *Cl. welchii* (Fig. 6.12), and the optimal temperature for the reaction was $37°$ C. The reaction was inhibited by periodate, iodoacetate cupric and fluoride ions, by the surfactant sodium lauryl sulphate, and by the chelating agent EDTA, but not by magnesium ions, or by lytic agents such as toluene, or with clostridia by formaldehyde or azide ions. No reduction was obtained if the reaction was carried out in phosphate buffer instead of peptone water. Preliminary screening studies (Table 6.8) showed that the anaerobic organisms (*Bacteroides fragilis, Cl. welchii, Cl.bifermentans,* lecithinase-negative clostridia and *Bifidobacterium* spp.) were more active than the aerobic *Esch. coli* and *Strep. faecalis.*

HIF—4

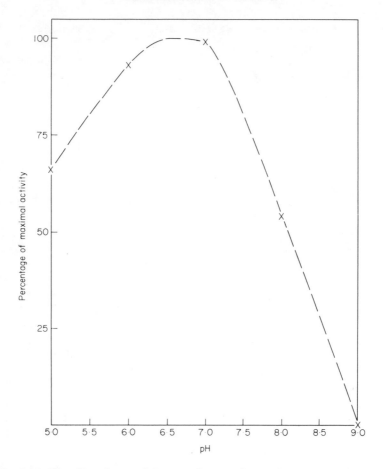

Fig. 6.12. The pH-optimum of the azoreductase of *Cl. welchii* and *Strep. faecalis.*

A wide range of azo dyes are used by the food industry as colouring agents. Most of these are sulphonated water soluble dyes but a number of oil soluble azo dyes have also been studied. Radomski and Mellinger (1962) studied the reduction of amaranth, ponceau SX and sunset yellow (Fig. 6.13) and demonstrated that the liver azo reductase was relatively unimportant on their metabolism, the dyes being almost entirely reduced by the gut bacteria. A strain of *Strep. faecalis* was isolated from faeces and shown to reduce acid yellow (Scheline and Lonborg, 1965). The hydrolysis of brown FK by rat intestinal contents and by several isolated strains of *Strep. faecalis* was investigated by Fore *et al.* (1967) and a number of azo dyes were hydrolysed by strains of *Proteus vulgaris* and *Esch. coli* (Roxon *et al.*, 1967).

TABLE 6.8

The reduction of salazopyrine by gut bacteria

Organisms tested		Activity of salazopyrine azoreductase[+]	
		Mean	Range
Esch. coli	(10)	0.389	0.095-0.918
Strep. faecalis	(9)	0.917	0.410-2.19
Lactobacillus spp.	(10)	12.990	0-50.72
Bacteroides fragilis	(9)	0.246	0.009-0.785
Eubacterium biforme	(5)	0.276	0.189-0.449
Bifidobacterium adolescentis	(4)	0.810	0-3.06
Clostridium bifermentans	(5)	14.554	0-64.56
Clostridium welchii	(5)	26.695	2.184-115.44
Lecithinase ⁻ve clostridia	(9)	7.406	0-22.25

Numbers in parentheses indicate the number of strains tested.

[+] Activity is expressed as the amount of substrate (nM) reduced by 10^8 cells per hour.

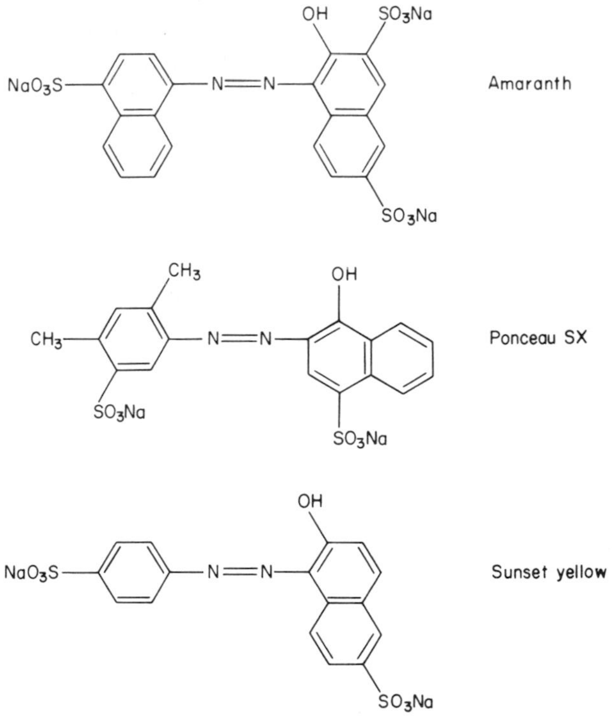

Fig. 6.13. The structure of amaranth, ponceau SX and sunset yellow.

In a systematic study of the hydrolysis of food colours by gut bacteria, Linnecar *et al.* (unpublished results) incubated 20 food dyes with a range of intestinal bacteria. All of the dyes were permitted for use in the U.K. Nineteen were azo dyes and the remaining one was the indigoid dye indigo carmine. The eight dyes amaranth, black 7984, black PN, carmoisine, fast red E, ponceau 4R, red FB and sunset yellow all have sulphonated aromatic nuclei on both sides of the diazo bond; they are highly water soluble and strongly ionized in an aqueous solution and they are all readily hydrolysed by gut bacteria to give highly polar amino or aminohydroxy-sulphonic acids as products. In contrast, the dyes orange G, orange RN, ponceau MX, red 6B, red 10B and red 2G which all give rise to at least one relatively non-polar (i.e. unsulphonated) metabolite are less readily degraded. It is the less polar metabolites which are potentially the more toxic. The two other less readily hydrolyzed dyes, tartrazine and yellow 2G, although giving only sulphonated metabolites, are azo derivatives of pyrazolone – a hetero-cyclic compound. In general the anaerobic organisms, the bacteroides, bifidobacteria and clostridia, hydrolysed the azo dyes more effectively than did the aerobic bacteria tested (*Esch. coli* and *Strep. faecalis*), in agreement with the results obtained with salazopyrine.

The significance of azo dye reduction by gut bacteria is hard to assess. It is unlikely that the highly polar sulphonated napthylamines, which are released by hydrolysis of most of the dyes, would be absorbed from the gut. There are however, reports of fission products of the dyes being excreted in free or conjugated form in the urine (Daniel, 1962), mainly in small rodents. The non-polar products are potentially toxic since they will be absorbed and may be metabolized by the liver to aryl N-hydroxyl-amines, which are postulated to play a role in bladder cancer.

V. Reduction of a nitro group, nitrate or nitrite

Nitrate reductase is an enzyme widely distributed in the bacterial world (Table 6.9) although the most active group of organisms is the *Esch. coli* group. The nitrate reductase activity has been extensively studied and is related to the amount of cytochrome b_1 in the bacterial membranes (Chang and Lascelles, 1963; Taniguchi and Itagaki, 1960). Taniguchi and Itagaki isolated a particulate nitrate reductase system, which included cyt. b_1 as an intermediary carrier from formate or DPNH to nitrate, from *Esch. coli* cells grown anaerobically in the presence of nitrate. The nitrate reductase is an anaerobic enzyme and is profoundly retarded even by a low oxygen pressure; however, it can function aerobically in the presence of a suitable respiratory substrate such as formate. When nitrate reduction is linked to formate oxidation the product is first nitrite then ammonia which is then incorporated into protein. The anaerobic reduction of nitrate to nitrite is

TABLE 6.9

Production of nitrate reductase by human intestinal bacteria

Organisms tested	Production of nitrate reductase	
	No. of strains tested	% reducing nitrate
Esch. coli	27	96
Strep. faecalis	21	19
Clostridium spp.	30	23
Bacteroides fragilis	17	35
Bifidobacteria	22	32

referred to as nitrate respiration, whereas the aerobic reduction linked to formate metabolism is called nitrate assimilation. Cells of *Esch. coli* grown anaerobically carry out nitrate respiration whereas those grown aerobically tend to carry out nitrate assimilation. Further work with *Esch. coli* by Cole and Wimpenny (1968) showed that at high nitrate concentration in anaerobic cultures the end product of nitrate reduction was nitrite (i.e. nitrate respiration) whereas at low nitrate concentrations a nitrite reductase was produced, giving ammonia as the end product (i.e. nitrate assimilation). Fewson and Nicholas (1961), working with *Pseudomonas aeruginosa*, isolated a particulate enzyme with a pH optimum of 7.4 (similar to that for *Esch. coli*). The enzyme activity was decreased as the oxygen tension during growth of the organisms increased, as with the *Esch. coli* enzyme, but whereas the latter enzyme required cyt. b_1 as electron carrier that from *Ps. aeroginosa* required cyt. c. Rogosa (1961) investigated the nitrate reductase produced by some strains of *Lactobacillus plantarum* and *L. fermenti*. In these organisms there was no requirement for anaerobiosis but there was an apparent requirement for a medium poor in fermentable carbohydrate. This was traced to its effect on pH, and it was shown that no nitrate reductase was produced when the pH fell below 5-5.5.

Nitrite reductase has received a little attention but has not been intensively studied. Rogosa (1961) reported that at pH 7.5 or above the nitrite reductase produced by *Staphylococcus aureus* effectively kept pace with the nitrate reductase so that no nitrite was detectable in the incubation mixture; here nitrogen was the end product of nitrate reduction. Cole (1968) has studied the nitrite reductase of *Esch. coli* and has shown that it is associated with cytochrome c reductase. They failed to separate the two activities by a range of purification steps, and postulated that "cytochrome c reductase" is a manifestation of the lack of specificity of nitrite reductase for an electron acceptor. The enzyme has a pH optimum of 7.9, which is compatible with the observations on the nitrite reductase of *Staphylococcus aureus*.

Many organisms produce nitrite reductase; in some cases the end product of nitrite is N_2, in others it is ammonia. Nitrate reduction is assayed routinely in the identification of bacteria by the addition of sulphanilic acid and α-naphthylamine. If nitrate is reduced to nitrite, the nitrite forms a diazonium salt with sulphanilic acid which then couples with the α-naphthylamine to form a red diazo dye. In the absence of dye formation it is then necessary to check that the nitrate has not been reduced to nitrogen or ammonia; this is done by adding a small quantity of zinc dust to the culture, which reduces nitrate to nitrite and the assay for dye formation is then repeated.

The reduction of nitro substituents by gut bacteria has been examined mainly with respect to chloramphenicol metabolism; certain organisms reduce the p-nitro group of chloramphenicol giving rise to an arylamine with no antibiotic activity. This is discussed later in the section on antibiotics. Egami *et al.* (1951), working with a cell-free enzyme from *Strep. haemolyticum* (i.e. *Strep. pyogenes*) observed that the nitro reductase acting on chloramphenicol was inhibited by nitrite and vice versa; from this they concluded that the two activities were carried out by the same enzyme. Saz *et al.* (1953, 1954a, b) worked extensively with the chloramphenicol nitro reductase of *Esch. coli*. They showed that in contrast to the streptococcal enzyme, their cell-free enzyme was not inhibited by nitrite and that *Esch. coli* nitrite reductase was not inhibited by chloramphenicol. The nitro reductase was relatively non-specific, acting on a wide range of substituted nitrophenyl compounds both acidic and neutral, and with the nitro group in the ortho meta or para position. Of the compounds tested, only dinitrophenol was not reduced and this inhibited the enzyme. The enzyme had a requirement for cysteine, DPN and a dicarboxylic acid (e.g. fumarate, malate, aspartate). It was inhibited by azide, cyanide, aureomycin and its metabolites but not by tetracycline. They postulated that the nitro group was reduced to a nitroso group, then to a hydroxylamino group and finally to the amine. The production of arylamines from aryl nitro compounds is of importance because of the potential toxicity of the product.

VI. Degradation of amino acids

Amino acids are metabolized by gut bacteria via deamination, decarboxylation and other miscellaneous reactions. The pathways of deamination have been considered earlier. Amino acid deaminases are produced optimally *in vitro* at alkaline pH values and evidently represent an attempt by the bacteria to buffer their environment; similarly amino acid decarboxylases are produced optimally at acid pH.

A. AMINO ACID DECARBOXYLASES

Berthelot (1910, 1911, 1918) described the decarboxylation by bacteria of a range of amino acids yielding the parent amine or phenolic amine. The decarboxylation of phenolic amino acids was also noted by Bouwman in 1923 and by Hanks and Koessler (1924). The enzymes were investigated systematically by Gale (1940a, b, 1941) who showed that each decarboxylase was specific for a single amino acid and that a third polar group (in addition to the α-amino and α-carboxyl groups) was necessary for decarboxylation. Thus, he found amino acid decarboxylases for arginine, ornithine, lysine, histidine, tyrosine, glutamic acid, aspartic acid and tryptophan but not for simple monoamino monocarboxylic acids. Later proline was added to the list of amino acids decarboxylated (Hawksworth, 1973). In addition, an amino acid decarboxylase active on leucine, iso-leucine, valine and nor-valine and α-amino butyric acid has been described (Haughton and King, 1961) the multiplicity of substrates being in contrast to the mono specificity described by Gale. Derivative formation of the α-amino group or the third polar group resulted in inactivation of the amino acid as a substrate for its decarboxylase, but the addition of a further polar group (e.g. the formation of hydroxylysine, hydroxyglutamic acid or hydroxyproline) only reduces and does not prevent the decarboxylation by the corresponding decarboxylase.

Decarboxylation of lysine, arginine, ornithine and glutamic acid are of interest taxonomically in the identification of the enterobacteriaceae. Consequently the decarboxylases have been screened extensively in these organisms, but much less so in the other families. Table 6.10 summarizes our knowledge; in general the enzymes have been reported in a few instances but in only limited cases have enough strains been investigated to allow us to say that they are generally present or generally absent.

Many of the decarboxylations have been demonstrated *in vivo* in the intestine. Harke and Koessler (1924) suggested that the free and acetylated histamine in urine was the result of gut bacterial action, and supported by Urbach (1949). Wilson (1954) measured intestinal and urinary histamine in normal rats and rats treated with a range of antibiotics (penicillin, aureomycin, phthalylsuphathiazole and chloramphenicol); the antibiotic-treated rats excreted only 45% of the amount of histamine excreted by normal rats. Harke and Koessler had demonstrated histidine decarboxylase in coliforms and in anaerobes; Wilson expressed the opinion that the numbers of these were drastically reduced in the gut of antibiotic-treated rats. Beaver and Wostmann (1962) investigated the levels of histamine and 5-hydroxytryptamine in conventional, germ-free and mono-contaminated mice and demonstrated that the levels of histamine in the gut wall and lumen was much lower in germ-free animals. Mono-contamination with a

TABLE 6.10

Production of amino acid decarboxylases by gut bacteria

Organism tested	Amino acid decarboxylation										
	Lys.	Arg.	Orn.	Glut. acid.	Hist.	Tyr.	Prol.	Trypt.	Leu.	Val.	Norval.
Enterobacteria											
Esch. coli	+	+	+	+	†	†	+				
Salmonellae	+	+	+	−	†	†	+		†		
Shig. sonnei	−	+	+	+							
other Shigellae	−	+	−	+							
P. vulgaris	−	−	−	+							
other Proteus	−	−	+	+					†	+	
Serratia	+	−	+	−						†	
Klebsiella	+	−	−	−							+
Streptococci											
Strep. faecalis	−	−	−	−	−	+	†				
Group A-F	−	−	−	−	−	†					
Strep. lactis	−	−	−		−	−					
Clostridia											
Cl. welchii	−	−	−	+	+	−	+				
Cl. septicum	−	+	+	−	−						
Cl. bifermentans	+	†	†	†	†	†	+				
Bacillus spp.	†	†	†		†	†	†	†			
Bacteroides fragilis	†	†	+				+				
Bifidobacteria	+	†	+				+				
Vibriocholera	+		+								
Staphylococci	−	−		−	−	−					
Pasteurella	−	−		−	−	−					
Pseudomonas	−	−		−	−	−					

+ = more than 10 strains tested most of which were +ve. − = more than 10 strains tested; † = individual strains reported +ve, but no screening results available.

strain of *Clostridium perfringens* which produced histidine decarboxylase resulted in high histamine levels in the caecal lumen but failed to restore the level in the gut wall. They showed that the caecum was the site of maximal bacterial production of histamine (as would be expected from the distribution of the flora down the gut). They could, detect no 5-hydroxytryptamine in the intestinal or caecal contents of germ-free or conventional rats or mice, but the levels in mucosal cells was higher in germ-free animals and could be increased in conventional animals by treatment with antibiotics.

The *in vitro* decarboxylation of phenolic amino acids by rat faeces and rat caecal and colonic contents has been shown to be an anaerobic reaction; the urinary excretion of tyramine can be reduced by treatment with antibacterial substances (Asatoor, 1968). It has been suggested that the urinary tyramine is entirely of bacterial origin (Awapara *et al.*, 1964; Perry *et al.*, 1966) but Asatoor has disputed this, since he found urinary tyramine in rats with ligated or canulated bile ducts after injection of tyrosine. These findings do not conclusively demonstrate the presence of tissue tyrosine decarboxylase; the biliary route is not the only route of entry into the gut, since Mandell and Rubin (1965) have shown that intravenously administered trytophan is secreted into the gut lumen by reverse transport. Possibly tyrosine reaches the gut flora by the same route. It seems likely, in view of the evidence, that the gut flora is the major, if not the only, source of urinary tyramine.

Decarboxylation of lysine and ornithine are the first steps in the formation of piperidine and pyrrolidine respectively. These secondary amines are produced in the gut and excreted in the urine; the amount is reduced to zero on treatment with neomycin (Asatoor and Simenhoff, 1965) or in germ-free animals (Hawksworth, 1973).

Many of the amines produced have physiological or pharmacological activities, and so their production *in vivo* could have important consequences. Histamine is a "pressor" substance, injection of small amounts resulting in a fall in blood pressure. In addition, it has a general inflammatory reaction leading to vasodilation, erythema, leucotaxis etc., and is known to stimulate stomach acid secretion. Tyramine is a depressor substance, and injection of small amounts results in increased blood pressure. The diamines cadaverine and putrescine, the products of lysine and ornithine decarboxylation, are weak pressor substances, whilst the monoamines tend to be depressors. Agmatine, the product of arginine decarboxylation, has an insulin-like activity. The amines produced in the gut are absorbed and enter the portal blood system and are "detoxified". The liver produces a monoamine oxidase which deaminates the monoamines thereby rendering them non-toxic. In hepatic cirrhosis this dextoxification may be inactive or ineffective; the amines will then, instead of being restricted to the portal blood system, freely circulate to exert their pharmacological effect. Perry *et al.* (1966) showed that treatment with monoamine oxidase inhibitors led to the appearance of 4 amines in the urine in addition to those normally present, and Melnykowycz and Johansson (1955) suggested that this might be the aetiology of hepatic coma associated with cirrhosis. This will be discussed later, together with the other possible effects of failure to detoxify amines in cirrhosis (Chapter 16).

B. MISCELLANEOUS OTHER REACTIONS

In addition to the general reactions of decarboxylation and deamination there are a range of reactions undergone by individual amino acids. Many of these involve splitting of the amino acid molecule, but there are examples of synthetic reactions in addition to these degradative processes.

Many of the complex amino acids (i.e. those other than the monoamine monocarboxylic amino acids) undergo fission reactions; for example tyrosine is split to release ammonia, phenol and pyruvate (Fig. 6.14) by *Cl.*

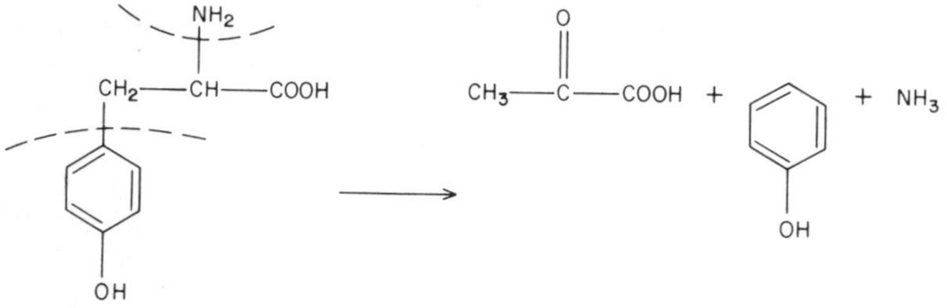

Fig. 6.14. The breakdown of tyrosine to yield phenol, ammonia and pyruvic acid.

tetanomorphum (Brot *et al.*, 1965) and by *Esch. coli* (Ichihara *et al.*, 1956). Arginine is hydrolysed by streptococci to yield ornithine, ammonia and carbon dioxide by the arginine dihydrolase system with the inter-medieate formation of citrulline (Fig. 6.15). This differs from the mamm-alian pathway; in the liver arginine is hydrolysed to ornithine with the removal of a molecule of urea and with no citrulline intermediate.

Tryptophan undergoes a variety of reactions, which will be considered later; two fissions reactions by gut bacteria (Fig. 6.16) are the production of indole, pyruvate and ammonia by *Esch. coli* (Gale, 1952) and the production of formyl kynurenine by oxidative opening of the heterocyclic ring. Indole production from tryptophan is a widely used diagnostic test (Table 6.11), the enzyme (or enzyme system) being widely distributed amongst both aerobic and anaerobic bacterial species. Urinary indole and

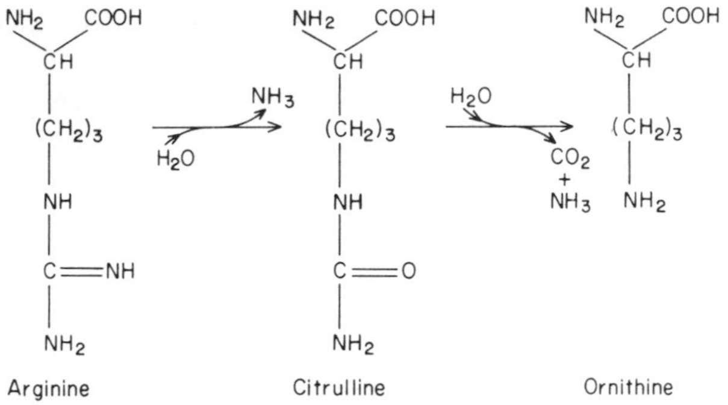

Fig. 6.15. The metabolism of arginine to ornithine via citrulline.

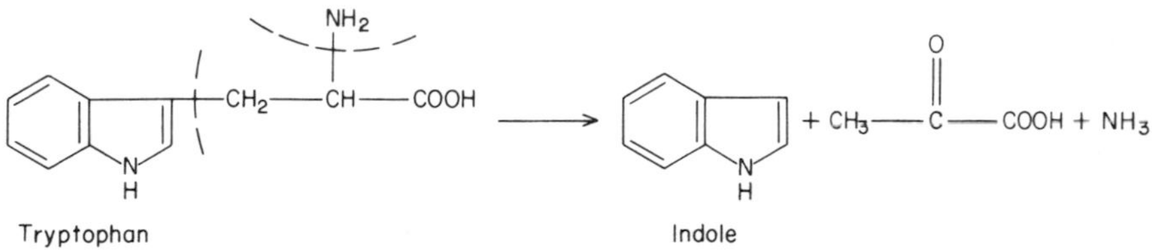

Fig. 6.16. The fission of tryptophan by bacteria to yield indole, ammonia and pyruvic acid.

TABLE 6.11

Production of indole from tryptophan by gut bacteria

	Indole +ve	Indole −ve
Enterobacteria	Escherichia	Salmonella
	Proteus (except	Klebsiella-Aerobacter
	P. mirabilis)	
	Providence	Serratia
	Some Shigellae	
Lactobacilli		All species
Streptococci		Strep. faecalis
		Strep. viridans
Bacilli	B. alvei	All other Bacillus spp.
Gram+non-	Prop. acnes	All other propioni-
sporing anaerobes		bacterium
		Eubacteria
		Bifidobacteria
Gram −non-	Fusobacterium (7/14	Butyrivibrio
sporing anaerobes	species)	
	B. melaninogenicus	Other Bacteroides spp.
	B. fragilis (2/4 sub-	
	species)	
	B. coagulans	

skatol are almost entirely of gut bacterial origin; early work by Distaso and Sugden (1919) demonstrated the hydrolysis of tryptophan by gut bacteria to yield indole and skatol. The production of formyl kynurenine is by a pathway common to bacterial and mammalian systems and is followed by a side chain oxidation, and further ring closure reactions.

In addition to these fission reactions, there are some examples of synthetic reactions, although involving metabolites of amino acid degradation rather than the amino acids themselves. Following the decarboxylation of lysine or ornithine, the diamines (cadaverine and putrescine) undergo oxidative deamination followed by ring closure (Fig. 6.9) to give the immediate precursors to the urinary cyclic secondary amines piperidine and pyrrolidine. The oxidative deamination is carried out by a range of organisms (Table 6.12), the cyclic unsaturated amine being trapped with o-aminobenzaldehyde (which forms a yellow addition complex with unsaturated amines of this type).

TABLE 6.12

Conversion of cadaverine to piperidine and putrescine to pyrrolidine by intestinal bacteria

	% of strains converting the diamine to the secondary amine	
	Cadaverine	Putrescine
Enterobacteria	0	0
Enterococci	0	0
Clostridia	50	63
Bacteroides	75	38
Bifidobacteria	63	25

VII. Production of phenols and phenolic acids from tyrosine

It was demonstrated by early workers that tyrosine is metabolized by the gut bacterial flora to yield a number of phenols (Baumann, 1879; Folin and Denis, 1915) including phenol itself, p-cresol and 4-ethylophenol. A quantitative relationship between protein intake and the amounts of certain phenolic compounds in human urine was demonstrated by Folin and Denis (1915) and Levine et al. (1941) and this was related to phenylalanine and tyrosine metabolism. An increase in dietary tyrosine leads to an increased excretion of urinary phenols (Bernhardt and Zilliken, 1959; Alam et al., 1967).

The production of phenols has been the subject of a recent in-depth study by Bakke (1969a, b, c, d). He has repeated and confirmed the early work showing that urinary simple phenols are produced from dietary proteins and in particular from dietary tyrosine, by the gut bacteria and that the treatment of rats with oral neomycin reduced the amount of urinary phenols to almost zero. Bernhardt and Zilliken (1959) produced a similar result with chlortetracycline.

The general concensus of opinion is that tyrosine is metabolized by the gut bacteria by the pathways shown in Fig. 6.17 (Williams, 1959; Kleiner and Orton, 1966; West *et al.*, 1966; Parke, 1968). Bacteria deaminate tyrosine reductively to phloretic acid (p-hydroxy-phenylpropionic acid) which is (a) decarboxylated to 4-ethylphenol, or (b) oxidized to p-hydroxy-phenylacetic acid which is then either decarboxylated to p-cresol or further oxidized to p-hydroxybenzoic acid the latter being decarboxylated to

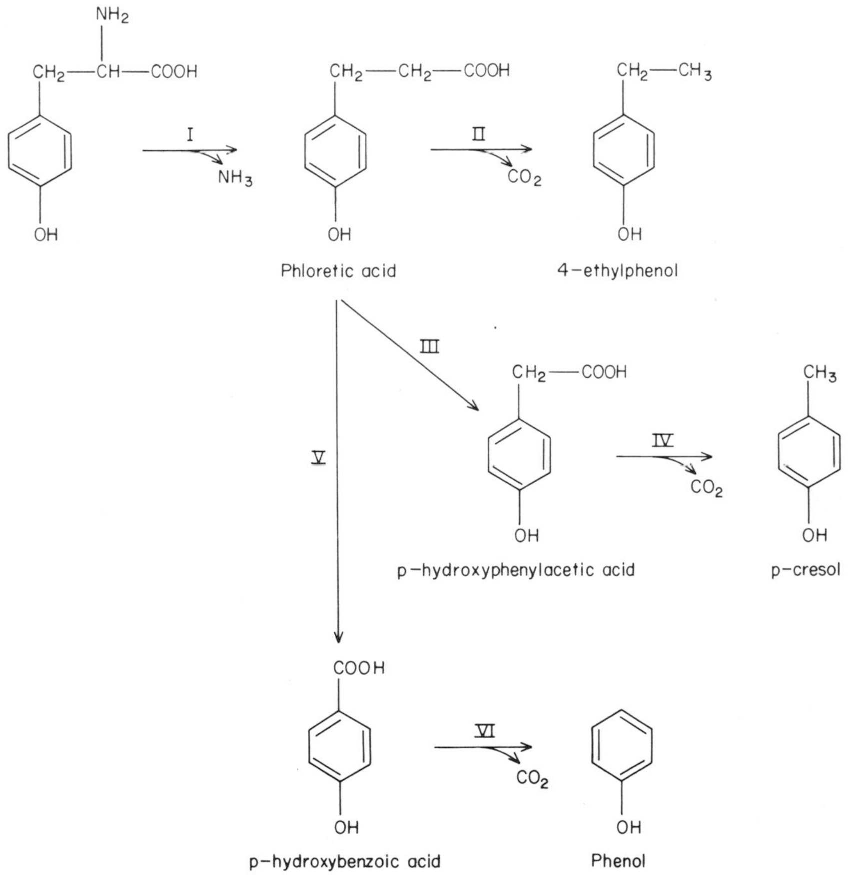

Fig. 6.17. Schematic diagram of the pathways of tyrosine metabolism by gut bacteria.

phenol. This would account for the major urinary phenols, but not all of the steps involved have been demonstrated *in vitro* with bacteria or with rat caecal contents. Bakke, working with rat caecal contents, has demonstrated the ready decarboxylation of p-hydroxyphenylacetic acid (step IV) and of p-hydroxybenzoic acid to phenol (step VI). He also found that rat caecal contents, when incubated with tyrosine, yielded phloretic acid (step I), p-hydroxyphenylacetic acid (step III), p-cresol (step IV) and phenol (step VI), leaving steps II and V unaccounted for. The lack of p-hydroxybenzoic acid (step V) was readily explained by its very rapid decarboxylation, but he was unable to demonstrate step II using rat caecal contents.

In addition to these major pathways, a number of additional reactions have been demonstrated. Scott *et al.* (1964) demonstrated that phloretic acid was dehydroxylated to phenylpropionic acid by sheep rumen contents. If this were a major reaction it would be expected that sheep would excrete only small amounts of urinary phenols; we have no information on how true this is. Harai (1921) demonstrated the formation of p-hydroxyphenylpyruvic acid by the oxidative deamination of tyrosine by *P. vulgaris.*

There is a possible role for urinary phenols in human disease. The phenols are produced in the gut, travel to the liver where some are detoxified, and then enter the general circulation before being excreted in the urine. Boutwell (1967) has shown that small amounts of phenol and p-cresol promote the development of benign and malignant tumours when repeatedly applied to mouse skin that has been initially exposed to an appropriate carcinogen. This co-carcinogenic effect may be relevant to human cancer. Certain phenols have been shown to be convulsant agents, and these include phenol and catechol (Angel and Rogers, 1968). Normally the phenols are detoxified to some extent by conjugation in the liver, but this breaks down in cirrhosis and the freely circulating phenols may be implicated in the hepatic coma associated with cirrhosis (Rogers *et al.,* 1955).

VIII. Metabolism of 3,4-dihydroxyphenylalanine (dopa)

Studies on the metabolism of dopa have shown a marked resurgence in recent years because of the publicity given to its possible role in the treatment of Parkinsonism. The data concerning its metabolism in man and animals are summarized in Fig. 6.18.

L-dopa is first metabolized to 3,4-dihydroxyphenylacetic acid (I), presumably via deamination followed by side-chain oxidation. This then undergoes p-dehydroxylation, decarboxylation or further side-chain oxidation. The deamination and removal of the p-hydroxyl group to give m-hydroxyphylacetic acid (II) was demonstrated by Booth *et al.* (1957) and by Deeds *et al.* (1957). Booth and Williams (1963a, b) then went on to

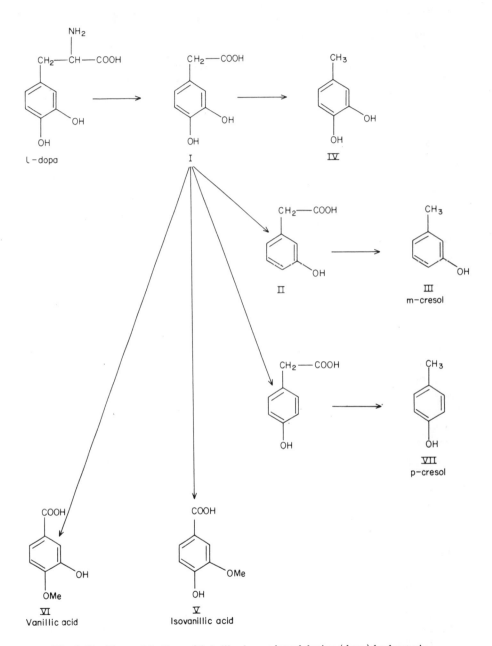

Fig. 6.18. The metabolism of 3,4-dihydroxyphenylalanine (dopa) by bacteria.

demonstrate the same reaction using rat faecal bacteria, and showed that the reactions were inhibited by aerobiosis and by several antibiotics. Sandler *et al.* (1969) isolated the same metabolite from the urine of humans with Parkinsonism being treated with large doses of L-dopa; the amount of metabolite decreased significantly on treatment of the patients with neomycin. O'Gorman *et al.* (1970) demonstrated that in man the metabolites of L-dopa include 3,4-dihydroxyphenylacetic acid (I), m-hydroxyphenylacetic acid (II), homovanillic acid (V) and homo-isovanillic acid (VI) in addition to the simple phenols m-cresol (III), p-methylcatechol (IV) and its O-methylated product, 4-methylguaiacol. Bakke (1971) was able to demonstrate all of these metabolites in the rat with the possible addition of p-cresol (VII). The O-methylation of simple phenols by rat intestinal bacteria had been demonstrated by Bakke (1970) and used to explain the formation of 4-methylguaiacol from 4-methylc-atechol. As in the human, the metabolism of L-dopa was inhibited in the rat with neomycin.

IX. Metabolism of tryptophan

The major metabolites of tryptophan produced by bacteria are shown in Fig. 6.19. Many of these are common to both bacterial and mammalian systems; a few are specifically bacterial. The production of indole is a specific bacterial reaction and has been described already. Similarly, tryptophan is not decarboxylated in the tissues and the urinary tryptamine is of gut bacterial origin. Suda *et al.* (1950) demonstrated that tryptophan was oxidized by *Pseudomonas* spp. to kynurenine, then anthranilic acid to catechol; this was called later the aromatic pathway. Stanier and Hayaishi (1951) reported that there was an alternative pathway through kynyrenine to kynurenic acid and onwards — the so called quinoline pathway. Kaihara and Price (1961) fed kynurenic acid to rabbits and got 70% of the dose dehydroxylated to quinaldic acid; no dehydroxylation of kynurenic acid given s/c was detected. Smaller amounts of dehydroxylation took place in cats and man. Similarly xanthenuric acid was dehydroxylated to 8-hydroxyquinaldic acid in rabbits (Lower and Bryan, 1969). Pretreatment of the rabbits with neomycin sulphate in amounts said to be sufficient to severly inhibit multiplication of the intestinal bacteria also severely inhibited the dehydroxylation step.

In addition to the common pathways and the bacterial pathways there are metabolites of tryptophan apparently produced only by mammalian pathways. Inevitably, then, there will be considerable interaction between the gut bacteria and the mammalian metabolites and, conversely, between tissue enzymes and bacterial metabolites. Thus, the 8-methyl ether of xanthenuric acid, which is a product of mammalian metabolism, is

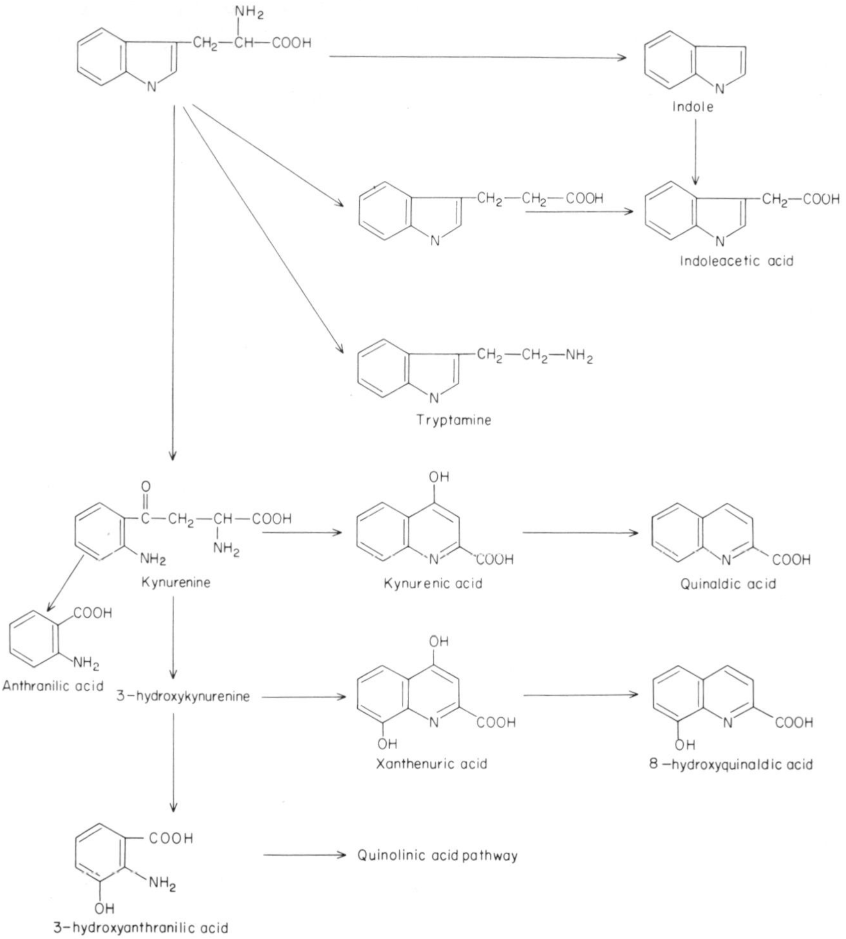

Fig. 6.19. The metabolism of tryptophan.

oxidatively demethylated by the gut flora. Lower and Bryan (1969) adminis-tered xanthenuric acid-8-methoxy ^{14}C and recovered $^{14}CO_2$ as the product of demethylation; the released xanthenuric acid was then further de-hydroxylated to 8-hydroxyquinaldic acid.

Complete destruction of the quinoline ring has been reported by Hayaishi *et al.* (1961); using a strain of *Ps. fluorescens* they obtained glutamic acid and alanine as degradation products.

Tryptophan metabolites present in urine have been implicated in bladder cancer by Bryan (1971), in particular 8-methoxyxanthenuric acid. The contribution of the gut flora to the pattern of metabolites is not clear and is generally not considered. The metabolic "indican" which is a tryptophan metabolite, is claimed by many to be a good indicator of bacterial colonization of the small bowel; this is strongly disputed by many others.

CHAPTER 7

Bile Acid Degradation

The bile acids secreted in human bile are substituted cholanic acids conjugated to taurine or glycine (Fig. 7.1). Those synthesized by the liver are cholic acid (3α 7α 12α-trihydroxy-5β-cholanic acid) and chenodeoxycholic acid (3α 7α-dihydroxy-5β-cholanic acid), and normal human bile contains, in addition to conjugates of these two primary acids, conjugates of a secondary bile acid, deoxycholic acid which results from the 7α-dehydroxylation of cholic acid. The bile salts play a role in fat

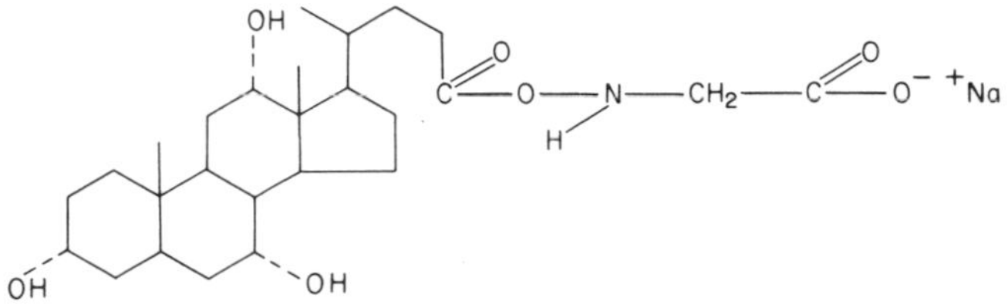

Fig. 7.1. Structure of the bile salt sodium glycocholate.

absorption, which is discussed later, and after their transit through the small intestine, are absorbed from the terminal ileum by an active transport mechanism (Lack and Weiner, 1961). Any free bile acids released may be absorbed by passive diffusion from the small or large intestine (Samuel *et al.*, 1968). The absorbed bile acids then return to the liver, via the portal blood system, where they are reconjugated and resecreted in the bile. In each cycle a proportion of the bile acid pool is lost and passed in the faeces; this loss is normally less than 5% of the total pool (Kern and Meihoff, 1970) but is increased in diarrhoea or in steatorrhoea.

The faecal bile acids are entirely deconjugated and contain, in addition to small amounts of primary bile acids, a wide range of secondary bile acids (Table 7.1), produced by bacterial oxido-reduction of the hydroxyl groups (yielding keto bile acids and the β-hydroxylated bile acids) and by bacterial dehydroxylation (Hill and Aries, 1971). Studies with germ-free and conventional animals show that the secondary bile acids present in the faeces and bile of conventional animals are absent from those of the

TABLE 7.1

The principal faecal bile acids. All are 5β-cholanic acids with oxygen functions at the 3,7 or 12-positions

Nature of substituent at position:			
3	7	12	Trivial name
αOH	α OH	α OH	Cholic acid (a)
α OH	α OH	—	Chenodeoxycholic acid (a)
α OH	—	α OH	Deoxycholic acid (b)
α or β OH	oxo	α or β OH	
α or β OH	—	α OH	
α or β OH	—	α or β OH	
α or β OH	—	oxo	
α OH	—	—	Lithocholic acid
β OH	—	—	Isolithocholic acid
oxo	—	—	
—	—	—	Cholanic acid

(a) Primary bile acids synthesized by the liver.
(b) Secondary bile acids present in large amounts in bile.

germ-free animals, confirming the bacterial origin of these metabolites. Colonization of germ-free rats with deconjugated and dehydroxylating strains of bacteria restores the secondary bile acids to the faeces (Gustafsson *et al.,* 1968). Further, the half-life of cholic acid in the bile acid pool is five times longer in germ-free than in normal rats (Gustafsson *et al.,* 1957).

The principal reactions involved in bile salt degradation in the gut are:

(a) hydrolysis of the amide bond to release the free bile acids. (Fig. 7.2a):

(b) oxido-reduction of the hydroxyl groups at C-3, C-7 and C-12 to give oxo-bile acids and those with β-hydroxyl groups — the inversion products (Fig. 7.2b), and

(c) dehydroxylation at C-7 and also, to a much smaller extent, at C-3 and at C-12 (Fig. 7.2c).

Until fairly recently these reactions had only been demonstrated in pure cultures of intestinal bacteria in a very few cases. However, there has been a considerable increase in our knowledge of this subject over the last few years.

I. Cholanoylglycine hydrolase

In 1955 Norman and Grubb reported the isolation of some clostridia and some enterococci capable of bile salt deconjugation, and in 1966 Drasar *et*

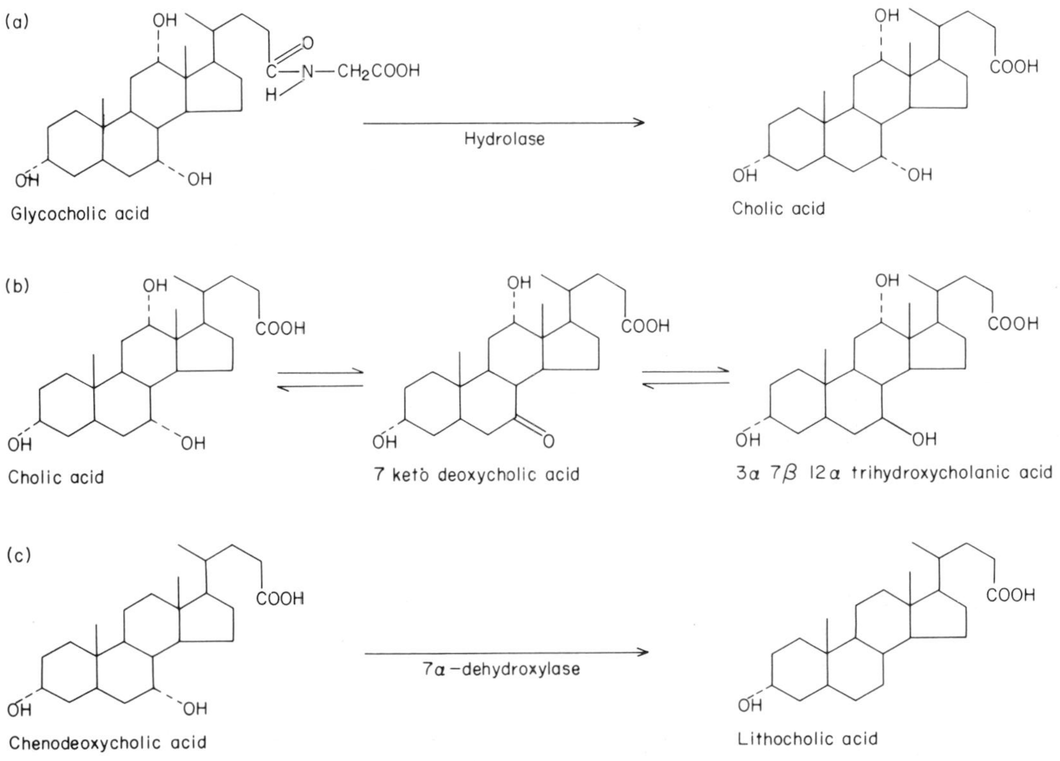

Fig. 7.2. The principle bile degradations carried out by the gut bacteria. (a) hydrolase; (b) 7α-hydroxy oxidoreductase, (c) 7α-dehydroxylase.

al. showed that a high proportion of strains of *Bacteroides* spp. and *Bifidobacterium* spp. were able to perform this reaction. Since then there have been a number of surveys of human faecal bacteria (e.g. Midtvedt and Norman, 1967; Hill and Drasar, 1968; Aries *et al.*, 1969; Shimida *et al.*, 1969) which have shown that most strains of *Bacteroides* spp., *Bifidobacterium* spp., *Clostridium* spp., *Strep faecalis* together with many strains of *Veillonella* spp. possess this enzyme when freshly isolated (Table 7.2).

TABLE 7.2

Deconjugation of bile acids by human intestinal bacteria

Organism	No. of strains tested	% of strains deconjugating glycocholic acid
Esch. coli	267	0
Enterococci	252	91
Strep. salivarius	82	0
Lactobacilli	48	0
Clostridia	130	95
Bifidobacteria	192	82
Bacteroides	54	79
Bacillus spp.	81	32
Veillonella spp.	92	48
Anaerobic sarcinae	12	67

Nair *et al.* (1967) isolated and characterized a cholanoylglycine hydrolase from a strain of *Clostridium perfringens* and since then cell-free hydrolases has been isolated by a number of groups (e.g. Hill and Drasar, 1968; Aries and Hill, 1970a; Yessair and Himmelfarb, 1970) and it is evident that there is more than one type of hydrolase. The enzyme isolated by Nair *et al.* (1967) from *Cl. perfringens* was an intracellular enzyme with a pH optimum of 5.6-5.8, was equally active on glycine and taurine conjugates and was equally active on conjugates of cholic, deoxycholic and chenodeoxycholic acids. These properties were shared by the hydrolases isolated from the two strains of *B. fragilis* and one *Cl. welchii* studied by Hill and Aries (1970a). *Cl. welchii* is another and more commonly used name for *Cl. perfringens*. The hydrolases isolated from another strain of *Cl. welchii* and from two strains of *Strep. faecalis* were more active on glycine than on taurine conjugates and more active on cholic than on deoxycholic acid conjugates (Table 7.3). The two strains of *Bifidobacterium* spp. studied did not produce an intracellular hydrolase but produced an extracellular enzyme specific for glycine conjugates. Regardless of the substrate specificity of the intracellular or extracellular enzyme, all 8

TABLE 7.3

Activity of hydrolase from various cell fractions

Source of enzyme		Activity of enzyme from various sites on two substrates					
		Intracellular		Wall/membrane		Extracellular	
		GD	TD	GD	TD	GD	TD
Strep. faecalis	E1	++	+	++	+	−	−
	E12	+++	−	++	−	−	−
Cl. welchii	CC20	+++	+++	++	++	−	−
	CC63	+++	+	++	++	−	−
B. fragilis	NCTC9343	+++	+++	++	++	−	−
	BV10	+++	+++	++	++	±	±
Bifidobacterium	18	−	−	++	++	+++	−
	29	−	−	++	++	+++	−

GD = glycodeoxycholic acid; TD = taurodeoxycholic acid; Activity is graded − to +++

strains possessed a wall-membrane bound enzyme which had no substrate specificity either with respect to the conjugating amino acid or with respect to the number of hydroxyl substituents on the bile moiety. The relative rates of hydrolysis of taurocholate, taurodeoxycholate, glycocholate and glycdeoxycholate are shown in Table 7.4.

TABLE 7.4

Substrate specificity of enzyme preparations from various strains of gut bacteria

Source of enzyme		Location of enyzme	Relative enzyme activity on various substrates (GC = 100)			
			GC	GD	TC	TD
Strep. faecalis	E1	Intracellular	100	100	50	50
	E12	Intracellular	100	100	0	0
Cl. welchii	CC20	Intracellular	100	100	100	100
	CC63	Intracellular	100	65	35	4
B. fragilis	9343	Intracellular	100	100	100	100
	BV10	Intracellular	100	100	100	100
Bifidobacterium	18	Extracellular	100	25	0	0
	29	Extracellular	100	25	0	0

GC = glycohoclate; GD = glycodeoxycholate; TC = taurocholate
TD = taurodeoxycholate

The pH optimum of the extracellular hydrolase produced by the bifidobacteria was somewhat higher than that of the intracellular clostridial enzymes, and was probably the enzyme found by Norman and Widstrom (1964) in filtered rat caecal fluid. The only membrane enzyme studied quantitatively (that of a strain of *Strep. faecalis*) had a pH optimum near to 7 (Hill and Drasar, 1968).

The hydrolases were specific for conjugates of 5β-cholan-24-oic acid; glyco-allodeoxycholate was hydrolysed very slowly and the conjugates of C-27 bile acids were hardly hydrolysed at all. Those hydrolases which were equally active on glycine and taurine would also hydrolyse conjugates containing alanine or aspartic acid as the conjugating amino acid, whilst those specific for glycine conjugates would not hydrolyse the synthetic conjugates.

Only 3 of the 8 hydrolases studied were inhibited by the addition of 8.5 mM free bile acid (Table 7.5). This product inhibition was exerted equally on all four conjugates tested. Added glycine or taurine (20 mM) had no inhibitory effect on the hydrolase and in fact tended to enhance the activity.

A range of inhibitors tested by Aries and Hill (1970a) showed that all 8

TABLE 7.5

Product inhibition of cholanoylglycine hydrolase by 8.5 mM free bile acid

Source of enzyme		% inhibition of hydrolysis of conjugates			
		GC	GD	TC	TD
Strep. faecalis	E1	0	0		
	E12	0	0		
Cl. welchii	CC 20	55	55	55	55
	CC 63	35	35	35	35
B. fragilis	9843	20	20	20	20
	BV10	0	0	0	0
Bifidobacterium	18	0	0		
	29	0	0		

GC = glycocholate; GD = glycodeoxycholate; TC = taurocholate; TD = taurodeoxycholate

enzymes preparations were inhibited by periodate, iodoacetate and cupric ions and by formaldehyde, but not by calcium, magnesium, azide or fluoride ions, EDTA or methiolate. The enzyme isolated by Nair *et al.* (1967) was inhibited by PCMB, iodoacetate, mercuric, cupric and zinc ions and activated on occasions by EDTA and by β-mercaptoethanol. Thus, all of the hydrolases investigated are inhibited by sulphydryl inhibitors and by heavy metals.

The hydrolases are constitutive enzymes and, when produced by an anaerobic organism, are only produced under extremely anaerobic conditions. The isolated enzyme is oxygen-sensitive and needs to be protected by the presence of a reducing agent such as cysteine or thioglycollate. Chromatography on G–200 Sephadex indicates a molecular weight for the enzyme of 50-100,000, although that isolated by Nair (1969) appeared to have a molecular weight in excess of 200,000. The enzyme could be purified on DEAE cellulose (Nair *et al.*, 1967; Aries and Hill 1970a).

Faecal bile acids are entirely deconjugated although those secreted in the bile are entirely conjugated. Thus there must be a high activity of hydrolase in the intestine in order for this reaction to be taken to completion. The widespread nature of the enzyme and the fact that such a high proportion of the non-sporing anaerobes produce the enzyme ensures this postulated high total activity in the gut.

II. Hydroxy-steroid oxido-reductases

In 1944, Hoehn *et al.* reported an oxidoreductase produced by *Alcaligenes faecalis* and active on the hydroxyl groups of cholic acid, and similar findings were reported by Norman and Bergman (1960) using strains of *Esch. coli* and *Cl. perfringens.* The latter workers found 7-oxo-deoxycholate as the main metabolite of cholic acid produced by rat caecal contents, but obtained small amounts of 3-oxo and 12-oxo bile acids. They examined a number of organisms for the ability to metabolize cholic acid and found a number of strains of *Cl. perfringens,* and 15/16 strains of *Esch. coli* positive (producing 7-oxo-deoxycholate) but no metabolites produced by strains of pseudomonas, *K. aerogenes, Staph. aureus, Staph. albus, B. subtilus,* aerobic and anaerobic streptococci, some diphtheroid strains and some strains of candida and streptomyces. Norman and Sjovall (1958) had previously identified keto bile acids as metabolites of cholic acid in the rat caecum did not demonstrate bacterial involvement.

In a survey of 55 strains of assorted species Midtvedt and Norman (1967) demonstrated that a number of them could convert cholic acid to 7-oxo-3α,12α-dihydroxycholanate, 3α-hydroxy-7,12-dioxo cholanate and 3,7,12-trioxocholanate; they also had some inversion of hydroxyl groups to the β-configuration presumably via an oxo-intermediate. In a survey of more than 1,100 strains freshly isolated from human faeces and assayed for their bile acid degradative abilities it was found that 7-hydroxysteroid oxidoreductase was extremely widespread (Table 7.6) with enzyme acting at the 3-position being somewhat less common and that acting at the 12-position being produced by approximately 10% of strains of the active species tested.

TABLE 7.6

Production of hydroxycholanoyl exidoreductases by human gut bacteria

Organism	No. present per g faeces	No. tested[+]	% dehydrogenating hydroxyl groups at position		
			3	7	12*
Enterobacteria	10^7	267	35	65	10
Enterococci	10^6	252	22	72	10
Strep. salivarius	10^6	82	0	0	0
Lactobacilli	10^6	48	0	0	0
Clostridia	10^5	130	45	88	10
Bifidobacteria	10^{10}	194	19	52	10
Bacteroides	10^{10}	54	24	60	10
Veillonellae	10^4	92	25	60	10
Anaerobic sarcinae		12		58	0
Bacilli		81	5	16	0

[+] All strains tested were from Ugandan or English faecal samples
* The percentages quoted are approximations; in those species which dehydrogenated the 12-hydroxyl group about 10% of strains were active.

The dehydrogenases could be purified by stepwise elution from DEAE cellulose with increasing concentrations of phosphate buffer solution, pH 7.0 (Aries and Hill, 1970b). The elution behaviour on G200 sephadex and on sepharose 6B suggested that the enzyme had a molecular weight of 50-1000,000. The dehydrogenases were inducible and were located in the cell cytoplasm; the enzyme isolated in cell-free form after Mickle disintegration of the cells was of high activity and was stable on storage at $-10°C$. All dehydrogenase preparations required NAD^+ or $NADP^+$ and oxygen; the enzymes were readily assayed therefore, by measurement of nucleotide reduction from the absorbance at 340 nM.

A. 7α-HYDROXYCHOLANOYL DEHYDROGENASE

Enzymes isolated from five strains were isolated and characterized by Aries and Hill (1970b); two of the strains were *Bacteroides fragilis,* two were *Cl. welchii* and the other an *Esch. coli.* The enzymes from the clostridial strains were $NADP^+$-dependent whilst those from the *Esch. coli* and the *Bact. fragilis* strains were NAD^+-dependent (Table 7.7). The greatest activity per cell was possessed by the strains of *Cl. welchii,* with the bacteroides showing least activity by a factor of 10-20. However, because of their numerical superiority this still means that the anaerobes produce 99% of the total faecal 7-hydroxycholanoyl dehydrogenase. The pH-optimum of the bacteroides enzyme is 1 pH unit lower than that of the clostridial enzyme and so the enzyme of the former will be more likely to be active at physiological pH values; their optimum of pH 9 is much higher, however, than that likely to be found in the gut. The pH-activity curves of the isolated enzymes show relatively sharp optima (Fig. 7.3) but suspensions of

TABLE 7.7

Some properties of the 7 α-hydroxycholanoyl dehydrogenases from five strains of gut bacteria

Source of enzyme		Nucleotide requirement	Enzyme activity per 10^9 cells	K_m (mM)	pH-optimum	Substrate specificity (activity on cholic chenodeoxycholic)
Esch. coli.	109	NAD^+	40	0.24	9.0- 9.4	1
Cl. welchii	49	$NADP^+$	61	0.25	9.8-10.2	1
	273	$NADP^+$	56	0.046	9.8-10.2	1
B. fragilis	9343	NAD^+	4	0.25	8.8- 9.3	0.6
	BV10	NAD^+	3	0.17	8.8- 9.3	0.7

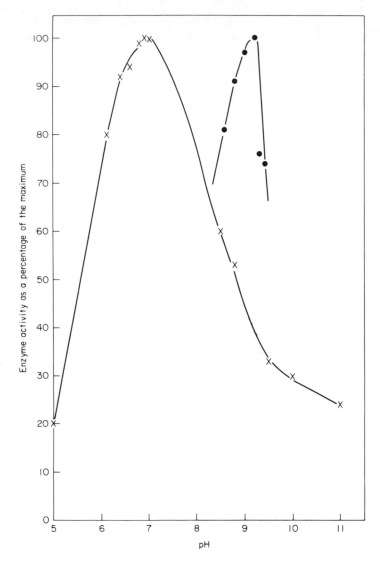

Fig. 7.3. pH optimum of 7αhydroxycholanoyloxioreductase of *B. fragilis* 9343.
x——x, reduction; ●——●, oxidation.

whole cells show fairly high dehydrogenase activity even at pH 7. The
dehydrogenases were true oxidoreductases since they catalysed the reverse
reduction step; the pH-optimum for this reaction was close to neutrality
(Fig. 7.3, Table 7.8).

Comparison of the ability to dehydrogenate the 7α-hydroxyl group of

TABLE 7.8

Some further properties of the 7 α-hydroxycholanoyl oxidoreductases of two strains of gut bacteria

		B. fragilis 9343	Cl. welchii CC49
pH-optimum	oxidation	8.8-9.3	9.8-10.2
	reduction	6.8-7.2	6.8- 7.2
K_m with cholic acid substrate		0.30 mM	0.48 mM
K_m with chenodeoxycholic acid		0.074 mM	0.43 mM
Percentage inhibition by excess substrate		16	0
% activity lost on storage (21 days, $-10°$C)		44	95
% activity lost on heating at $58°$C/30 min		3	100

3α,7α-dihydroxycholanoic acid and 3α,7α,12α-trihydroxycholanoic acid showed that the bacteroides enzymes were more active on the dihydroxy than in the trihydroxy substrate; the enzymes from the *Cl. welchii* strain and from the *Esch. coli* strain showed no such specificity. Further examination of one of the bacteroides strains showed that the K_m with the dihydroxy substrate was 0.074 mM compared with 0.30 mM with the trihydroxy substrate. In contrast the enzyme from one of the clostridial strains had a K_m of 0.48 mM with the dihydroxy and 0.43 mM with the trihydroxy substrates (Fig. 7.4, Table 7.8).

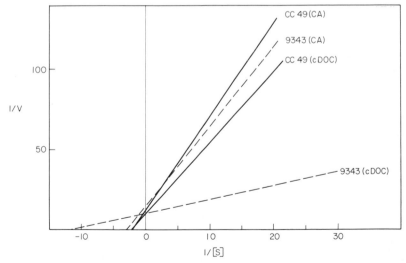

Fig. 7.4. Lineweaver-Burke plots for 7α-dehydrogenase from 9343 and CC49 acting on cholic acid (CA) and chenodeoxycholic acid (CDOC).

In addition to the difference in substrate specificity and in the pH optimum between the NAD^+requiring bacteroides enzyme and the $NADP^+$requiring clostridial enzyme, there were considerable differences in stability and in the response to high levels of substrates. Thus, after heating at $58°C$ for 30 minutes all of the activity of the clostridial enzyme was lost whilst 97% of the activity of the bacteroides enzyme still remained. Similarly after storage at $-10°C$ for three weeks only 5% of the activity of the clostridial enzyme remained compared with 56% of that of the bacteroides enzyme.

The activity of the clostridial enzyme was unaffected by wide ranges of substrate concentration, being as active on 16 mM cholic acid as on 1 mM. The bacteroides enzyme, in contrast, was rather less active on the higher substrate concentration and its activity was reduced by 16% by increasing the substrate concentration from 1 to 16 mM. The concentration of bile acids in faeces is approximately 4-5 mM, so that it is evident that even the bacteroides enzyme is unlikely to be significantly inhibited by substrate excess *in vivo*.

A range of inhibitors were tested on the 7-hydroxycholanoyl dehydrogenases. The enzyme reaction was partially inhibited by the presence of 3 mM periodate ion, 30 mM Cu^{++}, 30 mM Mg^{++} and 30 mM iodoacetate, but not by as much as 50 mM Cu^{++}, F^-, and N_3^-. The incomplete action of the inhibitors indicates that the enzyme does not possess readily denatured or complexed groups at the active site. The activity of the enzyme was considerably reduced when the free carboxyl group was methylated or conjugated with taurine or glycine.

Thus the enzyme has a requirement for a free carboxyl group and in the case of the bacteroides enzyme the presence of a 12α-hydroxyl group appears to interfere with enzyme-substrate interaction. The enzyme has a requirement for a nucleotide cofactor (NAD^+ or $NADP^+$) and for oxygen, presumably as a terminal electron acceptor.

B. 12α-HYDROXYCHOLANOYL DEHYDROGENASE

This is the dehydrogenase which is produced by fewest bacterial strains, and has been studied in a strain of bifidobacterium spp (Table 7.9). The enzyme activity/cell was similar to that of the other dehydrogenases studied, and the enzyme was slightly more active on 3α, 12α-dihydroxycholanic acid than on 3α, 7α, 12α-trihydroxycholanic acid. The pH-optimum of the 12-dehydrogenase (8.2-8.5) was the lowest of the dehydrogenases tested and virtually as close to physiological pH values as was that of the reduction reaction; thus of the hydroxycholanoyl dehydrogenases, only that active on the 12 position will be able, on pH criteria, to oxidize a relatively high proportion of its substrate groups. In the reverse reduction

TABLE 7.9

Properties of the hydroxycholanoyl oxidoreductases-isolated from 3 strains of gut bacteria and active on the 3α-and the 12α hydroxyl groups

Source of enzyme	Position of oxidized OH group	Enzyme activity per 10^9 cells	K_m (mM)	pH-optimum Oxidation	pH-optimum Reduction	Substrate specificity*
Cl. welchii CC377	3	30	0.086	10 -10.5	6.4-7.8	0.8
	7	11			6.5-7.0	0.8
Cl. welchii CC63	3	30		10.3-10.5		0.8
	7	20		9.4- 9.8		0.8
Bifidobacterium 33/5	3	20	0.28	10.5-11.2	6.4-7.8	0.9
	12	25	0.167	8.2- 8.5	5.8-6.4	0.9

* Ratio of activity on trihydroxy : dihydroxy bile acids

reaction some 12β-hydroxyl groups were produced although most of the product was in the 12α form. Thus, there may have been two enzymes present or, and more likely, the enzyme was relatively non-speific and although more active on 12α-hydroxyl groups, could act on and produce 12β-hydroxyl groups.

C. 3α-HYDROXYCHOLANOYL DEHYDROGENASE

Of the three dehydrogenases studied this was intermediate in abundance. Enzyme from three strains was studied; that from the two *Clostridium welchii* strains CC63 and CC377 was produced together with an enzyme active at the 7-position. The enzyme produced by Bifidobacterium 33/5 was produced together with an enzyme active at the 12-position. The properties of the enzyme preparation are summarized in Table 7.9.

Again the enzyme units per 10^9 cells and the K_m were of the same order of magnitude as those obtained for the 7α-dehydrogenase. The pH optimum of the 3-hydroxycholanoyl dehydrogenase was even higher than that of the enzyme active at the 7-position whilst the reverse reduction reaction had a broad pH optimum about neutrality. The reduction of 3-oxo groups produced hydroxyl groups in the α-configuration only: in our screening studies (Aries *et al.,* 1969a), however, we have detected 3β inversion products produced by many strains of human intestinal bacteria.

Because 3-hydroxyl groups in the α and β configuration are widely distributed in the family of steroids, it was of interest to note the specificity of the bacterial enzyme studied here. The enzyme would oxidize 3α-hydroxyl groups of the 5β-cholanic acid series, but had no action on the

3β-hydroxyl groups of 3β-hydroxy-5βcholestane, 3β-hydroxy-cholest-5-ene, or 3β-hydroxy-5β-cholanic acid (isolithocholic acid) or the 3α-hydroxyl groups of 3α-hydroxy-5α-androstan-17-one. The enzyme, therefore, appears to have a requirement for a 3α-hydroxyl group, a 5β-configuration for the steroid and a 24-carboxyl group.

D. SUMMARY OF PROPERTIES OF THE HYDROXYSTEROID DEHYDROGENASES

(1) Hydroxysteroid dehydrogenases have low activity on bile conjugates (or non-acid steroids) so that hydrolysis to release the free acid is a pre-requisite for their full activity in the gut.

(2) The enzymes are inducible, although there is a background enzyme level. The hydroxycholanoyl dehydrogenase activity is doubled by growth in the presence of 0.01% cholic acid substrate.

(3) Hydroxycholanoyl dehydrogenases all have pH-optima on the alkaline side of neutrality, with that of the 12-dehydrogenase being 8.2-8.5 and that of the 3-dehydrogenase being greater than 10 (that of the 7-hydrogenase is intermediate). Since the pH-optimum of the reverse hydrogenation is around neutrality it would be expected that the bulk of the oxygen functions would be in the hydroxyl form and with most of the oxo groups being at the 12-position.

The study of the substituents at C-7 gives misleading data due to the high activity of the 7α-dehydroxylase. In six countries studied, involving assays on 81 faecal samples, 14-31% of the oxygen functions at C-12 were in the oxo form (mean of 21%) compared with 2-9% of the oxygen functions at C-3 (mean of 5%) so that to this extent the results conform largely to those expected.

(4) The hydroxycholanoyl dehydrogenases maintain their optimal activity over a range of substrate concentrations up to 16 mM (the concentration in normal human faeces being 4-5 mM; the highest concentration found in our studies being 9.5 mM).

III. Hydroxycholanoyl dehydroxylases

In normal human faecal bile acids there is very little chenodeoxycholic acid and the amount of trisubstituted bile acid is less than 20% of the total (Hill and Aries, 1971). Thus, more than 80% of the faecal bile acids have been 7-dehydroxylated. The 7-dehydroxylation product from cholic acid is deoxycholic acid and much of the deoxycholate formed will be reabsorbed from the gut and recirculated; thus we cannot conclude that 80% of the faecal bile acids have been dehydroxylated in a single transit through the gut. Nevertheless, it is certain that a high proportion of the bile acids are dehydroxylated during their last passage from the ileum to the rectum. It follows, therefore, that either the 7-dehydroxylase is widespread in the human intestinal flora, or, alternatively is of phenomenally high activity. In general the dehydroxylase has not been detected in a high proportion of strains, but our studies have led us to conclude that a capacity to produce the dehydroxylase is, indeed, widely distributed.

In 1957 Linstedt fed labelled cholate to rats and recovered most of the label in the deoxycholate of the bile acids; he therefore concluded that deoxycholate is produced as a metabolite of cholic acid rather than being produced directly from cholesterol. Norman and Sjovall (1958) showed that amongst the metabolites of cholic acid produced on incubation with rat ceacal contents was deoxycholic acid. Norman and Bergman (1960) incubated cholic acid with rat caecal contents and obtained, amongst a range of other metabolites, deoxycholate. They showed that the dehydroxylation was performed mainly by the anaerobes but none of their isolated bacterial strains performed the reaction. In 1967 Midvedt reported the isolation of 8 strictly anaerobic non-sporing rod-shaped organisms capable of 7-dehydroxylating cholic acid (yielding deoxycholate) and chenodeoxycholate (to yield lithocholate). He partially identified his 8 strains and concluded that they all closely approximated to the family lactobacillus. Hill and Drasar (1968) reported the enzyme in small numbers of strains of *Bacteroides* spp., *Bifidobacterium* spp., *Clostridium* spp. and *Strep. faecalis.* We now believe that if freshly isolated cultures are used and grown in a well buffered medium containing added cysteine and kept at a pH above 6.5 in the presence of 0.01% cholic acid, then the dehydroxylase can be induced in 30-50% of strains of *Bacteroides, Bifidobacterium* spp., and *Clostridium* spp., together with smaller numbers of *Strep. faecalis* and *Veillonella* spp.

The conditions for production of 7α-dehydroxylase are rather more stringent than those for the production of other bile degradative enzymes and have been studied by Midvedt and Norman (1968) for their lactobacilli and by Aries and Hill (1970b) for *Bacteroides, Clostridium* spp., *Strep. faecalis* and a strain of *Esch. coli.* If the pH of the culture medium falls below 6.5 during the course of growth very little enzyme can be detected, so that a well buffered medium (e.g. Todd-Hewitt broth) is essential. The enzyme is entirely inducible, no enzyme being produced in the absence of cholic acid as substrate inducer. The cultures had to be grown under extremely anaerobic conditions which involved using medium which had been freshly steamed (to remove dissolved oxygen) and cooled with caps well screwed down prior to inoculation, the addition of a reducing agent to the medium (e.g. cysteine, thioglycollate, or whole blood) and very vigorous flushing of the growth vessel with hydrogen prior to the incubation in an atmosphere of hydrogen. In the absence of these rigorous conditions only a few of the more robust strains will produce the dehydroxylase and the vast majority of the strains will appear inactive. If the conditions are ideal for dehydroxylation then little keto acid formation should take place. Having grown a strain which is producing dehydroxylase the assay must also be performed under strictly anaerobic conditions. Because of these restrictions, the enzyme has not been studied in depth; however, enzyme from all strains studied appear to behave similarly. The dehydroxylase has a pH optimum between 7 and 8, acts equally well on cholic as on chenodeoxycholic acid, is inactive on the bile acid conjugates or on methyl esters of bile acids. The enzyme is inhibited by substrate in excess of 6 mM (i.e. in excess of the normal level found in human faeces). The enzyme is extremely labile in cell-free or cell-bound preparations and could not be stabilized or reactivated by reducing agents such as cysteine, thioglycollate or glutathione, or by the cofactors NAD^+, $NADP^+$, NADH, NADPH, FAD or FMN. The enzyme was completely inhibited by 30 mM Cu^{++} and by 3 mM periodate, and partially inhibited by 30 mM iodoacetate. There was no inhibition by F^-, N_3^-, Ca^{++}, Mg^{++} and EDTA. The inhibition suggest the presence of a liable or easily complexed group at the active site, possibly a sulph-hydryl group.

The enzyme is so labile that it could not be stabilized sufficiently to survive chromography on sepharose or on DEAE-cellulose. Consequently no estimate of the molecular weight has been made. The properties of the 7-dehydroxylases are summarized in Table 7.10.

TABLE 7.10

Summary of the properties of 7α-hydroxycholanoyl dehydroxylase

pH-optimum	7.0-8.0
Substrate specificity	Cholic and chenodeoxycholic acids are metabolized; conjugates or methyl esters not metabolized
Effect of substrate excess	Inhibited by more than 6mM substrate
Requirements for production	pH >6.5; strict anaerobiosis; presence of substrate
Effect of inhibitors	Inhibited by Cu^{++}, IO_4', iodoacetate; not by F^-, N_3^-, Ca^{++}, Mg^{++}, EDTA

As long ago as 1960, long before any strains of bacteria had been persuaded to dehydroxylate *in vitro* Samuelsson demonstrated that the 7-dehydroxylation proceeded via a Δ^6 intermediate (Fig. 7.5). In a previous paper (Samuelsson, 1959) he had eliminated the possibility of a 7-oxo intermediate. Using a double labelling technique he demonstrated that

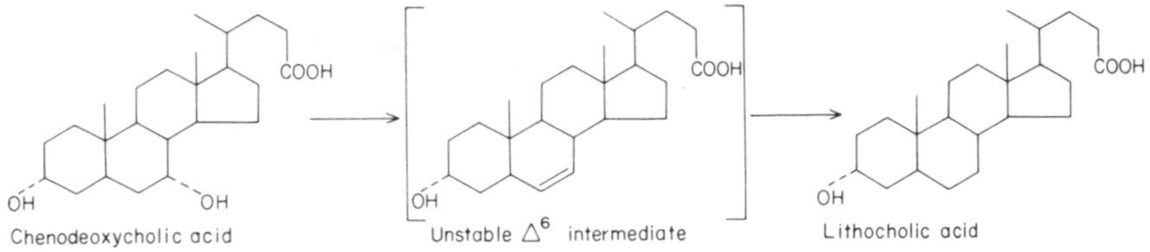

Fig. 7.5. Mechanism of dehydroxylation of cholic acid by gut bacteria.

there is a transelimination, with loss of the 7α-hydroxyl and 6β-hydrogen groups leaving a Δ^6 intermediate, followed by a reduction to deoxycholic acid. This was demonstrated *in vivo* in the rabbit intestine. There have been no reports, as yet, of a Δ^6 intermediate being detected in the *in vitro* system.

Since the 7-dehydroxylase is completely inducible this might explain the findings (Table 7.11) that the percentage of strict anaerobes able to 7-dehydroxylate increases with increasing faecal bile acid concentration. In the same way, that the degree (measured as the percentage mono+ unsubstituted bile acids) increases with increasing faecal bile acid concentration (Fig. 7.6).

TABLE 7.11

The relationship between the mean faecal bile acid concentration and the percentage of strains able to 7α-dehydroxylate

Country	Mean faecal bile acid concentration	Percentage of strains possessing 7α-dehydroxylase			
		Bacteroides	Bifidobacteria	Clostridia	*Strep. faecalis*
England	6.05	44	40	34	11
Scotland	6.13	56	56	45	40
U.S.A.	6.13	50	50	60	—
India	0.51	5	5	0	0
Uganda	0.45	33	4	6	3

From the faecal bile acids one would suspect the existence of a 3α-dehydroxylase. In fact this enzyme has yet to be reported, although cholanic acid reported to be present in human faeces by Ali and Kuksis (1965) and by Hill and Aries (1971), cannot be produced without such an enzyme. We have detected, however, a 12α-dehydroxylase producing chenodeoxycholic acid from cholic acid and lithocholic acid from deoxycholic acid. This enzyme has yet to be isolated, and, indeed, we have yet to find the correct reaction conditions which would allow us to reproduce the reaction; all observations of the reaction to date have been accidental while looking for other enzymes.

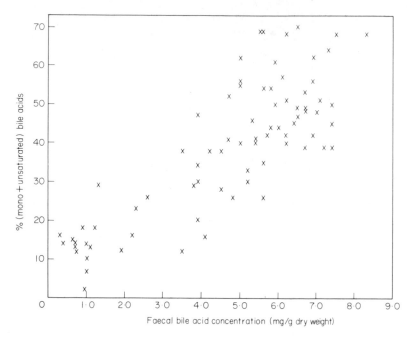

Fig. 7.6. Relation between the degree of degradation and faecal bile acid concentration.

Norman and Palmer (1964) fed labelled lithocholate to a patient undergoing cholecystectomy for non-obstructive cholelithiasis and isolated, amongst a number of metabolites, an unsaturated cholanic acid which was unidentified but might well have been the product of a 3-dehydration reaction.

Since the 7α-dehydroxylase is not produced when the pH falls below 6.5, the intestinal pH may be of critical importance. The faecal pH may not give an exact measure of the colonic or caecal pH, but will give an indication of comparative trends. The faecal pH of English people is much higher than that of the Indians or Ugandans tested (Fig. 7.7). Whereas the mean faecal pH of the English is 6.7 and 60% of the samples had a pH greater than 6.5, the mean pH of the Ugandan samples was only 5.7 and less than 10% of the samples had a pH greater than 6.5. Undoubtedly the colonic and caecal pH will be higher than that of the faeces but the results indicate that the colonic pH of the Ugandans and Indians is more acid than that of the English and may well be less favourable to dehydroxylase production. This may therefore provide a partial explanation of the higher degree of dehydroxylation of English, compared with Indian and Ugandan faecal bile acids.

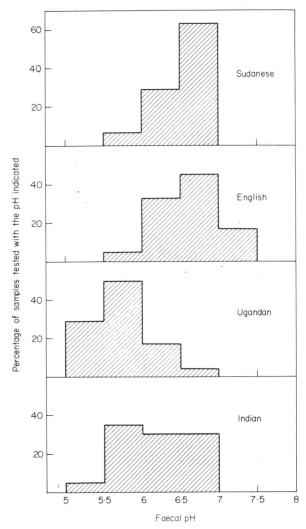

Fig. 7.7. Histograms of faecal pH of English, Indians and Ugandans.

Similarly, the 7α-dehydroxylase is only produced and is only active under extremely anaerobic conditions. The ability of the anaerobic bacteria to outgrow the anaerobes may well be an indication of the degree of anaerobiosis of the gut, and a plot of the log

$$\frac{\text{(no. of anaerobes)}}{\text{(no. of aerobes)}}$$

against the degree of dehydroxylase (Fig. 7.8) indicates a rough relationship between the two.

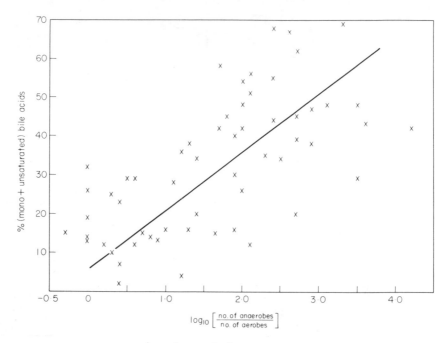

Fig. 7.8. Graph of log $\dfrac{\text{(no. of anaerobes)}}{(\text{ no. of aerobes })}$ against the percentage dehydroxylation of the faecal steroids.

IV. Bile acid degradation in the human intestine

Comparison of the faecal bile acids with those secreted in bile indicates that the following reactions take place:

(a) *Hydrolysis of the amide bond to yield free bile acids.* This reaction proceeds to completion indicating that the hydrolase is widely distributed in the gut flora. This has been demonstrated.

(b) *Hydroxycholanoyl dehydrogenation.* The dehydrogenases act only slowly on bile conjugates so that the hydrolase must act first to release the substrate for the dehydrogenases. In all cases the dehydrogenases have high pH optima whereas that of the reverse reaction is close to neutrality. Therefore the oxygen functions would be expected to be mainly in the hydroxyl form — that in the 3-position almost entirely so and that in the 12-position being somewhat less so. The picture at the 7-position would be expected to be much less clear cut due to the high activity of the 7-dehydroxylase. All of these expectations are fulfilled.

(c) *Dehydroxylation at the 7 and 3-position.* More than 80% of the faecal bile acids have undergone 7-dehydroxylation, indicating the widespread nature of the enzyme; this has been confirmed. The enzyme is inducible and is not produced when the pH falls below 6.5; both the low faecal bile acid concentration and the relatively acid pH may partly explain why the faecal bile acids of Ugandans and Indians are less dehydroxylated than are those of English people. The 7α-dehydroxylase is only produced and is only active under extremely anaerobic conditions and, if the ratio

$$\frac{\text{anaerobes}}{\text{aerobes}}$$

in the faecal flora is a measure of the degree of anaerobiosis in the gut then there is an indication (Fig. 7.8) that anaerobiosis might play a role in determining the degree of hydroxylation.

CHAPTER 8

Cholesterol Metabolism

Like the bile acids, cholesterol undergoes extensive bacterial metabolism during its transit through the large bowel. There are two major faecal metabolites of cholesterol (coprostanol and coprostanone) with smaller amounts of a third (cholestenone) also present (Mitchell and Diver, 1967; Grundy and Ahrens, 1969; Hill and Aries, 1971). The reactions are shown in Fig. 8.1, and quantitative data on the relative amounts of these metabolites are given in Table 8.1. In general, more than half of the faecal cholesterol is in the form of its hydrogenated metabolite coprostanol (5β-cholestan-3β-ol) whilst a further 5-10% is usually in the form of coprostanone; unmetabolized cholesterol accounts for 25-45% of the total faecal neutral steroid fraction. In studies with germ-free rats the faecal neutral steroids are entirely in the form of unchanged cholesterol (Kellogg and Wostmann, 1969) indicating that the intestinal bacteria are responsible for the degradation of cholesterol during its transit through the large bowel.

TABLE 8.1

Mean daily excretion rates of cholesterol and its metabolites by people living in various countries

		Daily excretion of neutral steroids (mg/day)				
Country	Reference	Cholesterol A	Coprostanol B	Coprostanone C	Total	$\dfrac{B + C}{A}$
England	1(150)	140	285	25	450	2.22
Scotland	1(150)	120	280	20	420	2.49
	2	68	208	37	313	3.60
U.S.A.	1(150)	145	270	25	440	2.03
	3	135	—	—	447	2.31
Uganda	1(500)	29	32	4	65	1.25
India	1(500)	24	29	7	60	1.40

References: 1. Hill *et al.* (1971a). 2. Mitchell and Diver. (1967). 3. Connor *et al.* (1969).

Figures in parentheses indicate the mean faecal mass assumed in the calculation.

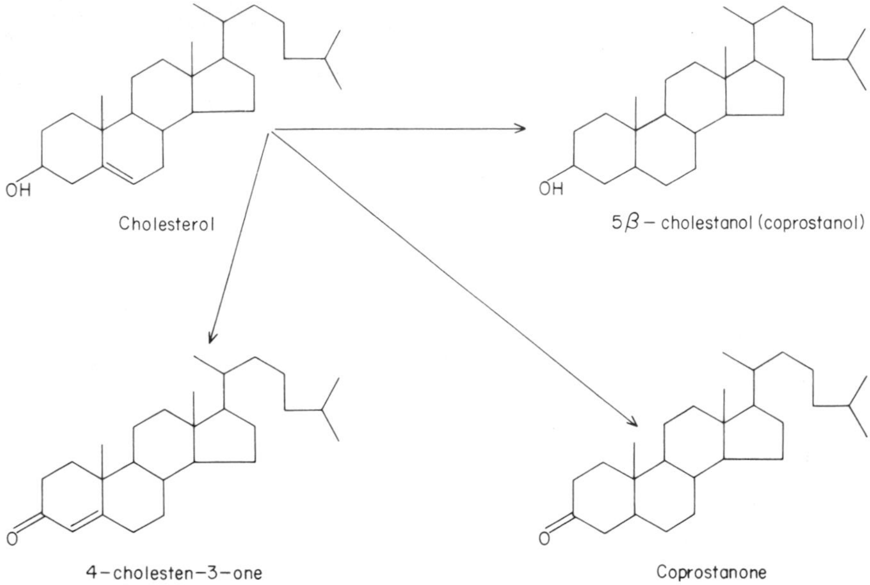

Fig. 8.1. The inter-relationship between cholesterol and its principal faecal metabolites.

Cholesterol is subject to enterohepatic circulation, being absorbed from the small bowel and returned to the liver via the portal blood system to be re-secreted in the bile. Coprostanol is not absorbed from the gut and so it might be suspected that bacterial reduction of the cholesterol nucleus might result in an increased faecal excretion of neutral steroid. In fact this does not appear to be so. Kellogg and Wostmann (1969) demonstrated that the rate of faecal excretion of cholesterol and its metabolites was the same in germ-free as in conventional rats. Danielsson (1960) showed that in the rat the metabolism of cholesterol occurred after the cholesterol had passed the absorptive regions of the gut and that the bacteria were only degrading that part of the cholesterol pool which was to be lost in the faeces anyway. Thus the metabolism of cholesterol by gut bacteria appears to play no part in the overall cholesterol metabolism of the host.

I. Reduction of cholesterol to coprostanol

The conversion of cholesterol to coprostanol has been the subject of much study and there is a wealth of early literature demonstrating the role of the gut bacteria in this reaction (for example, Rosenheim and Starling, 1933; Schoenheimer and Sperry, 1934; Anchel and Schoenheimer, 1938; Rosenheim and Webster, 1941). Rosenheim and Webster (1943) showed that treatment of rats with sulphonamide antibiotics to repress the gut flora inhibited the production of coprostanol.

Since more than 50% of the faecal cholesterol has undergone this reduction, the enzyme catalysing the nuclear hydrogenation of cholesterol must be of high activity in the intestine. Nevertheless, attempts to demonstrate such a reaction using pure strains of bacteria have not been very successful. Snog-Kjaer *et al.* (1956) showed that, provided a suitable culture medium was used, the reaction could be demonstrated with mixed cultures of faecal anaerobic bacteria. Their culture medium was a 5% suspension of calf-brain which had been exhaustively extracted with acetone until no more cholesterol could be detected in the extract. A solution of essential mineral salts was then added to this suspension together with the cholesterol substrate. The results of Snog-Kjaer *et al.* were supported by those of Coleman and Bauman (1957). We have attempted to demonstrate reduction of cholesterol to coprostanol by pure strains of bacteria using a wide range of culture media and have had success only with the Snog-Kjaer medium. When grown in the extracted calf-brain medium we could get up to 80% conversion of cholesterol to coprostanol using pure strains of *Bacteroides* spp., *Bifidobacterium* spp. and *Clostridium* spp. (Table 8.2).

TABLE 8.2

Reduction of cholesterol to coprostanol by pure strains of human intestinal bacteria

Bacterial species	Number of strains tested	Percentage of strains producing coprostanol[+]
Esch. coli	20	0
Strep. faecalis	20	0
Bacteroides spp.	18	67
Bifidobacterium spp.	12	75
Clostridium spp.	20	45

There has been some debate concerning the mechanism of this reduction and two major pathways have been postulated (Fig. 8.2). Mechanism A involves a direct reduction of the C5-6 double bond; mechanism B involves oxidation of the 3β-OH group and isomerization to give 4-cholesten-3-one, which then undergoes nuclear reduction to 5β-cholesten-3-one followed by oxo-reduction to give coprostanol. There is much evidence for the individual steps in mechanism B in the early literature but Rosenfeldt and Gallacher (1964) concluded that mechanism A was the major pathway for coprostanol formation. A recent study by Bjorkhem and Gustafsson (1971) has yielded results which, in contrast to those of Rosenfeldt and Gallacher,

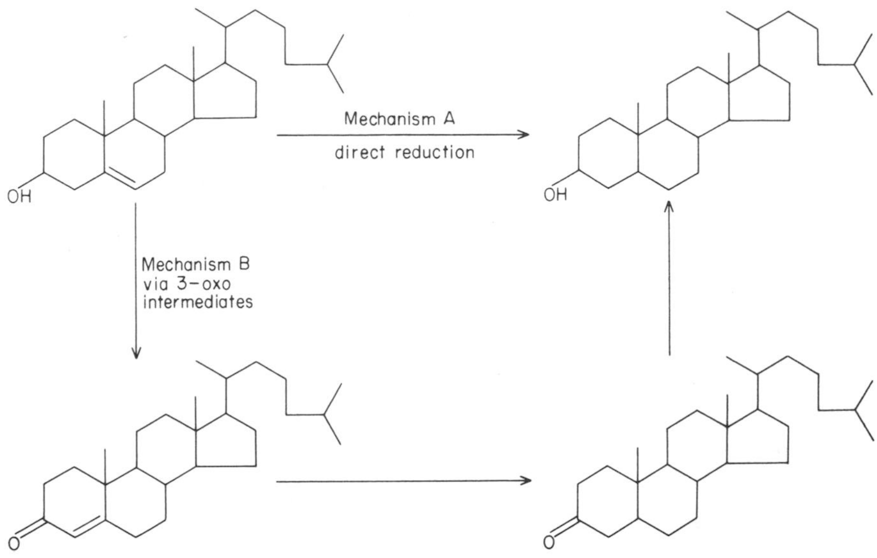

Fig. 8.2. The suggested mechanisms for the reduction of cholesterol to coprostanol.

indicate that both mechanisms are of equal importance. It is possible that different organisms may utilize different pathways and that the rat caecal contents used by the two groups of workers may have differed in the relative proportions of the two types of organisms.

We have found little evidence for the production of coprostanone from cholesterol, but the reaction is a significant, though minor one, in the gut. Bjorkhem and Gustafsson (1971) showed that coprostanone is readily reduced by rat caecal contents to coprostanol and possibly our *in vitro* conditions strongly favour this reaction, thereby minimizing the evidence for the formation of coprostanone. The hydroxy-steroid oxido-reductases described in Section III were specific for acid steroids but undoubtedly the gut bacteria produce similar enzymes active on the neutral steroids.

Production of coprostanol by the intestinal bacteria is dependent not only on the presence of bacteria able to reduce cholesterol, but also on the generation of the conditions necessary for the production of or the action of the enzyme. This is evident from the data that we have obtained on the effect of diet on the faecal steroid composition (Hill, 1971b; Crowther *et al.*, 1973). While living for thirty days on a diet containing less than 30 g fat per day the faecal neutral steroids of a volunteer contained a progressively decreasing proportion of bacterial metabolites (Table 8.3) during the third and fourth weeks, although there was no decrease during the first two weeks. Throughout the period there was no gross alteration in

TABLE 8.3

Ratio of bacterial metabolites of cholesterol to undefraded cholesterol in faeces of people on low fat diets

Nature of the low fat diet	Subject	Ratio (coprostanol + coprostanone/cholesterol in faeces					
			Period in weeks on the low fat diet				
		Pre-diet	2	4	10	20	Post-diet
Solid	a	1.61	1.90				2.28
	b	1.03	1.03				1.07
	c	1.79	1.55	1.15			1.72
	d	1.60	1.59				2.90
Liquid	a	1.33	0.07				1.13
	b	1.33	0.67				1.22
	c	1.90	0.11				1.50
Starvation	a	1.50	1.04	1.04	0.37	0.18	—
	b	1.57	0.56	0.25	0.33	0.30	—

the faecal bacterial flora or in the daily production of faeces. In volunteers living on a liquid diet designed for astronauts and containing all essential nutrients, there was a rapid and considerable reduction in the amount of coprostanol and in the proportion of neutral steroids as bacterial metabolites in their faeces (Table 8.3). Here there was a rapid decrease in the number of enterococci which paralleled the decrease in the amount of coprostanol (Fig. 8.3) although our *in vitro* studies did not reveal any cholesterol reduction by these organisms. Similarly the faecal neutral steroids of two obese patients living on a starvation diet for a long period of time contained a reduced proportion of coprostanol which paralleled the decrease in the number of enterococci (Fig. 8.4). Here the situation was less clear cut because although there was a good correlation between the amount of coprostanol formed and the number of enterococci found in faeces, there were many other changes in the faecal bacterial flora.

Although these studies of individuals indicate a correlation between the number of faecal enterococci and the degree of metabolism of cholesterol, a plot of the percentage of neutral steroids as coprostanol against the number of enterococci per gram of faeces from more than 50 people (each point being the paired data from a person) showed no relationship (Fig. 8.5). This, together with the fact that in our *in vitro* studies the enterococci tested all failed to reduce cholesterol to coprostanol, would indicate that the correlation found in the dietary studies were fortuitous. The people living on the low-fat or no-residue diets were living on a low

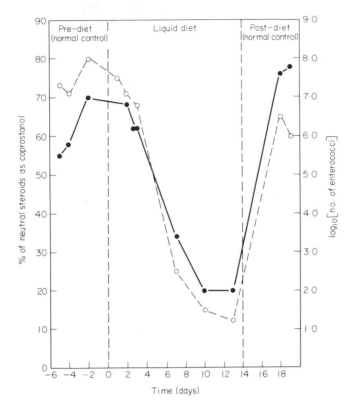

Fig. 8.3. The effect of a liquid diet on the numbers of enterococci per gram faeces and on the percentage reduction of cholesterol to coprostanol in faeces of healthy volunteers. ●——●. $\log_{10}$ (No. of enterococci); ○— — —○, per cent of neutral steroid as coprostanol.

cholesterol diet and it is known that this results in a decreased faecal excretion of cholesterol (Dietschy, 1969) and this, indeed, happened after a lag period of two weeks. It is possible, therefore, that this is an example of enzyme induction and that the amount of nuclear hydrogenase is dependent on the substrate concentration. However, this is not borne out by a comparison of the amount of cholesterol reduction with the faecal neutral steroid concentration in people living on a normal British diet (Fig. 8.6). Similarly, although the degree of metabolism of the faecal bile acids could be correlated with $\log_{10}$ (anaerobes/aerobes), no such correlation was found with the metabolism of the neutral steroids (Fig. 8.7). As yet we have no clear evidence concerning the factors controlling cholesterol reduction in the gut.

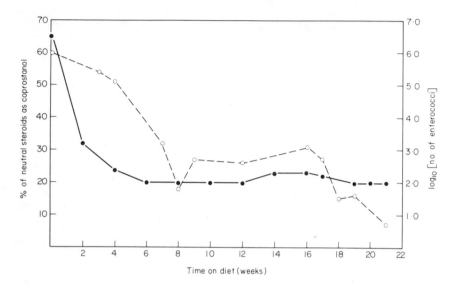

Fig. 8.4. The effect of prolonged starvation of an obese patient on the number of enterococci per gram faeces and on the percentage of neutral steroids as coprostanol. ●——●, log $_{10}$ (No. of enterococci); ○— — —○, per cent of neutral steroids as coprostanol.

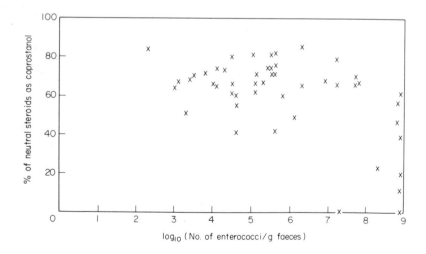

Fig. 8.5. The relation between the number of enterococci per gram faeces and the percentage of neutral steroids as coprostanol.

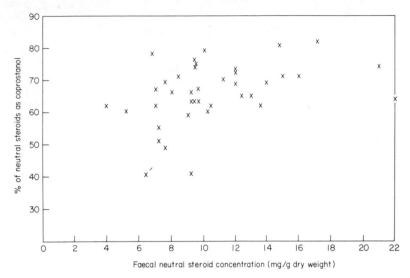

Fig. 8.6. The relation between the total faecal neutral steroid concentration and the percentage of neutral steroids as coprostanol.

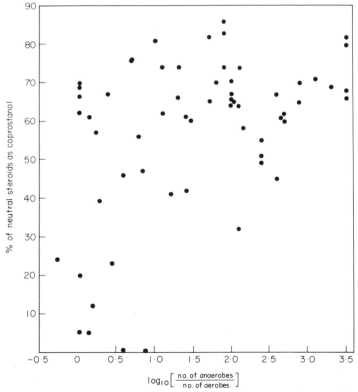

Fig. 8.7. The relation between the percentage of faecal neutral steroids as coprostanol and the ratio of anaerobes/aerobes.

II. Cholesterol side chain cleavage

Evidence that side chain cleavage of the cholesterol molecule takes place in the human gut is sparse. Grundy *et al.* (1968) showed that up to 40% of the intestinal cholesterol may be degraded to non-steroidal moieties during transit through the large bowel. Connor *et al.* (1968) obtained results similar to those of Grundy *et al.*; in 5/6 of their patients there was little loss of cholesterol from the large bowel but in the remaining patient the losses at time exceeded 50% of the total cholesterol entering the caecum. They were unable to find the cause for this loss, but side chain removal would yield a neutral steroid readily absorbed from the large bowel and excreted in the urine.

There have been a number of studies of side chain cleavage using *Nocardia* spp. (Sih *et al.*, 1968), *Mycobacterium* spp. (Peterson and Davies, 1964) *Azotobactor* spp. (Horvath and Kramli, 1947) and *Proactinomyces* spp. (Turfitt, 1948) which suggest a variety of mechanisms for the reaction. Horvath and Kramli (1947) claimed the isolation of methylheptanone, indicating cleavage at C-17 with removal of the side chain *in toto* (Fig. 8.8a). Turfitt obtained isocaproic acid as the product of side chain

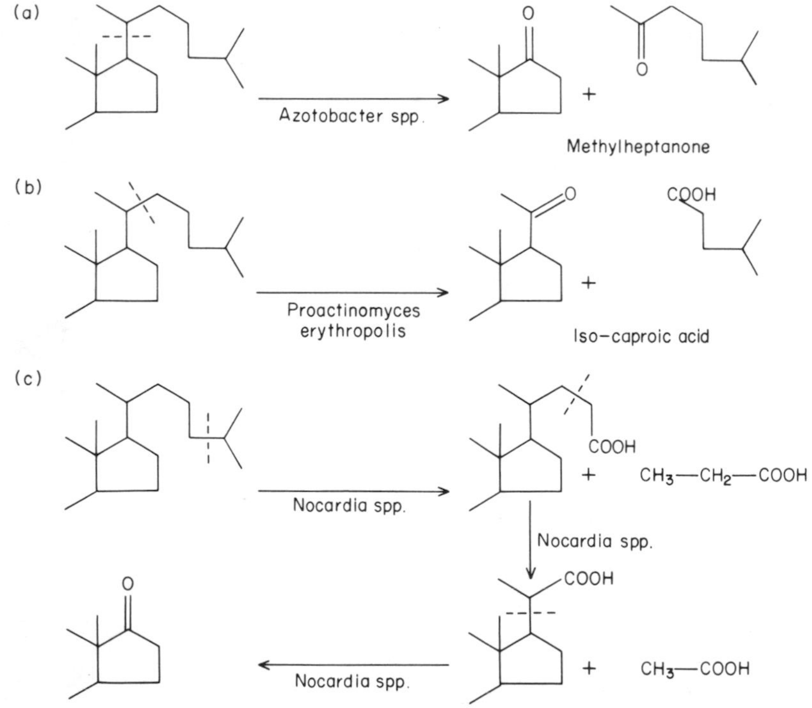

Fig. 8.8. The pathways for cholesterol side-chain cleavage by bacteria.

cleavage indicating cleavage between C-20 and C-22 (Fig. 8.8b), whilst Sih *et al.* (1968a, b) obtained impressive evidence for a stepwise removal of the side chain (Fig. 8.8c) although the evidence was incomplete. From cholesterol, propionic acid and 3-oxo-1,4-choladien-24-oic acid was obtained. When lithocholic acid was incubated with the same strain, acetic acid and a C-22 acid (a bis-norcholanic acid) were obtained. The conversion of a C-22 acid into a 17-oxo-steroid with the removal of propionic acid was also demonstrated, as was the overall conversion of C-27 cholesterol to a 17-oxo-steroid. However, although the overall reaction has been demonstrated and the individual steps C-27 → C-24 → C-22 → C-17 have also been shown, they have yet to produce a series of intermediates which are both products of the previous and substrates for the next reaction in the chain. Very little has been done in this field with organisms that might be considered normal inhabitants of the human gut. Hill *et al.* (1971) reported the metabolism of 4-cholesten-3-one to oestrone via a 10-demethylation and side chain cleavage; in addition, numerous other phenolic steroids were detected, presumably representing various stages of side chain degradation.

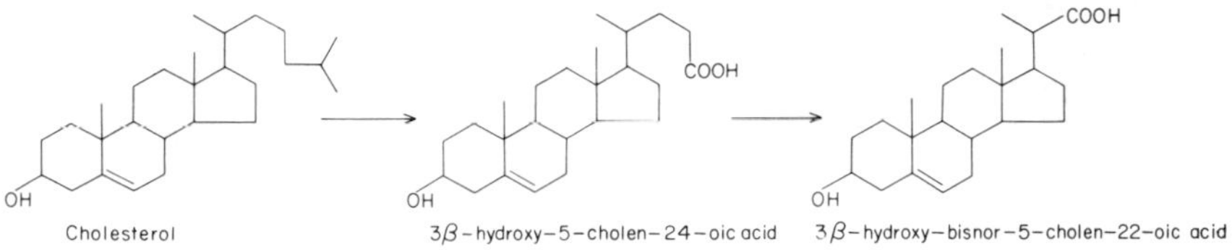

Cholesterol   3β-hydroxy-5-cholen-24-oic acid   3β-hydroxy-bisnor-5-cholen-22-oic acid

Fig. 8.9. The metabolism of cholesterol to 3β-hydroxy-bisnor-5-cholenic acid.

If the pathway postulated by Sih *et al.* is used by gut bacteria, then one of the intermediates would be related to bis-nor-Δ^5-cholenic acid (Fig. 8.9) which has been shown by Lacassagne *et al.* (1966) to be carcinogenic. Its possible role in the aetiology of colon cancer is discussed elsewhere in this book.

CHAPTER 9

Nuclear Dehydrogenation of Steroids

Although the nuclear dehydrogenation of steroids by intestinal bacteria has been little studied, the production of the responsible enzymes by soil organisms has received considerable attention and, indeed, dehydrogenation of ring A by bacteria is one of the most extensively studied reactions of steroid chemistry. The reason for this is that the products are of great clinical interest and therefore of great commercial importance to the pharmaceutical industry. For example, the dehydrogenation of cortisone to prednisone (Fig. 9.1) is accompanied by a great increase in anti-inflammatory activity.

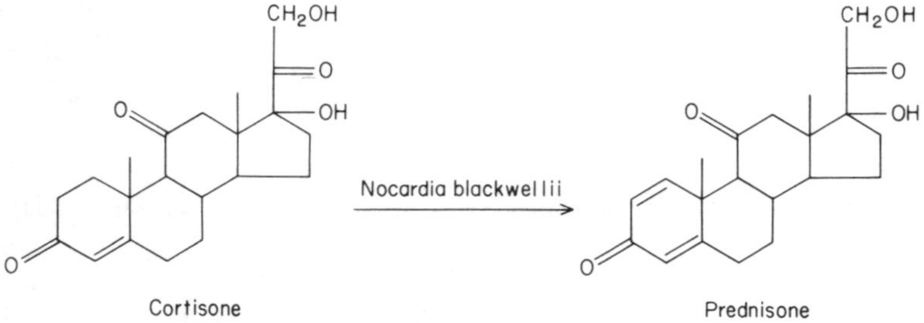

Fig. 9.1. Dehydrogenation of cortisone to prednisone.

There is some evidence that nuclear dehydrogenation takes place in the intestine. Bile acids having the 5α configuration (the allo-bile acids) have been isolated from the faeces of humans (Haslewood, 1967). The bile acids synthesized by the liver have the 5β configuration and Kallner (1967) has shown that the intestinal bacterial flora is responsible for the inversion at C-5 via a 3-oxo-4-cholen-24-oic acid intermediate (Fig 9.2). Norman and Palmer (1964) fed C^{14}-labelled lithocholic acid to ileostomy patients and obtained a number of metabolites, one of which was an unidentified unsaturated bile acid.

There are four principle types of reaction by which double bonds may be introduced into the steroid nucleus by bacterial action (Hill, 1971a). They are:

1. Introduction of a double bond conjugated to an oxo group.

2. Introduction of a double bond via a dehydration reaction.
3. Removal of the C—10 methyl group, which allows the keto-enolization of 1,4-dien-3-oxo steroids to the phenolic form.
4. Introduction of a double bond conjugated with other double bonds (rather than with an oxo group as in type 1).

These will be discussed in turn.

I. Introduction of a double bond conjugated to an oxo group

This is the nuclear unsaturation reaction which has been most widely studied and is exemplified in Fig. 9.2 — the inversion at C—5 of the bile acids. Reactions of this type have been demonstrated with a range of

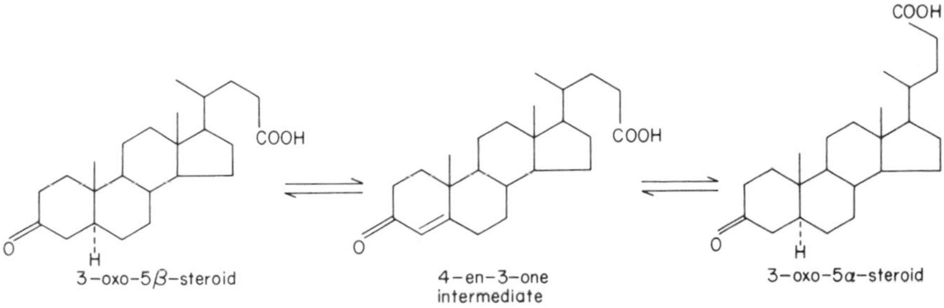

Fig. 9.2. Interconversion of the 5β cholanic acids and their 5α analogues via a Δ⁴ intermediate.

non-intestinal organisms, e.g. *Nocardia blackwellii* (Stoudt *et al.*, 1958), *Pseudomonas testosteronii* (Levy and Talalay, 1959a, b; Davidson and Talalay, 1966), *Alcaligenes faecalis* (Wix *et al.*, 1968), *Bacillus sphaericus* (Capek *et al.*, 1966) *Streptomyces rubescens* (Hayakawa *et al.*, 1958) and *Arthrobacter simplex* (Hayakawa *et al.*, 1969). We have demonstrated the presence in the human intestinal flora of organisms able to perform both Δ^1- and Δ^4-dehydrogenation reactions in conjugation with a 3-oxo group, the active organisms being opalescent-negative clostridia. (Aries and Hill, 1970; Aries *et al.*, 1971) and *Clostridium welchii*. In all cases the reaction has been demonstrated only in ring A of the steroid molecule and has yet to be demonstrated in rings B, C and D.

There are some notable differences between the dehydrogenases isolated from intestinal bacteria and those isolated from non-intestinal organisms. For example, the clostridial enzymes were both specific for 5β steroids, and for a $\Delta^{1,4}$-steroid to be formed it was necessary for the Δ^1 enzyme to act first before the Δ^4 enzyme had removed the assmetry from C—5 (Fig. 9.3). In contrast the Δ^1 dehydrogenases described by Levy and Talalay (1958b), Wix *et al.* (1968), Stoudt *et al.* (1955), and by Ringold *et al.* (1963) acted

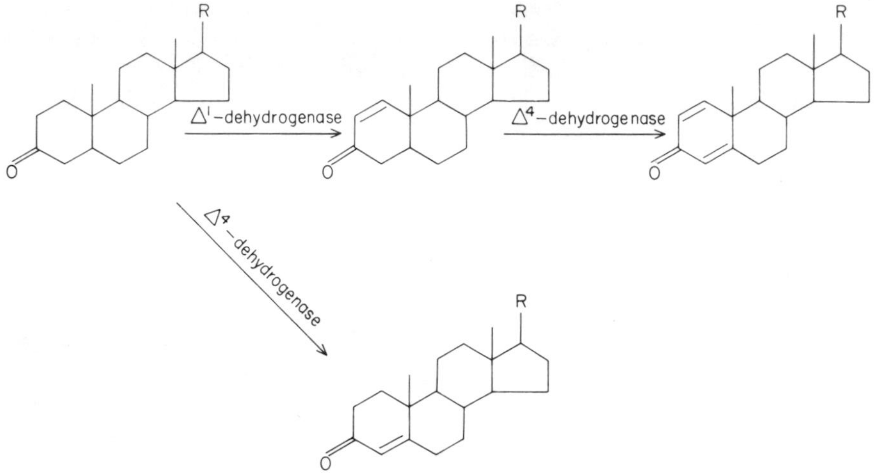

Fig. 9.3. Introduction of a double bond into ring A in conjugation with a 3-oxo group by human faecal clostridia.

in 5α-3-oxo and on Δ^4-3-oxo steroids. Unless the protoplast membrane of the clostridia was damaged, no Δ^1-dehydrogenation took place because the bacterial protoplast membrane was impermeable to the substrate. This would present no real problems *in vivo* since clostridia are highly autolytic organisms. Permeability to the substrate apparently presents no such problems to the soil organisms used industrially. On the other hand, there are many similarities. For example, all of the Δ^1- and Δ^4-dehydrogenases studied have been able to use artificial electron acceptors and all had pH optima above pH 7.

Reduction of a C4-5 double bond was more readily demonstrated with human intestinal bacteria. Such an enzyme was demonstrated with a high proportion of the opalescent-positive and opalescent-negative clostridia, bacteroides and bifidobacteria tested (Table 9.1). All of the active clostridial strains tested produced with the 5β-configuration, whereas most of the bacteroides strains gave products with the 5α-configuration.

II. Nuclear dehydration reactions

Samuelsson (1960) demonstrated that the 7-dehydroxylation of cholic acid to yield deoxycholic acid was a 7-dehydration, yielding an unstable Δ^6-intermediate which rehydrogenates to deoxycholic acid (Fig. 9.4). A reaction of this type, a 3-dehydration, may well have given rise to the unsaturated unsubstituted cholanic acid isolated by Norman and Palmer (1964) as a metabolite of lithocholic acid.

TABLE 9.1

Production of 4-andresten-3,17-dione from 5β-androstan-3,17-dione by gut bacteria

Bacteria tested	Production of 4-en-3-one	
	No. of strains tested	% positive
Bacteroides fragilis	50	0
Bifidobacteria	50	0
Escherichia coli	50	0
Streptococcus faecalis	50	0
Clostridium spp.		
(a) opalescent +ve	100	3
Cl. welchii	26	11
Cl. bifermentans	59	0
others	16	0
(b) opalescent —ve	394	35
Cl. paraputrificum	112	93
Cl. indolis	49	33
others	233	7

In addition to these whole-animal studies, there is a wealth of evidence in favour of nuclear dehydration of steroids by soil organisms. Hayakawa *et al.* (1958) have demonstrated the production of metabolites with 4-en-3-oxo and 4,6-dien-3-oxo structures from cholic acid, and they have postulated that the degradation of cholic acid may be via the pathways illustrated in Fig. 9.5, which involves a C6-7 dehydration reaction in conjugation with a 4-en-3-oxo group. This implies that the 7-dehydroxylase enzyme is not specific for 5β steroids. We have demonstrated a similar reaction with intestinal bacteria giving rise to 4,6-dien-3-oxo bile acids (Goddard and Hill, 1973). If we assume that all bacterial 7-dehydroxylases produce Δ^6- intermediates, then these unsaturated steroids may be formed, albeit transiently, by a wide range of intestinal bacteria.

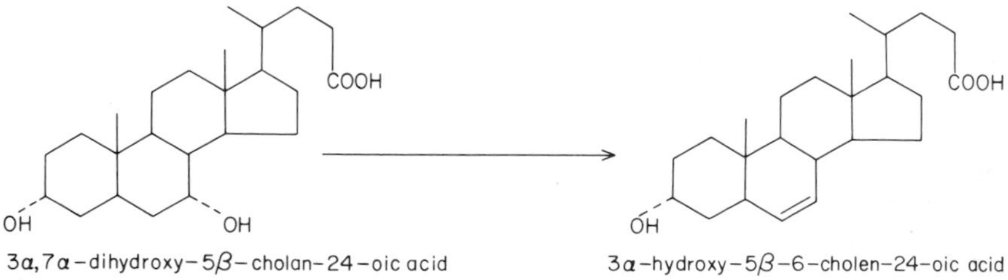

3α,7α–dihydroxy–5β–cholan–24–oic acid   3α–hydroxy–5β–6–cholen–24–oic acid

Fig. 9.4. Introduction of nuclear double bonds via a dehydration reaction.

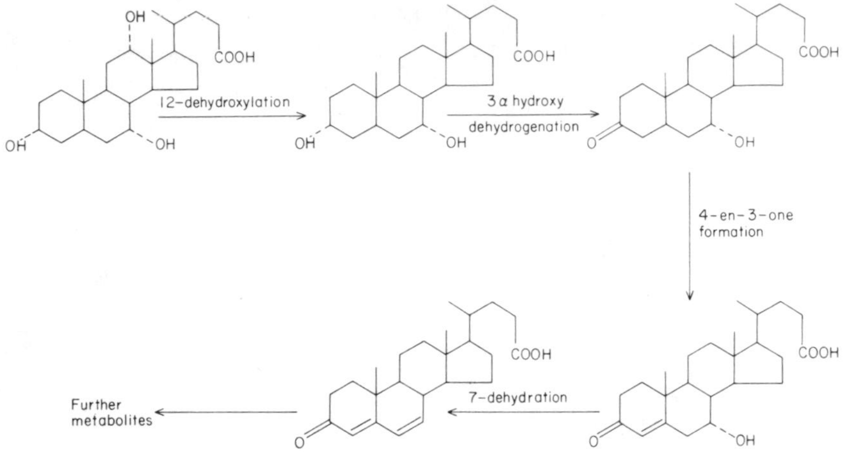

Fig. 9.5. Pathway postulated by Hayakawa *et al.* (1969) for the degradation of cholic acid by *Arthrobacter simplex*.

III. Removal of the C-10-methyl substituents

This reaction in itself does not give rise to nuclear desaturation. However, in the presence of the 10-methyl groups, a 1,4-dien-3-oxo-steroid is unable to undergo keto-enolization. In the biosynthesis of oestrogenic steroids by mammalian cells, the 10-methyl group is removed via an oxidative pathway (Fig. 9.6) and this pathway is also followed by *Bacillus cyclo-oxidans* and by *Pseudomonas testosteronii*. The keto-enolization of ring A following 10-demethylation has been demonstrated using human intestinal strains of clostridia (Goddard and Hill, 1971; 1972a) using principally strains of *Cl. paraputrificum*.

The mechanism differs from that followed by the mammalian system in two ways. Firstly, only 4-en-3-oxo steroids could act as substrates and no demethylation of 1,4-dien-3-oxo steroids was detected. Secondly, the methyl group was not oxidatively removed, but there was a nett transmethylation from C–10 to the oxygen function at C–17 (Fig. 9.7). The mechanisms of this nett transmethylation has not been determined. Due to the distances involved this is probably not an intermolecular rearrangement (Fig. 9.8a).

It is possible that this is a simple demethylation which happens to occur at the same time as a 17-O-methylation (Fig. 9.8b) but this is unlikely since these strains do not give rise to 17-O-methyl ethers under any other circumstances tested. It is more likely that the methyl group is taken up by a carrier molecule (Fig. 9.8c), and transferred to a suitable receptor group (in this case, the 17-oxygen function). In the case of 3-oxo-4-cholen-24-

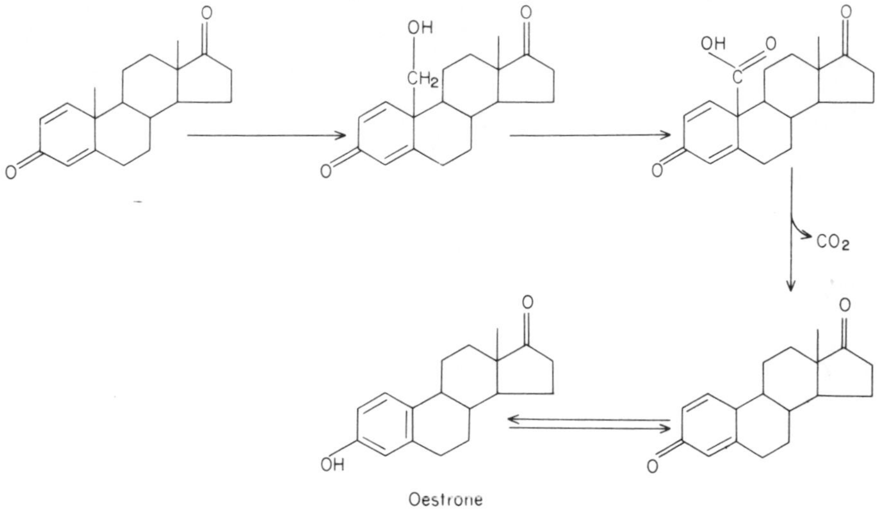

Fig. 9.6. Oxidative demethylation of 1,4-androstadien-3,17-dione.

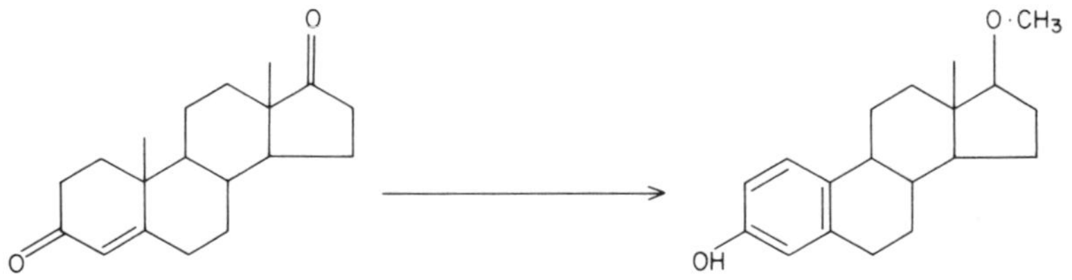

Fig. 9.7. 10-demethylation of 4-androsten-3,17-dione linked to a Δ^1-dehydrogenation and a 17-O-methylation by human intestinal clostridia.

oic acid the receptor group is the carboxylic group. In all three mechanisms the demethylation step is accompanied by a C1-2 dehydrogenation; note that in this case the C1-2 dehydrogenase has no requirement for a 5β configuration in contrast to the dehydrogenation conjugated to a 3-oxo group but unaccompanied by demethylation. Investigation of other substrates throws a little more light on the mechanism of demethylation. When 4-cholesten-3-one was used as substrate the product was 3-hydroxy-1,3,5 (10)-cholestatriene, indicating that there is no absolute requirement for a receptor group and thereby ruling out an intermolecular re-arrangement. When 3-oxo-4-cholen-24-oic-acid was the substrate this nett trans-methylation yielded a 24 ester as mentioned above. On the mechanism in Fig. 9.8b, we would now have to postulate a coincidental 24-methyl ester

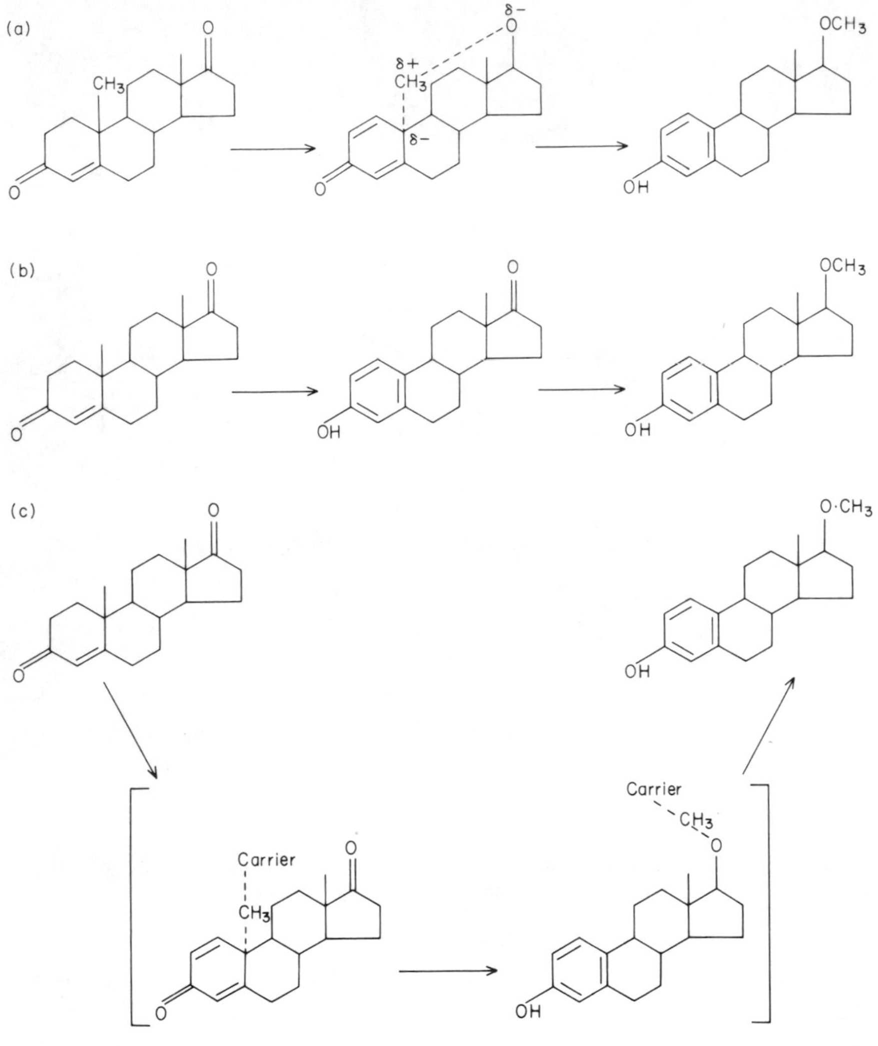

Fig. 9.8. Possible pathways for the formation of 17-methoxyoestradiol from 4-androsten-3,17-dione. (a) Intermolecular rearrangement; (b) demethylation followed by 17-O-methylation; (c) transmethylation via a methyl-carrier.

formation as well as a coincidental 17-O-methyl ether formation accompanying 10-demethylation; a 24-methyl ester however, would be the expected product of mechanism (c). In order to shed further light on the mechanism of this reaction it would be necessary to sythesize a substrate molecule with a C^{14} label on the 10 methyl substitutent; then on mechanism (c) the label should be transferred to the C—17 oxygen function whilst on mechanism (b) the label would be lost.

Although this reaction has been demonstrated *in vitro*, it has still to be demonstrated *in vivo*. Any 17-methoxyoestradiol formed in the gut would be absorbed by passive diffusion and excreted eventually in the urine. The simple task of looking for 17-methoxyoestradiol in human urine is complicated by a number of factors which make such a task difficult. Urinary oestrogens are conjugated as sulphates at the 3-position and as glucuronides in the 17-position. It is usual, therefore, to subject the excreted oestrogens to acid hydrolysis to release the free steroids; the conditions necessary to hydrolyse an O-sulphate linkage would be more than sufficient to hydrolyse the 17-O-methyl group making it unlikely that any bacterial metabolite could be detected. Secondly, the concentration of 17-methoxyoestradiol would be very low, presenting considerable problem in extraction and detection. The third major problem is that the liver produces an active O-demethylating enzyme which would reduce the amount of 17-methoxyoestradiol and replace it with oestradiol indistinguishable from the normally circulating hormone.

IV. Introduction of a nuclear double bond conjugated to other double bonds

Reactions of this type have been demonstrated with soil organisms but, as with the other nuclear dehydrogenation reactions, examples of such reactions carried out by gut bacteria are rare.

Sih *et al.* (1968) isolated 3-hydroxy-19-norbisnorchola-1,3,5(10),9 (11)-tetraen-22-oic acid as a degradation product of cholesterol, possibly via the pathway illustrated in Fig. 9.9. Formation of this metabolite

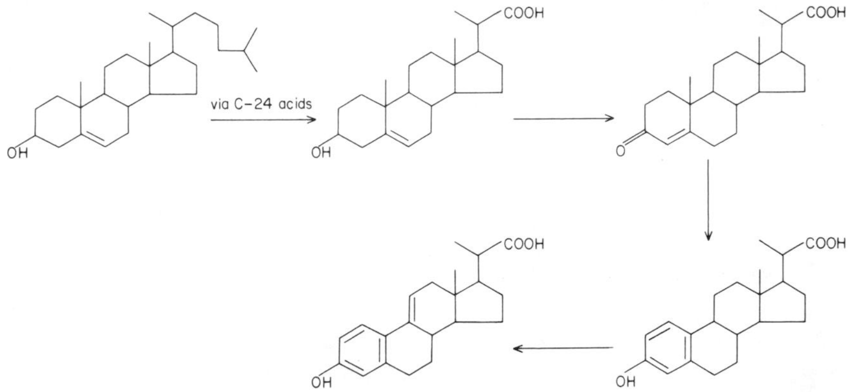

Fig. 9.9. The conversion by *Norcardia restrictus* of cholesterol to 3-hydroxy-19-nor bisnorchola-1,3,5 (10), 9 (11)-tetren-22-oic acid.

involves the insertion of a double bond in the 9-11-position in conjugation with the aromatic ring A of the steroid nucleus. Similarly, Korn *et al.* (1969) using a strain of *Acanthamoeba castallanii*, demonstrated the aromatization of ring B of 7-dehydrocholesterol. In this reaction the 10-methyl group migrated, possibly to the 6-position, followed by the formation of a 9-10 double bond to complete the aromatization of ring B (Fig. 9.10). The organism used is unlikely to inhabit the normal human gut

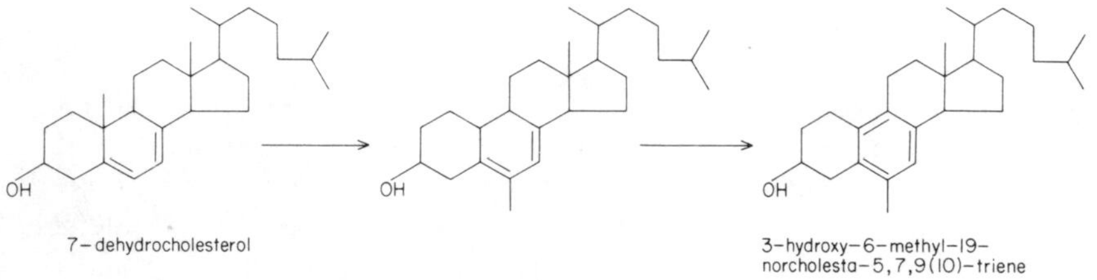

7—dehydrocholesterol

3—hydroxy—6—methyl—19—
norcholesta—5,7,9(10)—triene

Fig. 9.10. Aromatization of ring B of 7-dehydrocholesterol by *Acanthamoeba castellanii* to give 3-hydroxy-6-methyl-19-norcholesta-5,7,9 (10)-triene.

but the substrate molecule, 7-dehydrocholesterol, is secreted by the human intestinal mucosal cells and is a normal component of the faecal neutral steroids (although the amount is not certain). It is often confused with 4-cholesten-3-one since it gives a strong positive Liebermann-Burchardt reaction.

The single example of this type of reaction being carried out by human gut bacteria is the formation of dihydroequilenin from 4,6-androstadien-3-one-17β-ol (Goddard and Hill, 1972). This involves demethylation at the 10 position followed by dehydrogenation of the C8-9 bond in conjugation with the rest of rings A and B (Fig. 9.11). This reaction was demonstrated

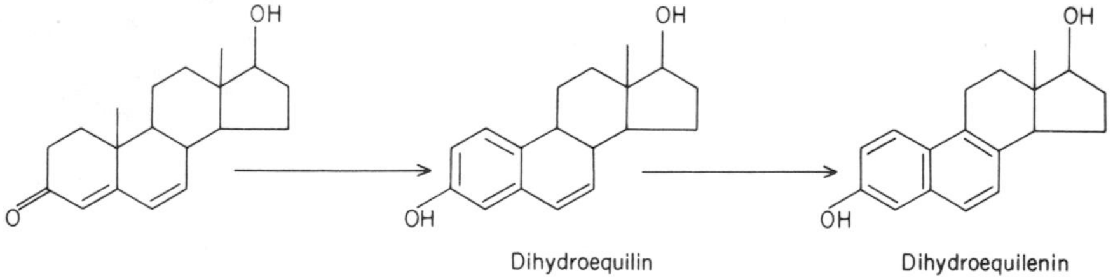

Dihydroequilin

Dihydroequilenin

Fig. 9.11. Metabolism of 4,6-androstadien-3-one-17β-ol by *Cl. butyricum* to dihydroequilin, then dihydroequilenin.

using the strain of *Cl. paraputrificum* described previously as being able to transmethylate from C—10 to the oxygen function at C—17. Using the agar plate method described by Vezina *et al.* (1969) a large number of organisms were screened for this reaction sequence (Table 9.2) and the

TABLE 9.2

Nuclear dehydrogenation of steroids

Genus	Proportion of strains able to convert 5β3one →4en-3one and 4en-3one →phenolic steroids
Bacteroides fragilis	0/100
Gram-positive non-sporing anaerobes (bifidobacteria and eubacteria)	0/100
Esch. coli	0/100
Strep. faecalis	0/100
Clostridium welchii	3/100
Other lecithinase-positive clostridia	0/100
Clostridium paraputrificum	60/69
Clostridium indolis	10/29
Clostridium chauvei	1/27
Clostridium felsinium	0/21
Other lecithinase-negative clostridia	5/107

results confirmed by the TL C procedure described by the same authors. To date, all of the strains found to be able to carry out this reaction have been of the species *Cl. paraputrificum*, or *Cl. indolis*.

CHAPTER 10

The Metabolism of the Major Non-steroidal Biliary Components

I. Introduction

Normal human bile contains four major components, these being cholesterol, the bile acids, the bile pigments and lecithin (Table 10.1). All four undergo extensive enterohepatic circulation. In addition to these major components the bile, in its capacity as a major route of excretion, contains small amounts of a wide range of excretory products in the form glucuronide or sulphate conjugates, or in the form of non-conjugated (usually polar) compounds. The factors controlling the biliary excretion of compounds has been studied extensively by Smith (1966) and by Hirom *et al.* (1972); the metabolism of the glucuronides has been described in Chapter 5, and of the sulphates in Chapter 12.

TABLE 10.1

The major components of normal human bile

Constituents	Concentration (g/100 ml)	
	Hepatic bile	Gall-bladder bile
Water	97-98	82
Total solids	2.3-3.3	16.6
pH	7.15	7.3
Steroids- bile acids	0.65-1.4	8.6
- cholesterol	0.08-0.21	0.23
Lipids - phospholipid	0.10-0.57	3.7
fatty acids	0.16-0.41	2.4
Bile pigments	0.017-0.071	0.003-1.78
Protein	0.14-0.27	0.45
Total sugar	0.03-0.09	0.24
Inorganic ions (Na^+, K^+, Ca^{++}, Cl^-, HCO^-_3)	0.6-0.9	0.5-1.1

II. Bile pigment metabolism

The bile pigments are the end product of the catabolism of haemoglobin and of haem-containing enzymes. They are derived from bilirubin via the pathways outlined in Fig. 10.1. Approximately 200-300 mg of bilirubin are produced each day and excreted in the bile. This excretion is dependent on the conjugation of bilirubin by the liver, probably more than 90% being converted to the glucuronide and about 10% to the sulphate. If the liver fails to conjugate the bilirubin, it is not excreted, and jaundice results.

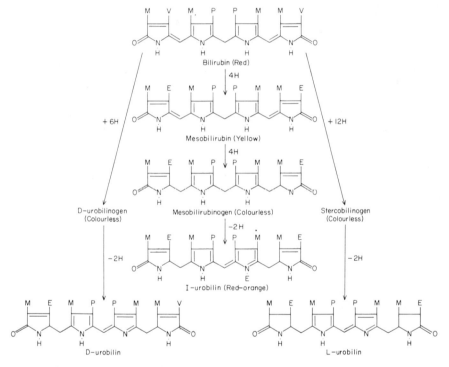

Fig. 10.1. Schematic diagram showing the inter-relationship between the faecal metabolites of bilirubin. M = methyl; E = ethyl; P = propyl; V = vinyl.

Following secretion into the small intestine, the bilirubin glucuronide is metabolized by the bacterial flora, either hydrolytically to release free bilirubin, or reductively to form the urobilinogens. Bilirubin glucuronide is poorly absorbed from the gut whereas free bilirubin is readily absorbed from the small and large intestine (Lester and Schmid, 1963a). The resultant enterohepatic circulation of bilirubin in humans was demonstrated by Lester and Schmid (1963b) to be relatively insignificant; only 5% of a dose of labelled bilirubin glucuronide was absorbed indicating that hydrolysis was, as would be expected, much less than in the rat (see Chapter 5).

In addition to hydrolysis, the bilirubin glucuronide is also subjected to reduction either before or after hydrolysis. As early as 1892, von Muller postulated that the gut bacteria were responsible for the production of urobilinogen from bilirubin, and the reaction was demonstrated using mixed faecal bacteria by Watson et al. (1958). No urobilinogens are formed in germ-free rats (Gustafsson and Kanke, 1960); when these animals were re-contaminated with an unidentified strain of Clostridium spp. urobilinogens were excreted, and in larger amounts if the animals were contaminated with both Esch. coli and the clostridial strain. Using a range of other contaminating organisms, mainly aerobic, they obtained no urobilinogen. Further evidence of bacterial involement in urobilinogen formation was obtained by Watson (1963) who showed that treatment of rats with broad spectrum antibiotics resulted in greatly reduced excretion of urobilinogen in faeces and in urine.

In the same paper, Watson reported production of urobilinogen from bilirubin by a pure strain of clostridial species. Troxler et al. (1968) studied the reaction further using disrupted cells and showed that the reaction involved a membrane-bound enzyme together with soluble cofactor(s) and required anaerobic conditions (which probably explains why most of the organisms tested by Gustafsson and Lanke failed). The enzyme was more active on mesobilirubin than on bilirubin itself; Watson et al. (1958) had shown that a better yield of mesobilirubinogen was obtained using conjugated bilirubin as substrate rather than free bilirubin.

The urobilinogen produced by bacterial metabolism is absorbed from the gut and excreted either in the bile or in urine. Only about 20% is absorbed (Lester and Schmid, 1965), most being passed in the faeces without recycling. Curiously, the urobilinogen does not need to be conjugated before excretion but is rapidly and efficiently transferred to the bile in its free state (Lester and Klein, 1966). Further investigation showed that bilirubin and mesobilirubin were both excreted as conjugates whilst mesobilirubinogen and i-urobilin were both excreted unchanged.

The urobilinogens are colourless products of bilirubin metabolism but are readily oxidized non-enzymically to the highly pigmented urobilins, which are the principal pigments of urine, and together with bilirubin, of bile and faeces.

III. Metabolism of phospholipids

Phospolipids, bile acids, bile pigments and cholesterol are the four major components of bile; of these the phospholipids are probably the least subjected to bacterial metabolism, and this is due to the high activity of pancreatic phospholipase which largely removes the substrate before it reaches the heavily bacterially colonized region of the gut. Nevertheless, many bacterial species produce phospholipases and, in the case of clostridia, these have important toxic properties and are also useful in diagnostic bacteriology.

There are four phospholipases, designated A, B, C and D (Fig. 10.2). Phospholipase A removes the α-acyl group yielding lysophosphatide; Phospholipase B is a lysophospholipase removing the remaining acyl group from lysophosphatides; thus both phospholipases A and B hydrolyse ester linkages to release fatty acids. Phospholipases C and D hydrolyse the

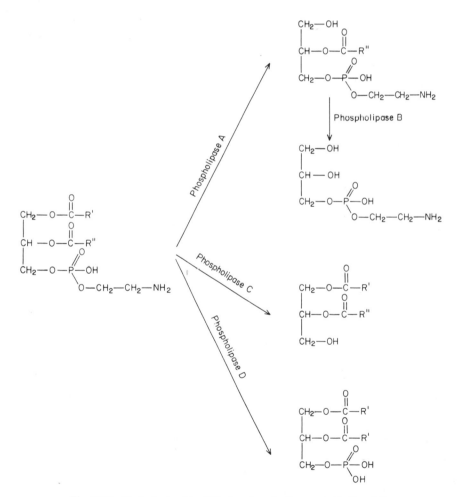

Fig. 10.2. Hydrolysis of lecithin by phospholipases A, B, C and D.

phosphate ester linkages, C releasing phosphoryl choline and a diglyceride, D releasing choline and a diacylphosphatidic acid. The high activity pancreatic enzyme is a phospholipase A; phospholipase D is rare outside the plant kingdom. Although many bacterial species produce phospholipases, few have been extensively studied and characterized. Prominent among those well characterized are the clostridial phospholipases.

Clostridium welchii produces a phospholipase which was shown to be identical to the α-toxin. It was demonstrated by Nagler (1939) that *Cl. welchii* produced a factor causing opalescence in serum, and that the opalescence was inhibited by anti-α-toxin antibody. The serum opacity factor was later shown to be identical to the egg-yolk factor by Macfarlane *et al.* (1941). The egg-yolk factor causes an aggregation of egg-yolk; by splitting lipovitellin the subtle balance which maintains the egg-yolk emulsion is upset and lipid substances are precipitated. In liquid medium this is manifest as a heavy yellow precipitate, on solid medium an opalescence is formed around the colony. The phospholipase was shown by Macfarlane and Knight (1941) to be a phospholipase C, releasing choline phosphate from lecithin. It has a pH-optimum of 7-7.6, requires Ca^{++} or Mg^{++} (although high concentrations of Mg^{++} are inhibitory), is inhibited by fluoride, citrate and phosphate ions and is inactivated by sodium lauryl sulphate and other surface active agents.

Cl. welchii is clinically important as one of the causative agents of gas gangrene and α-toxin plays an important role in the aetiology of this disease. Since lecithin is such a vital component of cell membranes, phospholipases tend to cause membrane disruption; α-toxin is both a haemolytic and a necrotic agent causing considerable tissue damage. The identificaton of a α-toxin as a phospholipase C is almost unique as an example of a toxic action being demonstrably due to a specific enzyme action.

Phospholipase C is produced by a range of clostridial species including *Cl. bifermentans, Cl. sordelii, Cl. sporogenes* and *Cl. haemolyticum.*

Although many organisms produce serum opacity and egg-yolk splitting factors superficially similar to those produced by the clostridia, it is by no means certain that any of these are phospholipases and it is probable that many are not. It has been demonstrated that the egg-yolk factor of *Staph. aureus* is not due to a phospholipase but to a lipase active on triglycerides or fatty acid esters (Shah and Wilson, 1965). Similarly the serum opacity factor of *Strep. pyogenes* which acts on the α-lipoprotein component of serum (Krumwiede, 1954) does not split lipovitellin, and appears to enhance the serum factor which transfers fatty acids from lecithin to cholesterol yielding lysolecithin and cholesterol esters (Rowan and Martin, 1963). An opalescence was also formed in aged serum which was not due to cholesterol esterification. No free fatty acid was released during the course of this reaction (Hill and Wannamaker, 1968) and it appears that this factor may well be active on the protein component of lipoprotein rather than on the lecithin fraction. Thus demonstration of a serum opacity reaction or an egg-yolk reaction unsupported by more definitive data on the nature of the substrate and products gives no indication of the nature of the responsible factor.

There is some data indicating that phospholipase C may be widespread through the bacterial world. Asatoor and Simenhoff (1965) showed that urinary dimethylamine is derived from endogenous lecithin, which is hydrolysed to release choline and the latter is N-dealkylated as described in Chapter 6. Hawksworth (1970) showed that bacteroides, bifidobacteria, clostridia and enterococci, which could produce dimethylamine from both choline and from lecithin, also give a positive egg-yolk reaction. Although no choline was demonstrated as the proximate metabolite of lecithin, it is reasonable to postulate that the organisms released choline from lecithin prior to N-dealkylation, indicating the presence of a phospholipase C or D. The phospholipases of *Esch. coli* have been investigated by Proulx and van Decnen (1966, 1967) and Fung and Proulx (1969). They demonstrated the presence of phospholipase A, phospholipase C and lysophospholipase. Lysolecithin was converted to glycerophosphate by a soluble enzyme fraction. The lysophospholipase and phospholipase C were active on phosphotidyl-ethanolamine as well as on phosphatidylcholine and unlike the phospholipase A, were not favoured by the addition of deoxycholate.

They also demonstrated a lysophosphatidyl acylase (the reverse action of phospholipase A), in the particulate fraction of the same organisms; this enzyme has also been demonstrated in *Salmonella minnesota* by Mulder *et al.* (1965).

In addition to these few examples of phospholipases there have been suggestions of many more. For example, many gut bacteria produce haemolysins and it has been suggested that some of these might be phospholipases (Berheimer and Schwartz, 1965). Although this seems likely, the mode of action of haemolysins like those of the serum opacity factors and egg-yolk factors, are largely unexplored and should provide a fertile field of study.

CHAPTER 11

Metabolism of Antibiotic Compounds

Most antibiotic-resistant organisms achieve their resistance either (a) by alteration in cell permeability, thereby preventing the antibiotic from reaching its target site, or (b) by an alteration on the target site preventing binding of the antibiotic or expression of its mode of action. In only a few instances is resistance generally achieved by enzymatic attack on the antibiotic molecule, the two notable examples being choramphenicol and penicillin resistance. In addition there are some individual examples of organisms metabolizing antibiotics to yield inactive metabolites.

I. Chloramphenicol metabolism

Chloramphenicol (Fig. 11.1) is an antibiotic which inhibits protein synthesis. The antibiotic binds to the 50s ribosome, so preventing the

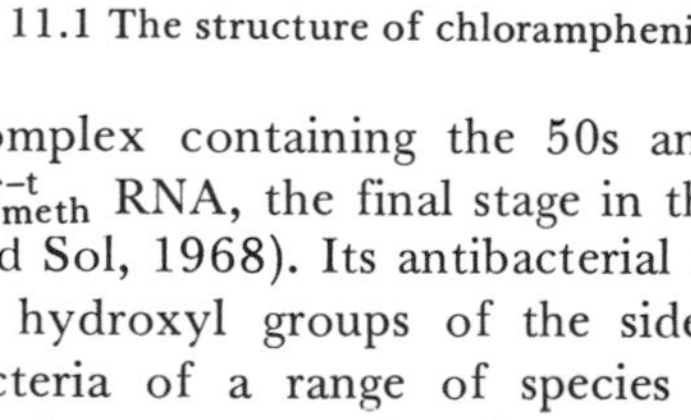

Fig. 11.1 The structure of chloramphenicol.

formation of the complex containing the 50s and 30s ribosomes, the messenger RNA and f_{meth}^{-t} RNA, the final stage in the initiation of protein synthesis (Lengyel and Sol, 1968). Its antibacterial activity is abolished by esterification of the hydroxyl groups of the side chain, and chloramphenicol-resistant bacteria of a range of species have been shown to acetylate the hydroxyl groups to give first the mono- and then the diacetate. Such an acetylation has been demonstrated with *Esch. coli*, *Klebsiella* spp., *Shigella* spp., *Proteus* spp., *Staph. epidermidis* and *Staph. aureus* (Sompolinsky *et al.*, 1968; Garber *et al.*, 1968; Shaw, 1967; Suzuki *et al.*, 1966; Okamoto and Suzuki, 1965; Suzuki and Okamoto, 1967, and Shaw *et al.*, 1970).

Okamoto and Suzuki (1965) demonstrated that the resistance to chloramphenicol associated with resistance factors in *Esch. coli* was due to antibiotic inactivation with acetylation of the hydroxyl groups mediated by acetyl-CoA. The 3-hydroxyl group (a primary alcohol group) is acetylated first, followed by the acetylation of the 1-hydroxyl group (a secondary alcohol group) as shown in Fig. 11.2. Both the mono- and diacetyl

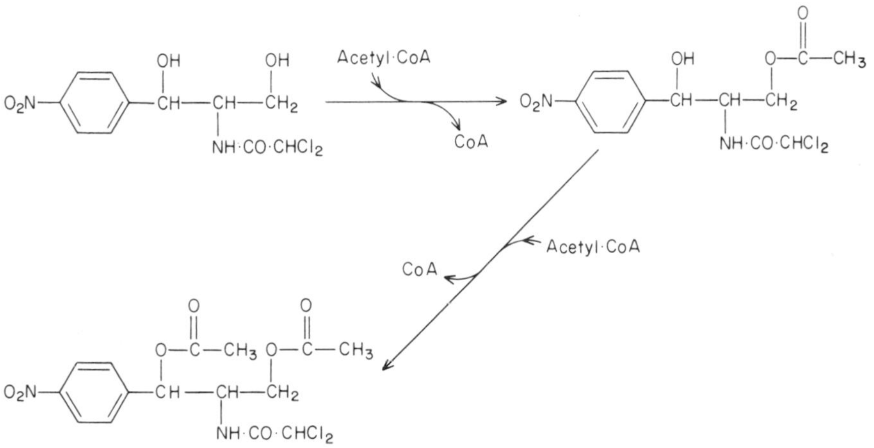

Fig. 11.2. The acetylation of chloramphenicol.

derivatives are inactive as antibiotics and the acetylation is extremely rapid (this would be essential for the mechanism to be the major route of chloramphenicol resistance in bacteria). The acetylated products bind only weakly to the 50s ribosome and so fail to interfere with the protein synthetic system. Most enteric bacteria resistant to chloramphenicol possess R-factors and those examined inactivate chloramphenicol by acetylation; strains which are sensitive to the antibiotic or which are resistant but possess no R-factor, do not acetylate (indicating that there are further, as yet undiscovered, routes to resistance). The chloramphenicol resistant strains of *Staph. aureus* and *Staph. epidermidis* that have been investigated have been shown to possess an extra chromasomal plasmid controlling resistance and acetylation (Suzuki *et al.*, 1966; Shaw and Brodsky, 1968; Shaw *et al.*, 1970). The acetylation by a purified enzyme preparation from *Esch. coli* at the 1 and 3-positions had a pH optimum of 7-8 which was sharp for the acetylation of the secondary alcohol group but broad for that of the primary alcohol group.

Whereas the acetylation is very rapid and leads to virtually complete inactivation of the chloramphenicol the other degradative reactions (Fig. 6.3) undergone by this antibiotic are relatively slow and lead to incomplete inactivation; these reactions are therefore of no importance in bacterial resistance to the antibiotic and are of more importance in providing a possible explanation of the pharmacological side effects of chloramphenicol treatment.

Glazko *et al.* (1949, 1952) showed that the nitro group was reduced to an amino group during transit through the gut and that 10-25% of a dose of chloramphenicol was excreted as the arylamine (Fig. 11.3a). Chloramphenicol nitro reductase has been demonstrated in a number of organisms including *Proteus vulgaris, B. subtilus* and *B. mycoides* (Smith and Worrel, 1949, 1950) and in *Esch. coli* (Saz and Slie, 1954a, b). The enzyme is not specific for chloramphenicol (Saz and Slie, 1954a, b) but acts on p-nitrobenzoic acid and a range of other aromatic nitro compounds. Because of the slowness of the reaction it can play little part in expressing the antibiotic resistance of the organisms.

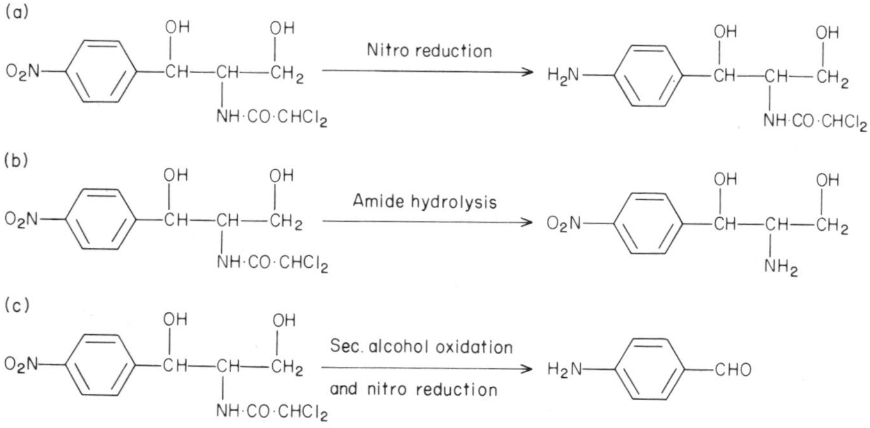

(a)

O_2N—⟨ ⟩—CH(OH)—CH(OH)—CH$_2$(NH·CO·CHCl$_2$)   Nitro reduction ⟶ H_2N—⟨ ⟩—CH(OH)—CH(OH)—CH$_2$(NH·CO·CHCl$_2$)

(b)

O_2N—⟨ ⟩—CH(OH)—CH(OH)—CH$_2$(NH·CO·CHCl$_2$)   Amide hydrolysis ⟶ O_2N—⟨ ⟩—CH(OH)—CH(OH)—CH$_2$(NH$_2$)

(c)

O_2N—⟨ ⟩—CH(OH)—CH(OH)—CH$_2$(NH·CO·CHCl$_2$)   Sec. alcohol oxidation and nitro reduction ⟶ H_2N—⟨ ⟩—CHO

Fig. 11.3. The minor metabolites produced by gut bacteria from chloramphenicol.

The antibiotic may undergo two forms of side chain cleavage. The amide bond may be hydrolysed to yield substituted amino propane diols (Fig. 11.3b); this reaction has been demonstrated in strains of *Esch. coli, P. vulgaris, B. substilus* and *B. mycoides* (Smith and Worrell, 1950) and has been demonstrated *in vivo* by Thompson *et al.* (1954). Holt (1967) has shown that the amide hydrolase was also able to remove the side chain from penicillin (i.e. has the properties of penicillin amidase) so that the enzyme must be relatively non-specific. The side chain may also be cleaved by oxidation of the secondary alcohol group (Smith and Worrell, 1950); since there was parallel nitro-reduction the product was p-amino benzaldehyde (Fig. 11.3c). This reaction has, again, been demonstrated with *Esch. coli, P. vulgaris, B. subtilus,* and *B. mycoides.*

Chloramphenicol undergoes extensive enterohepatic circulation and this is of major importance both in the treatment of intestinal infection and in the metabolism of the antibiotic possibly leading to undesirable side effects. The enterohepatic circulation of drugs in general has been discussed more fully in Chapter 5, Section 5. Orally administered chloramphenicol is sufficiently hydrophobic to be readily adsorbed from the small intestine and travels via the portal blood system to the liver where it is "detoxified" (chloramphenicol is an efficient inhibitor of mammalian protein synthesis in addition to its action on the bacterial protein synthetic system) by acylation to the 3-glucuronide and, to a much smaller extent, the 1,3-diglucuronides. Both of these hepatic metabolites are inactive as antibiotics. The glucuronides are then excreted via the bile into the small intestine, and are sufficiently hydrophilic to be poorly absorbed. Microbial β-glucuronidase releases the active antibiotic from the conjugate but also facilitates its reabsorption from the gut. Thus a single dose of chloramphenicol passes through the gut several times before final elimination from the body; this increases its efficacy in the treatment of small bowel infection, but also allows the various side reactions to take place and a variety of minor metabolites are formed. The major metabolites of chloramphenicol excreted in the urine are the 3-glucuronide and the arylamine produced as a result of amide hydrolysis. Some of the arylamine undergoes nitro reduction to yield the diamine; both the arylamine and diamine are conjugated by the liver prior to excretion.

The poor absorption of chloramphenicol ester from the gut is utilized in the treatment of infant diahrroea and of adult large bowel infection; the antibiotic is administered as the succinate (which is antibiotically inactive) and is hydrolysed to release the active antibiotic by bacteria. Thus the antibiotic reaches the infected region and is there released in its active form (Glazko *et al.*, 1958) after passage through the small intestine without being removed by absorption.

II. Metabolism of sulphonamide antibiotics

The sulphonamide antibiotics act by interfering with bacterial folic acid synthesis and were the first group of antibiotics to be introduced into general therapeutic use. Since folic acid is not synthesized in the human, sulphonamides have no major effect on mammalian metabolism and have a truly selective effect on the bacterial flora. The original sulphonamides, prontosil and neoprontosil, were azo dyes which had no *in vitro* antibacterial effect but were nevertheless active *in vivo*. The explanation was that the azo linkage was hydrolysed (Fig. 11.4) by the gut flora yielding the active agent sulphanilamide (Spink *et al.*, 1940). Azo reductase is an enzyme widely distributed amongst the gut bacterial flora and has been discussed elsewhere (Chapter 6, Section 4).

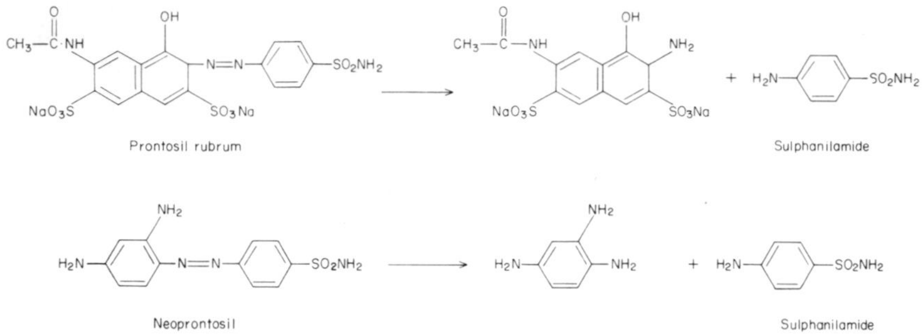

Fig. 11.4. The hydrolysis of prontosil and neo-prontosil to yield sulphanilamide.

A similar bacterial hydrolysis has been utilized in the development of sulphonamides for use in the treatment of enteric infection; in general the sulphonamide has been conjugated to an acid moiety via an amide bond with the free amino acid group. This yields a product with no antibacterial activity but of sufficient polarity to enable it to reach the large bowel without being absorbed; it then undergoes hydrolysis to release the active antibiotic. Thus succinylsulphathiazole is inactive *in vitro* but is hydrolysed by the gut bacteria to release the active sulphathiazole (Welch *et al.*, 1942; Scheline, 1968b), as is phthalylsulphathiazole (Goodman and Gilman, 1965; Scheline, 1968b).

N-acetylsulphiaoxazole was shown to be hydrolysed by strains of *Esch. coli, Strep. faecalis* and *L. acidophilus* by Uno and Kono (1961) but bacteria failed to hydrolyse N^4-acetylsulphadiazine (Pakte and Shirsat, 1961) or N-acetylsulphonamide (Scheline, 1968b). Salazopyrin is a conjugate of salicyclic acid and sulphadiazine and is used extensively in the treatment of ulcerative colitis; it is hydrolysed by gut bacteria to release salicylic acid (which may have an anti-inflammatory effect on the lesion) and a sulphonamide which might be active on any organism involved in the aetiology of the colitis.

III. Metabolism of the penicillins

Penicillin inhibits cell wall synthesis by interfering with the formation of peptide cross-links in the mucopeptide network (Strominger *et al.*, 1968). Resistant organisms inactivate the antibiotic either by hydrolysis of the β-lactam ring or by hydrolysis of the amide linkage of the side chain (Fig. 11.5). The β-lactamase has been demonstrated in a range of Gram −ve organisms including *Esch. coli, Proteus* spp. and *Aerobacter aerogenes,* and a range of Gram +ve bacteria including strains of *Bacillus* spp. *Staph. aureus* and *Staph. albus*. A similar range of organisms has been shown to produce

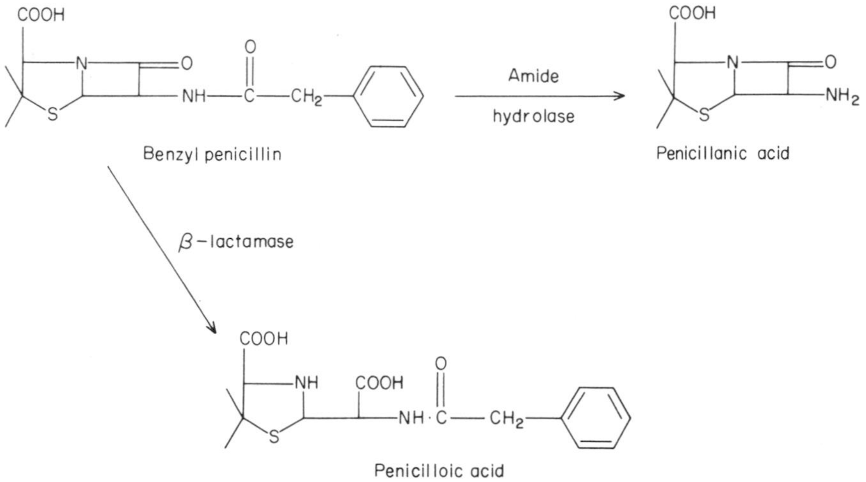

Fig. 11.5. The hydrolysis of benzylpenicillin by penicillin amidase and by β-lactamase.

the amidase. The family of penicillins differ in the nature of the side chain and this confers varying degrees of resistance to penicillinase (Table 11.1), with ampicillin, cloxacillin and methicillin being resistant to β-lactamase; there have been reports of β-lactamases which hydrolyse ampicillin (Sawai et al., 1970).

Although a large proportion of the gut bacteria produces penicillinase, this is a very minor metabolic reaction of the gut flora since the penicillinase-sensitive penicillins are not used extensively in the treatment of intestinal infection. Furthermore, the penicillins when used in the treatment of non-intestinal infections do not reach the bacterially colonized regions because they are absorbed from the small intestine or inactivated by stomach acid (when used, for example, in the treatment of oral infections).

IV. Inactivation by bacteria of streptomycin and other aminoglycosides

Streptomycin is an aminoglycoside antibiotic which interferes with protein synthesis by modifying the 30s ribosome sub-unit and, by inducing misreading of the m-RNA, thereby results in the formation of "nonsense" proteins with no biological activity. In general, streptomycin resistance in bacteria is due either to change in the 30s ribosome sub-unit preventing the antibiotic activity, or to a change in cell permeability. In a few cases, however, resistance is via antibiotic inactivation. Okamoto and Suzuki (1965) showed that a strain of Esch. coli with an R-factor conferring resistance to a number of antibiotics inactivated streptomycin.

TABLE 11.1

The susceptibility of synthetic penicillin with various side-chains to the action
of β-lactamase

Structure of the side-chains	Name	Sensitivity to β-lactamase
1. $-CH_2-$⟨phenyl⟩	Benzylpenicillin	S
2. $-H$	6-aminopenicillanic acid	R
3. ⟨2,6-dimethoxyphenyl, OCH$_3$ / OCH$_3$⟩	Methicillin	R
4. $-CH_2-O-$⟨phenyl⟩	Phenoxymethylpenicillin	S
5. $-CH_2-$⟨phenyl⟩ with NH_2	Ampicillin	S
6. $-C-C-$⟨2-chlorophenyl, Cl⟩ with CH_3, C, O, N (isoxazole ring)	Cloxacillin	R

The specific enzyme system was isolated and characterized by Yamada *et al.* (1968). They showed that in R^+ cells the enzyme was produced constitutively and had a requirement for a univalent cation, probably NH_4^+, the divalent cation Mg^{++} and ATP. The pH optimum was 7.5-8.5 and the enzyme was only active on streptomycin or closely related compounds; the other aminoglycosides tested, neomycin, kanamycin, gentamycin and paramomycin were not inactivated by the enzyme. The reaction product contained streptomycin, AMP and total phosphate in the molar ratio 1: 1: 1. They concluded that the enzyme was streptomycin adenylate synthetase, the reaction product being shown in Fig. 11.6. In contrast to streptomycin itself, this product was only weakly bound to ribosomes and was so unable to influence the synthesis of protein. Subsequently other strains have been isolated possessing R-factors for an adenylate synthetase

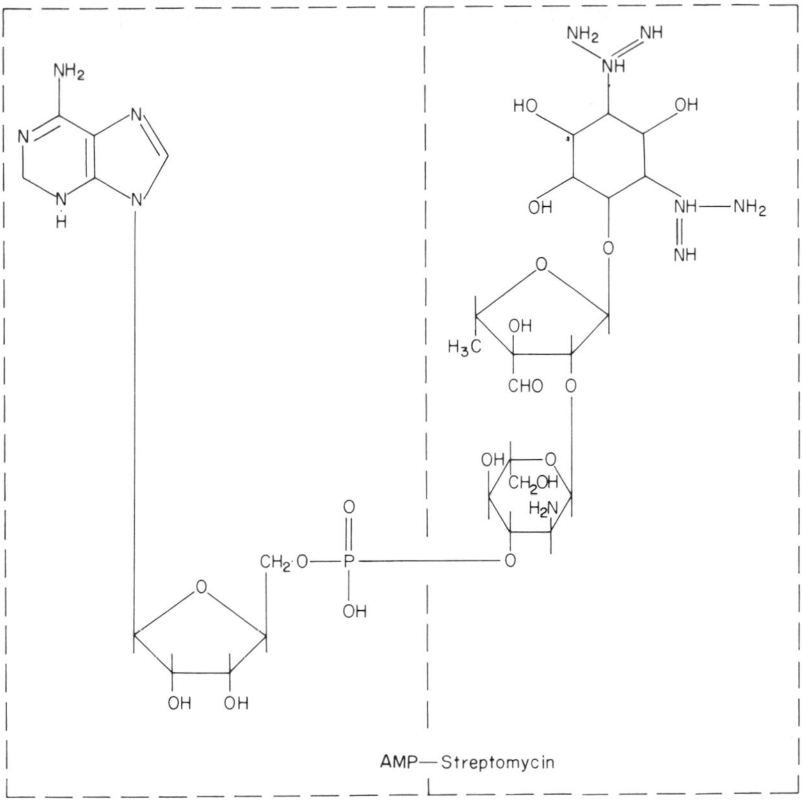

Fig. 11.6. The product of the action of streptomycin adenylate synthetase on streptomycin.

active on a number of aminoglycosides and this enzyme is now the basis of an assay system for gentamycin.

Strains of *Esch. coli* carrying R-factors for aminoglycosides possess, in addition to the streptomycin adenylate synthetase already described, three other enzymes, conferring aminoglycoside resistance. One phosphorylates streptomycin at the position involved in adenylation; a second phosphorylates neomycin, kanamycin and a number of other aminoglycosides (Ozanne *et al.*, 1969); the third acetylates kanamycin (Okamoto and Suzuki, 1965) neomycin and gentamycin (Benveniste *et al.*, 1971). Okamoto and Suzuki (1965) showed that kanamycin was inactivated by a pathway involving acetylation mediated by acetyl CoA. This reaction was further investigated by Benveniste and Davies (1971); they demonstrated that the acetylation took place at the amino group of the 6-amino-6-

deoxy-glucose component of the aminoglycoside. A wide range of other aminoglycosides were N-acetylated in the same position but normally this did not result in inactivation although the N-acetylated forms of neomycin B and gentamycin C_{1a} had reduced activity.

CHAPTER 12

Other Metabolic Reactions

I. Hydrolysis of sulphate esters

Many foreign compounds are metabolized to their ethereal sulphates by the liver as an aid to excretion as part of the general detoxification mechanism of the body. However, very few of these sulphates are excreted in the bile, the usual route being renal excretion, e.g. most urinary estrogens are excreted as the 3-O sulphate as are most phenolic compounds in general. Thus, it is likely that the gut flora is normally exposed only to sulphates of exogenus origin and not to endogenous sulphates. It is not surprising, therefore, that there have been few reports of aryl-sulphatase activity in the gut bacteria. Thus sulphuric acid esters of phenols having laxative properties are not hydrolysed in the intestine (Pala *et al.*, 1966). Scheline (1968b) also reported that p-nitro-catechol sulphate was not metabolized by rat caecal contents. We were unable to demonstrate sulphatase activity in *Esch. coli.*, *Strep. faecalis.*, *Clostridium* spp., *Bacteroides* spp., and *Bifidobacterium* spp. (twenty strains of each) isolated from rat faeces using nitro-phenyl sulphate as substrate (unpublished results).

However, there have been three reports of sulphatase activity in the gut. Dodgson *et al.* (1953, 1956) reported the presence of arylsulphatase activity in the human intestine using nitro phenyl sulphate as substrate and as the enzyme source. it has also been reported by Stemmel (1954) that human faeces hydrolysed sodium oestrone sulphate to free oestrone. Further, Closen *et al.* (1959) showed that rat intestinal bacteria possess an aryl-sulphatase capable of hydrolysing the sulphuric acid ester of 3,5,3'-tri-iodo-*l*-thyronine. Taurine is metabolized by the gut bacteria to free sulphate; taurocholate labelled with S^{35} was fed to volunteers and was hydrolysed in the gut to release taurine which was further metabolized, evidently, since free labelled sulphate was excreted in the urine (Hofmann, personal communication).

In addition to the examples of hydrolysis of C-sulphonates and O-sulphates cited above the hydrolysis of the N-sulphonate, cyclamate (Fig. 12.1) is worthy of mention. Cyclamate, cyclohexylamine N-sulphonate, was used extensively until its ban in 1971 as an artificial

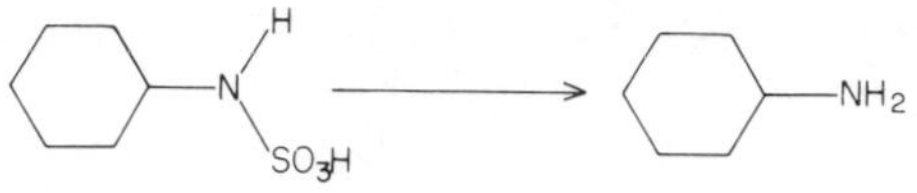

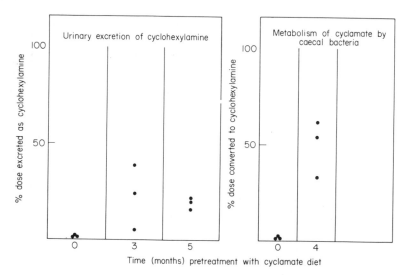

Fig. 12.1. The hydrolysis of cyclamate.

sweetening agent and was thought initially to be unmetabolized in the body. In 1966, however, it was shown by Kojima and Ichibagase to be metabolized by some to cyclohexylamine, the latter product of N-desulphonation being excreted in the urine. This has been confirmed by many groups but the percentage breakdown reported varied considerably from study to study. This has been explained to some extent by the results of Renwick and Williams (1969) who showed that both the percentage of rats able to hydrolyse cyclamate and the percentage of substrate metabolized by any individual rat could be increased by prolonged feeding of cyclamate to the animals; these results have been largely confirmed by Wallace *et al.* (1970). Further, when the animals were given no cyclamate for 5 days, the ability to break it down was lost. The picture was clarified still further by Drasar *et al.* (1972) who showed that the ability of the gut flora to metabolize cyclamate directly correlated with that of the whole animal (Fig. 12.2); thus the effect of prolonged feeding of cyclamate would seem to promote the emergence of a flora able to hydrolyse the N-sulphonate linkage. To round off the picture, they were able to demonstrate the

Fig. 12.2. Relation between the metabolism of cyclamate in the whole rat and the metabolism of cyclamate by the gut flora of the same animal.

hydrolysis of cyclamate not just by caecal contents but also by isolated pure strains of *Strep. faecalis.*

In the light of the paucity of examples, it is likely that either the sulphatase activity of gut bacteria is substrate specific (explaining the failure to demonstrate the enzyme using conventional laboratory sulphatase substrates) or else is relatively rare and only demonstrable in animals which happen to have large numbers of an active strain.

II. Ester and amide hydrolysis

There are a large number of isolated examples of ester hydrolysis by gut bacteria, including the hydrolysis of antibiotic esters, glucuronic acid esters and cholesterol esters.

The drug carbenoxalone, which is used in the treatment of peptic ulcers, is the hemi-succinate of 18β-glycyrretic acid (enoxalone) and, when fed to rats, is hydrolysed to glycyrretic acid which is then metabolized in the liver to the 3-sulphate, the 30-glucuronide and the 3,30-diglucuronide (Parke *et al.*, 1963; Iveson *et al.*, 1966). When administered intraperitoneally, on the other hand, only metabolites of carbenoxalone were detected (Dekanski *et al.*, 1970). The conclusion is that in the rat alimentary tract carbenoxalone undergoes ester hydrolysis with removal of the succinic acid moiety; evidence obtained using doubly-labelled substrate suggests that the hydrolysis is brought about by bacteria in the rat stomach. In man and in the squirrel monkey this hydrolysis occurs on a much reduced scale, with 70-80% of the drug being secreted unhydrolysed in the faeces (compared with only 12-36% in the rat).

Chlorogenic acid is the quinic acid ester of caffeic acid and is hydrolysed by rat intestinal organisms (Scheline, 1968a); the caffeic acid is then further metabolized to m-hydroxyphenylpropionic acid (Fig. 12.3) via a dehydroxylation reaction following hydrogenation of the aliphatic double bond (Booth and Williams, 1963a). Acetyl-digitoxin, in which the terminal digitoxose sugar residue is O-acetylated, is hydrolysed to digitoxin by intestinal bacteria; similarily acetyl digitoxin is deacetylated by intestinal bacteria, in particular by isolated strains of *Strep. faecalis* (Hawksworth *et al.*, 1971).

Amide hydrolases produced by gut bacteria and already described include those acting on the bile acid conjugates, the sulphonamides, chloramphenicol and penicillin. In addition, hippuric acid, the glycine conjugate of benzoic acid, is hydrolysed by the gut bacteria (Hulsman and van Eps, 1967). Hydrolysis of hippurate is one of the tests used in the classification of non-pyogenic streptococci (Colman, 1969). In addition, Scheline (1968b) has shown that rat caecal organisms hydrolyse the amide bond in p-acetamidobenzoic acid, whilst Sjaastad (1966) showed that human faecal organisms released histamine from N-acetyl histamine.

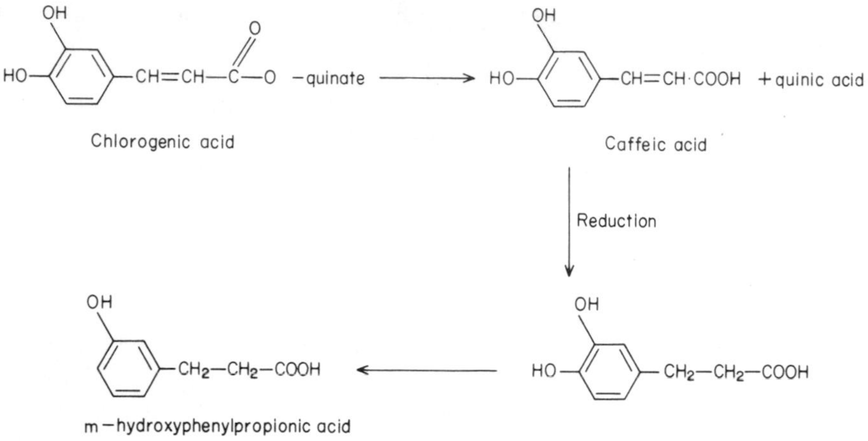

Fig. 12.3. The metabolism of chlorogenic acid and caffeic acid by rat intestinal bacteria.

III. Aromatization reactions

The aromatization of alicyclic compounds has been known for more than a century (Lautemann, 1863), the principal example being the metabolism of oral quinic acid to benzoic acid or hippuric acid (Fig. 12.4). In man 60% of

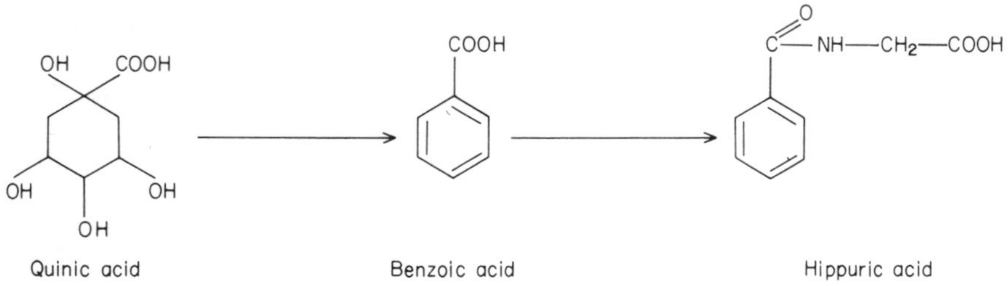

Fig. 12.4. The aromatization of quinic acid.

an oral dose of quinic acid is excreted as hippuric acid in the urine and a similar high proportion is aromatized in other old world primates, the baboon, rhesus monkey and green monkey, but a relatively small proportion is aromatized in new world primates, lemurs and the common laboratory animals (Williams, 1970a). Quinic acid is present in tea, coffee, fruits and vegables (a cup of coffee may contain as much as 150 mg quinic acid either free or as a component of chlorogenic acid) and is aromatized when taken orally but not when taken parenterally. The aromatization is inhibited by the action of neomycin in man (Cotran et al.,

1960) and in the rat. In the latter animal a higher rate of aromatization occurs if quinic acid is replaced by shikimic acid (Asatoor, 1965) and this too is abolished by neomycin treatment of the rats. Other aromatic metabolites of quinic and shikimic acid are catechol and vanillic acid; catechol was later shown to be a product of quinic acid metabolism by rat gut bacteria (Booth and Williams, 1963b) and a possible rationalization of these products is illustrated (Fig. 12.5).

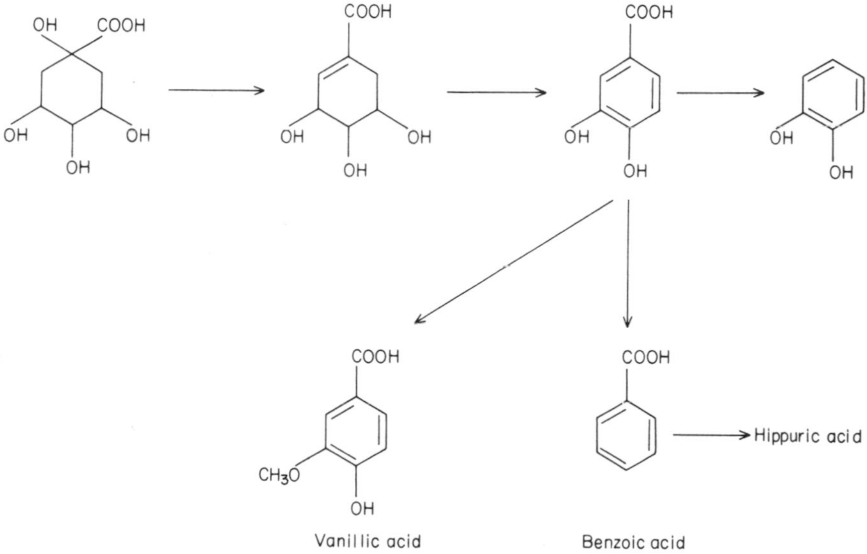

Fig. 12.5. The metabolites of quinic acid and their possible routes of production.

IV. Reduction of double bonds

The reduction of the aliphatic double bond in caffeic acid was cited in the previous section and has been demonstrated with faecal homogenates from the rat and from man. This type of metabolic reaction is probably of most significance in the gut in the reduction of cholesterol to coprostanol (Chapter 8) and in the metabolism of fatty acids.

Approximately 70% of plant fatty acids are unsaturated (Garton, 1963) and the metabolism of these acids has been studied using rumen and large intestinal organisms. Ricinoleic is reduced to hydroxy stearic acid in both the rat and human intestine (Watson, 1965). Kepler and Tove (1967), studying the hydrogenation of linolenic acid (18:3) showed that this acid was first isomerized to the conjugated triene acid before being reduced to the unconjugated diene linoleic acid (18:2) Mills *et al.* (1970), using rumen micrococcus, demonstrated the further reduction of linoleic acid (18:2) to oleic acid (18:1) but could find no evidence of complete reduction to the saturated stearic acid 18:0). These results were in agreement with those obtained by Kemp and White (1968). Pearson *et al.* (1972) using human intestinal bacteria demonstrated the production of hydroxystearic acid from oleic acid, and postulated that this was an intermediate in the reduction of oleic to stearic acid. They also found evidence for the hydroxylation of oleic acid to ricinoleic acid; this suggested that the pathway was oleic → ricinoleic → hydroxystearic → stearic acid. The reaction was most readily demonstrated with strains of *Strep. faecalis,* and was also carried out by clostridia, bacteroides and bifidobacteria. Ricinoleic acid is a component of castor oil and it has been suggested that the hydroxy fatty acids in general are purgatives and that ricinoleic and hydroxystearic acids are the active components of castor oil.

V. Dehydroxylation reactions

The dehydroxylation of bile acids, of quinic acid and of a range of phenolic compounds has been referred to at various points previously and has been extensively discussed by Scheline (1968a) and by Smith (1966). Some examples of bacterial dehydroxylations are shown in Fig. 12.6.

Cholic acid and chenodeoxycholic acid both undergo 7-dehydroxylation, a reaction carried out mainly by anaerobic bacteria and then only under highly anaerobic conditions. This is a dehydration reaction yielding an unsaturated product which then rehydrogenates readily. This reaction is discussed more fully in Chapter 7. Quinic acid is also probably dehydroxylated via a dehydration reaction giving rise to an unsaturated product as illustrated in Fig. 12.5. It is probable that this is the mechanism of dehydroxylation of many aliphatic hydroxylated compounds.

The dehydroxylation of the phenolic acids is, on the other hand, very unlikely to follow the above type of pathway and is more likely to be a straightforward substitution of a hydrogen for a hydroxyl group. A number of phenolic acids undergo dehydroxylation in the gut, including the 3,4-dehydroxyphenyl series of acids. The members of this series studied include 3,4-dihydroxybenzoic acid (protocatechuic acid), 3,4-dihydroxyphenylacetic acid (homoprotocatechuic acid), 3,4,-dihydroxyphenylcinnamic acid (caffeic acid) and 3,4-dihydroxyphenylalanine (*dopa*). All four compounds are dehydroxylated in the para-position by gut bacteria; there is little evidence of meta-dehydroxylation which must therefore be considered at most as a minor reaction. The evidence that these reactions are carried out *in vivo* in the whole animal by gut bacteria is based on the difference in yield of product when the substrate is given orally compared with parenterally, and on the effect of neomycin (which virtually abolishes

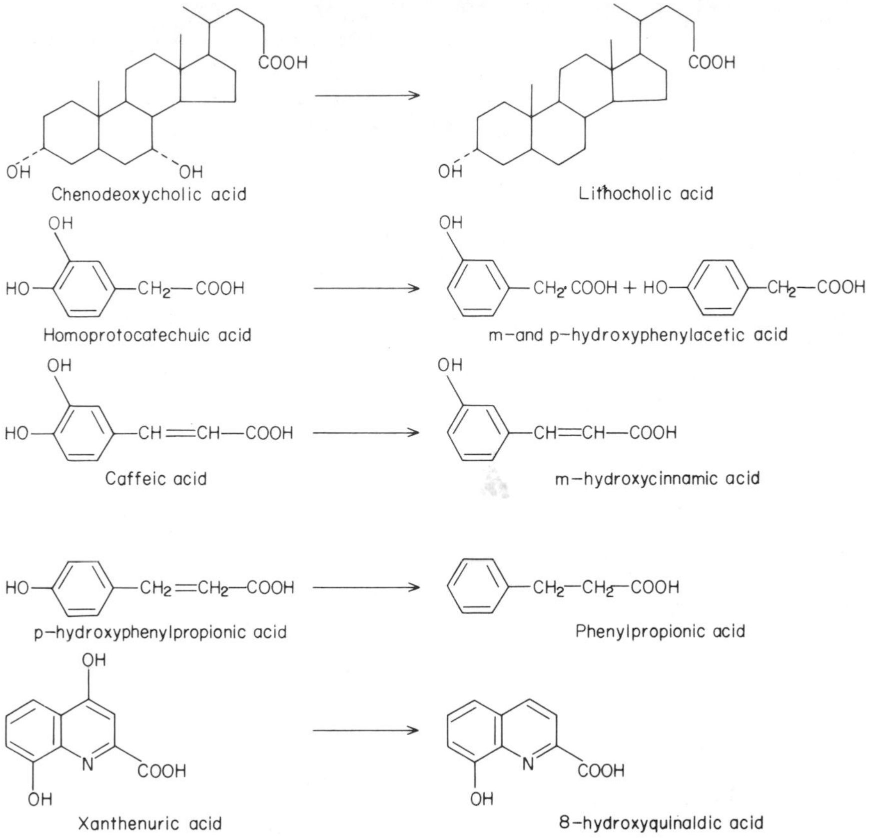

Fig. 12.6. Some examples of dehydroxylation reaction carried out by gut bacteria.

the reaction). The metabolism of the four substrates has been demonstrated by Dacre and Williams (1968) with protocatechuic acid, Dacre *et al.* (1968) and Scheline *et al.* (1960) with homoprotocatechuic acid, Booth *et al.* (1957) with caffeic acid and Deeds *et al.* (1957) with *dopa*. The dehydroxylation of caffeic and homoprotocatechuic acids was inhibited by aerobiosis (in agreement with the findings on the dehydroxylation of cholic acid); the extent of dehydroxylation increased with increased side-chain length. The carboxyl group was not essential, since pyrogallol was very readily dehydroxylated.

The dehydroxylation of quinaldic acid derivatives has been discussed with respect to the overall metabolism of tryptophan in Chapters 6 and 16. Thus kynurenic acid and xanthenuric acid both undergo 4-dehydroxylation to yield quinaldic acid and 8-hydroxyquinaldic acid respectively when given to animals (Takehashi *et al.*, 1956; 1958). The ability to carry out this reaction was abolished by treatment with neomycin but was restored when treatment with the antibiotic was discontinued.

The dehydroxylation of tryosine and phloretic acid has been referred to in the section on tyrosine metabolism in Chapter 6.

VI. Decarboxylation reactions

Normal human urine contains a wide range of phenolic compounds and it is likely that many of them are the products of bacterial decarboxylations in the gut of phenolic acids from dietary sources. The diet is known to be rich in phenolic acids.

A number of such decarboxylations have been demonstrated (Table 12.1) and the decarboxylation of simple phenolic acids has been studied extensively by Scheline (1966, 1967, 1968b) using rat caecal microorganisms. He concluded that the presence of a *para*-hydroxyl group

TABLE 12.1

Decarboxylation of phenolic acids by gut bacteria

Phenolic acid	Product
4-hydroxybenzoic acid	Phenol
4-hydroxyphenylacetic acid	4-cresol
4-hydroxyphenylpropionic acid	4-ethylphenol
4-hydroxycinnamic acid	4-vinylphenol
3,4 dihydroxybenzoic acid	Catechol
3,4 dihydroxyphenylacetic acid	4-methylcatechol
Caffeic acid	4-vinylcatechol
Gallic acid	Pyrogallol

is essential for the reaction. Thus p-hydroxybenzoic acid was readily decarboxylated but the ortho- and meta-hydroxy analogues were not metabolized. The decarboxylation of protocatechuic acid was investigated by Dacre and Williams (1968) who showed that the reaction rate was reduced by substituents in the meta- position and abolished by ortho-substituents. In the study of a series of phenolic carboxylic acids it was found that whilst phenylacetic and cinnamic acids were readily decarboxylated the phenylpropionic acid analogues were unmetabolized. In this series the presence of a *para*-hydroxy group was again essential.

A number of these reactions have been demonstrated in the gut of whole animals, the techniques usually being dependent on showing that

(a) the reaction occurs more extensively to oral than to parenteral doses of the substrate;

(b) the reaction occurs less extensively in animals whose gut flora had been extensively reduced by antibiotic treatment;

(c) alternatively, the reaction could be shown to occur in conventional but not in germ-free animals.

The first type of approach is exemplified in the study of the study of the decarboxylation of protocatechuic and gallic acids (Scheline, 1966), whereas the second approach, using germ-free animals, was used in the study of the decarboxylation of orotic acid (Windmeuller *et al.*, 1965).

There has been little work using isolated organisms. Peppercorn and Goldman (1971) studied the metabolism of caffeic acid by human gut bacteria and showed that it was decarboxylated to 4-vinylcatechol by a strain of *Strep.faecium.* Indahl and Scheline (1968) have also shown that the decarboxylation of p-hydroxycinnamic acid can be carried out by *Bacillus* spp. isolated from rat caecal contents.

The decarboxylation of amino acids has been discussed in Chapter 6. The role of the simple phenols produced by microbial decarboxylations in human cancer is considered in Chapter 15.

VII. Metabolism of intestinal mucin

The intestinal epithelial cells continuously secrete a mucin which forms a barrier between the luminal contents and the epthelial tissue. It performs a variety of functions which include protection of the epithelium from bacterial toxins and catabolic enzymes (by acting as a molecular sieve) and as a lubricant for intraluminal movement of solid matter (Wold *et al.*, 1972). A characteristic feature of germ-free animals is the accumulation of large amounts of mucous material in the gut and, in particular, in the vastly distended caecum (Linstedt *et al.*, 1965; Loesche, 1969). This is thought to be because the gut flora normally degrades the mucin to small molecular weight material in the conventional animal.

Linstedt *et al.* (1965) produced some evidence for the degradation of intestinal mucins by gut bacteria. They measured the hexosamine and nitrogen contents of stools and caecal contents of germ-free and conventional rats fed on a semi-synthetic laboratory diet. The hexosamine content of the caecum of germ-free rats was 40 times that in conventional rats and was in the form of high molecular weight water soluble material. Incubation of this material with the caecal bacteria of a conventional rat resulted in hydrolysis of the mucin to low molecular weight material.

The intestinal mucins are glycoproteins. The carbohydrate part (accounting for 80% of the total) contains galactose, mannose, fucose, arabinose, xylose, N-acetyl glucosamine, N-acetylgalactosamine and sialic acid; the peptide moiety contains serine, threonine, aspartic acid and glutamic acid as the major acid together with smaller amounts of proline, glycine and alanine and very small amounts of the other amino acids (Wold *et al.,* 1971). Hoskins and Zamcheck (1968) analysed stools of conventional and germ-free rats for proteins, hexoses, hexoamines, methyl pentoses, sialic acids and blood group A, B and H antigens, after first separating the material into dialysable and non-dialysable fractions. The average daily excretion of non-dialysable carbohydrates by germ-free rats was 6-10 times greater than that by conventional rats. ABH antigens were detected only in the stool of germ-free animals and only in the non-dialysable fraction. They concluded that microorganisms normally degrade gastro-intestinal mucins, particularly the carbohydrate portion which probably constitutes a source of nutrition for intestinal bacteria. In particular, they consider destruction of the ABH antigens as a measure of mucin degradation and, in an accompanying paper (Hoskins, 1968) the examination of stool material for ABH group-destroying enzymes revealed that these were absent from stools of germ-free animals but present in those of conventional animals, and were produced by an anaerobic culture of stool bacteria.

There have been no studies of pure cultures of gut bacteria for mucin-degrading enzymes, but sialidase is known to be produced by enterobacteria and in very large amounts by *Vibrio cholerae.*

SECTION III

The Significance of Gut Bacteria

Some Problems in Relation to the Intestinal Flora

The intestinal flora may be regarded as an "organ" of the body (Csáky, 1968); if this designation is accepted the flora is potentially the most metabolically active of all the organs. Mammalian cells do not approach the growth rates of bacterial cells nor are they able to metabolize so wide a range of chemicals. Further, the flora is able to adapt more rapidly than other organs to metabolic pressure. Adaptation can occur both by induction of enzymes in bacterial cells and by replacement of bacterial species in the intestine during ecological succession in response to metabolic changes (Drasar *et al.,* 1970; Williams *et al.,* 1971).

Although, the growth potential of the flora would enable it to consume the body in less than a day, in fact, the growth of the flora is slow, 2 or 3 divisions a day (Gibbons and Kapsimalis, 1967) and its influence is exerted largely through the breakdown of body secretions and foreign compounds and the effect of its presence on intestinal structure and immune systems. For example, the deoxycholate in human bile is entirely a bacterial product (Chapter 7) and the half-life of C^{14} cholic acid in germ-free rats is five times larger then in normal animals (Gustafsson *et al.,* 1957). Similarly the mucosal surface area in the germ-free intestine is less than normal and the body defence systems under developed (Gordon and Pesti, 1971).

The distribution and metabolic potential of the flora has been described previously. The significance of much of this data has been examined within the context of the relevant chapters. This section attempts to examine some specific problems not dealt with elsewhere.

CHAPTER 13

Malabsorption

Defects in the absorption of nutrients contribute to the pathology of many intestinal diseases. Most malabsorption is not bacterial in origin although the gut flora may contribute to some of the overt symptoms. This chapter is concerned with bacteria as a cause of malabsorption and the role of the gut flora in malabsorption of other types. No attempt will be made to review all aspects of malabsorption, for comprehensive coverage, the reader is referred to Avery Jones *et al.* (1968) and Dawson (1971).

Digestion and absorption is a two-phase system. Within the intestinal lumen intestinal enzymes and other secretions such as bile salts, prepare the food for absorption. The intestinal mucosa is the organ of absorption and contains specific transport systems for some molecules. Table 13.1 summarizes some aspects of absorption.

For efficient digestion and absorption an adequate supply of luminal enzymes and secretions, together with an intact mucosa are essential.

TABLE 13.1

Some aspects of absorption

	Intestinal lumen		Absorptive cell	
	Digestive secretion	Products	Brush border	Cell interior
Starch	α Amylase	{ Monosaccharides { Disaccharides	Active transport Disaccharide-ase	Monosaccharides Monosaccharides
Protein	Proteases	{ Amino acids { { Di and Tri- { peptides	Active transport { Active transport { { peptidases	Amino acids Di and Tri- peptides Amino acids
Triglycerides	Lipase Bile salts	Mixed Micelles	Tri, di and mono glycerides fatty acids, glycerol	
Vitamin B_{12}	Intrinsic factor	B_{12}—I.F. complex		Vitamin B_{12}

Bacteria could interfere with digestion by degrading enzymes and secretions, or by competing with the body for food-stuffs. These mechanisms probably account for the malabsorption of fat, protein and vitamin B_{12} in the blind loop syndrome (Table 13.2). Studies on germ-free animals have shown that the bacteria can influence the mucosa and some studies in patients with an abnormal flora suggest that similar changes may occur in human disease (Dyer and Hawkins, 1972); however, the importance of such changes remains conjectural.

TABLE 13.2

Bacteria as the cause of malabsorption

Substance malabsorbed	Bacterial action on the small intestine	Notes
All substances	Reduction of the absorptive capacity of the mucosa	Germ-free animal studies and some "blind loop" cases suggest that bacteria affect the mucosa. May be significant in "tropical intestine".
Protein	Disruption of enterohepatic circulation of Urea nitrogen	"Blind loop" patient studied by Jones *et al.* (1969).
Fat	(a) Deconjugation of bile salts decreasing effective concentration. (b) Degradation of bile salts increasing faecal loss	Cause of steatorrhoea in blind loop syndrome
Vitamin B_{12}	Competition of free B_{12} by *Escherichia coli* and for Complexed B_{12} by some *Bacteroides fragilis.*	Cause of B_{12} malabsorption in Blind loop syndrome
D-xylose	Utilization of D-xylose by intestinal flora	"Blind loop" patient studied by Goldstein *et al.* (1970)

I. Post pathogen malabsorption

Absorption may be impaired during acute diarrhoea due to pathogenic bacteria (Lindenbaum, 1965) but such malabsorption seldom persists after recovery from the acute disease (Gorbach *et al.,* 1970; Giannella *et al.,* 1971). Acute malabsorption has received comparatively little attention. Chronic malabsorption due to bacterial action has only been demonstrated unequivocally in the blind loop syndrome. Giannella *et al.* (1971) reported on a case of salmonelosis whose malabsorption persisted after the eradication of the infection, presumably due to a mucosal lesion, and this finding suggests that post-pathogen malabsorption should be studied further.

II. The blind loop syndrome

The blind loop or stagnant loop syndrome, which is characterized by vitamin deficiency, steatorrhoea and weight loss, can result from a number of structural abnormalities, including intestinal strictures, fistulae, diverticuli and static afferent loops resulting from Polya partial gastrectomy (Table 13.3). The metabolic effects of the blind loop can be alleviated by oral antibiotics, or by surgical measures to restore continuity and prevent stagnation of intestinal contents.

TABLE 13.3

Conditions predisposing to the development of the blind loop syndrome

Gastric surgery	Gastro jejunostomy	
	Partial gastrectomy (Billroth II)	
Other surgery	Oesophogeal replacement by colon	
	Entero-anastomosis	
Intestinal diseases and abnormalities	Diverticulosis	
	Strictures:	Congenital
		Crohn's disease
		Tuberculosis
	Adhesions:	Postoperative
		Postinfective
	X-irradiation of intestine	
	Scleroderma	
	Gastro-colic fistula	
	Entero-colic fistula	
Others	Diabetis mellitus	

The vitamin B_{12} deficiency associated with a "blind loop" is not rectified by administration of B_{12} either alone or with intrinsic factors (Stammers and Williams, 1963; Tabaqchali et al., 1966a; Starzl et al., 1961). When B_{12} is administered with tetracycline, absorption improves (e.g. Naish and Capper, 1953; Polacheck et al., 1961). Surgical treatment of the loop also improves absorption (e.g. Siurala and Kaipainen, 1953; Watkinson et al., 1959). Similar effects can also be demonstrated in experimental animals (e.g. Donaldson, 1962; Donaldson et al., 1962; Bishop, 1963).

Steatorrheoa associated with a blind loop is, like B_{12} malabsorption, improved by antibiotics (e.g. Naish and Capper, 1953; Wirts et al., 1959; French, 1961), or by surgical correction of the loop, in both man and experimental animals (Wirts et al., 1965; Donaldson, 1965).

Vitamin C, D, K and B_2 deficiencies have been recorded. The vitamin K deficiency may be sufficiently serious to cause spontaneous bleeding (Starzl et al., 1961; Badenoch, 1960). Serious protein deficiency has also been reported (Naish and Capper, 1953; Krikler and Schrive, 1958; Jones *et al.*, 1969). This deficiency also seems to respond to antibiotics (Jones *et al.*, 1969).

A. ALTERATIONS IN THE BACTERIAL FLORA OF THE SMALL INTESTINE IN THE BLIND LOOP

The malabsorption that occurs in the Blind Loop Syndrome is not due to any particular pathogenic bacterial species but rather to the redistribution within the intestine of bacteria normally found in the large intestine. The flora of intestinal contents from patients with the "Blind Loop Syndrome" tends to resemble that of faeces but to be more diluted (Table 13.4). Such a flora is not diagnostic of the "Blind Loop Syndrome" since a similar flora can be demonstrated in intestinal contents from patients without malabsorption (Chapter 4). It may be that the total number of bacteria in the small gut is of importance but such information has not been obtained. The study of the concentrations of the various bacteria present has proved less valuable than was at first hoped.

B. THE MECHANISM OF B_{12} MALABSORPTION IN THE BLIND LOOP SYNDROME

The reason for the failure to absorb vitamin B_{12} is unknown but the mechanism most favoured is that of direct competition between the host and bacteria for available B_{12} (Tabaqchali and Booth, 1970). Bacteria isolated from blind loops have been shown to take up B_{12} (Doig and Girdwood, 1960) even, though less well, in the presence of intrinsic factor (Booth and Heath, 1962). Radioactively labelled vitamin B_{12} administered to patients with blind loops or to animals with experimentally produced blind loops is bound to that fraction of intestinal contents capable of being deposited by centrifugation. Although this particulate fraction consists principally of bacteria the identity of the organisms responsible is uncertain. Of the bacteria present in blind loops both *Escherichia coli* and *Bacteroides fragilis* are able to bind B_{12} *in vitro*; however, the organisms may also be capable of vitamin synthesis (Donaldson, 1970; Schjonsby *et al.*, 1972).

C. STEATORRHOEA IN THE BLIND LOOP SYNDROME

The steatorrhoea seems unlikely to be due to a direct competition between the host and the bacteria, since the uptake of radioactive triolein by bacteria is negligible (Donaldson, 1965). Thus an indirect mechanism is postulated, for example, the hydrolysis of conjugated bile salts by bacteria colonizing the blind loops (Dawson and Isselbacher, 1960). Free bile acids

TABLE 13.4

Bacterial flora of the small intestine in patients with the blind loop syndrome. Intestinal fluid from the region of the blind loop

Condition	Log$_{10}$ bacteria/ml intestinal fluid					Reference
	Enterobacteria	Bacteroides	Streptococci	Lactobacilli	Gram^{+} non-sporing anaerobes (e.g. Bifido-bacteria/Eubacteria)	
Billroth II Partial gastrectomy	8.7	9.6	6	5.6	N	Polter et al. (1968)
Multiple small intestinal diverticulli	5	6	3	N	N	
Blind loop of Ileum	8	9	N	N	N	Drasar and Shiner (1969)
Multiple duodenal and jejunal diverticulosis	8	4	6	6	7	
	8	8	7	4.5	6	[+]Gorbach and Tabaqchali (1969)
	8	6	5	5	5	
Entero-enteric fistula	7.7	9.3	2	6	N	Jones et al. (1969)
Jejunal diverticulosis	6	8	N	N	7	

[+] Counts estimated from diagrams; N = not detected

have been demonstrated in the jejunal juice of patients (Donaldson, 1965; Tabaqchali and Booth, 1966) and in blind loops in experimental animals. Many types of bacteria are able to degrade bile salts (Chapter 7). Bacteria able to hydrolyse bile acid conjugates have been isolated from patients with the Blind Loop Syndrome. Antibiotic treatment of such patients leads to a reduction in the steatorrhoea accompanied by an eradication of the deconjugating bacteria (Drasar and Shiner, 1969). Bacteroides are probably the most important group of bacteria involved in the deconjugation of bile acids in the blind loop syndrome, (Drasar *et al.,* 1966; Gorbach and Tabaqchali, 1969; Donaldson, 1970; Tabaqchali and Booth, 1970).

Conjugated bile acids are important stimulators of the enzymatic processes accompanying fat absorption (Senior, 1964); free bile acids are less effective both in the formation of micelles and as enzyme stimulators, while free deoxycholic acid inhibits pancreatic lipase (Fritz and Melius, 1963; Hofmann, 1965; Borgstrom, 1964). The concentration of conjugated bile salts in the jejunum of patients who have blind loops associated with steatorrhoea may be lower than the critical concentration required to form micelles (Tabaqchali and Booth, 1966, 1967, 1970; Krone *et al.,* 1968).

The interaction of bacteria with bile salt metabolism is not restricted to the hydrolysis of bile acid conjugates. The formation of insoluble metabolites such as lithocholic acid probably also plays a role since the formation of such substances will lead to an increased rate of loss from the bile salt pool. In any individual patient the occurrence of steatorrhoea is probably the resultant of the complex interaction between bile salt deconjugation and further degradation by the flora, the absorption and reconjugation of the soluble free acids and the synthesis by the liver of fresh cholic and chenodeoxycholic acid to replace bile salts lost through degradation to non-absorbable substances. Steatorrhoea would result when liver synthesis was unable to compensate for loss from the intestine thus producing a reduction in the size of the bile salt pool available for use in fat absorption.

The hypothesis that bile salt degradation is the cause of the steatorrhoea has been challenged (Goldstein, 1971). The feeding of cholestyramine, an ion exchange resin that binds salts, produces only a mild steatorrhoea, whereas the steatorrhoea associated with blind loops may be very severe. However, congenital lack of bile salts results in a severe steatorrhoea (Ross *et al.,* 1955), and it may be that bacteria are more effective than cholestyramine in reducing the bile salt pool.

D. OTHER DEFECTS IN THE BLIND LOOP SYNDROME

The mechanisms involved in the deficiences of the vitamins B_2, C, D and K have not been examined. Vitamin D absorption does, however, require the participation of bile salts and their metabolism by bacteria may account for cases of osteomalacia in the blind loop syndrome (Thompson, 1967; Tabaqchali and Booth, 1970).

Protein malnutrition may occur in the Blind Loop Syndrome; the suggested mechanism postulates the degradation of enterohepatically circulated urea and the conversion of dietary protein to urea by the small intestinal bacteria (Jones et al., 1969).

Bacterial disruption of steroid metabolism can effect not only fat metabolism but also growth and maturity. In children with the Blind Loop Syndrome there may be retardation of growth and sexual development (Neale, 1968; Bayes and Hamilton, 1969; Tabaqchali and Booth, 1970).

III. Malabsorption and malnutrition in the tropics

Malabsorption and malnutrition occur widely in tropical regions. There is some suggestion that the intestinal flora may be involved in these conditions. In this discussion the role of bacteria in the malabsorption found in normal people resident in the tropics, the so-called "tropical intestine" (Editorial, 1972) and the group of diseases grouped together as "Tropical Sprue" is examined. Other aspects of the problem are reviewed in a recent symposium (Klipstein, 1968) and in the communication of a Wellcome Trust Study Group (Wellcome Trust, 1972).

A. THE TROPICAL INTESTINE

Residents in tropical countries, whether indigenous or expatriate, tend to have an intestinal mucosa and D xylose absorption that is regarded as "abnormal" in comparison with normal people in Western Europe and North America (Sprinz et al., 1962; Russel et al., 1966; Schenk et al., 1968; Klipstein et al., 1968; Bayles et al., 1968; Sheehy et al., 1968; Lindenbaum, 1968; Jeejeebhoy et al., 1968; Baker and Mathan, 1968; England, 1968). The cause of the abnormalities is unknown. On transfer to a temperate climate the intestinal structure and function adopts the normal values of the local population even for ethnic groups of tropical origin (Gerson, et al., 1971; Lindenbaum et al., 1971).

Bacteria can influence the morphology of the intestinal mucosa. The migration of villus cells from the crypts to the tips of the villi takes four days in germ-free mice as compared with two days in normal animals (Khoury et al., 1969). Similar variation has been reported by Abrams et al. (1963). The mucosa of germ-free pigs is regular and similar to that in normal people but that of normal, bacterially colonized pigs is much more irregular (Kenworthy and Allen 1966a, b). The small intestine in these animals is much more extensively colonized than that in man resident in

Western Europe and North America (Smith, 1965). It may be that the small intestine in tropical residents without disease is more heavily colonized than that in other people.

The normal tropical residents studied by Gorbach *et al.* (1969) and Bhat *et al.* (1972) yielded more bacteria from the small intestine than would be expected from normal English. If this changed distribution of bacteria is general it may be that this contributes to the changed mucosal morphology. Animal models of intestinal infection suggest that some mucosal damage is caused by pathogenic bacteria (e.g. Takeuchi *et al.*, 1965) – the significance of such changes is uncertain. Similarly xylose absorption by germ-free mice is more efficient than that of their conventional counterparts.

Although the supposition that the "tropical intestine" results from the unusual distribution of bacteria within the small intestine of tropical residents is firmly based, other evidence suggests that the bacterial distribution may result from nutritional deficiencies (Klipstein *et al.*, 1970; Gorbach *et al.*, 1970). Animal models of human protein malnutrition in rhesus monkeys suggest that protein limitation can cause mucosal abnormalities (Deo *et al.*, 1965). However, work in rats is more equivocal; while some workers claim no effect (Brunser *et al.*, 1968), others demonstrate a decreased mitotic activity of crypt cells (Hopper *et al.*, 1968); the time course of the studies may be crucial.

B. TROPICAL SPRUE

Many workers have reported on patients whose disease responded to antibiotic therapy (Table 13.5). The response to short-term therapy is generally only symptomatic and long-term therapy as much as six months, is necessary for improvement of the absorptive defect. The response of expatriates has in general been much more consistent than that of the indigenous inhabitants of the tropics. If this disease is really of bacterial origin the mechanism of malabsorption must be explained.

No specific pathogen associated with tropical sprue has been reported. However, Gorbach *et al.* (1970) isolated strains of *Escherichia coli*, that produced enterotoxin from patients with tropical sprue. Moreover, field studies on sprue have demonstrated that epidemic spread compatible with the involvement of an infective agent can occur (Mathan and Baker, 1968) and the indication of clusters of cases occurring in single houses is also suggestive (Fraser, 1968).

Bacteria cause several gastrointestinal diseases; however, these are usually acute while tropical sprue is a chronic disease. Furthermore, although malabsorption occurs during bacterial disease this does not, or rather has not been reported to persist after recovery from the disease (Lindenbaum,

TABLE 13.5

The response of patients with tropical sprue to anti-microbial therapy

	Area	Number patients treated	Number patients responding	Reference
European	India	400	400	Elder (1947
expatriates	Hong Kong	7	7	French, Gaddie and Smith (1956)
	S. E. Asia	11	11	O'Brien and England (1966)
Indigenous	Puerto Rico	12	6	Sheehy and Perez-Santiago (1961)
populations		17	17	Guerra, Wheby and Bayless (1965)
		4	4	Klipstein, Schenk and Samloff (1966)
		1	1	Klipstein (1966)
		16	9	Maldonado et al. (1969)
	Haiti	8	4	Klipstein (1968)
		8	8	Klipstein et al. (1968)
	India	70	30	Chuttani et al. (1968)
		22	14	Jeejeebhoy et al. (1968)
		2	2	Gorbach et al. (1969)
		Not specified	Very few	Baker and Mathan (1968)
	Nigeria	5	5	Falanje (1970)

1965). However, the recent work of Mitchell and Rees (1970) suggests that a transmissible agent may be associated with Crohn's disease while the evidence that Whipple's disease can be treated with antibiotics provides some support for the concept of chronic intestinal disease caused by bacteria. Salmonella diarrhoea can produce persistent malabsorption in occasional patients (Giannella et al., 1971); the prevalence of infection in the tropics leads to the supposition that sprue results from persistent infective disease in a malnourished population.

Interest in the Blind Loop Syndrome (Section II above) has led to speculation as to the possibility that sprue might be due to a redistribution of the normal flora. The Blind Loop Syndrome is a malabsorption syndrome caused by colonization of the small intestine resulting from anatomical abnormalities. The process does not involve specific pathogens but rather a change in location of bacteria normally present in the intestine. Such changes in the bacterial distribution occur in association with small intestinal diverticuli and as a result of intestinal surgery. In people suffering from the Blind Loop Syndrome the loop and at least part of the small intestine contains increased numbers of bacteria, at least 10^5 organisms per ml, both aerobic and anaerobic bacteria occur, prominently Enterobacteria and Bacteroides; the flora is qualitatively similar to faeces though more dilute (Krone *et al.*, 1968; Polter *et al.*, 1968; Drasar and Shiner, 1969; Tabaqchali and Booth, 1970).

Although abnormalities of the small intestinal flora have been reported in patients with sprue, the abnormalities are similar to those reported in normal tropical residents (Bhat *et al.*, 1972). Gorbach *et al.*, 1969 showed that a "blind loop flora" occurs in the ileum of people with tropical sprue and suggested that this caused malabsorption. The patients studied by these workers responded rapidly to antibiotic therapy; however, as noted previously, the responses of most patients treated with antibiotics has been slow; the response of patients with blind loops is usually rapid. Furthermore, the lower ileum is colonized in some normal people (Chapter 3). One is left with the problem of defining the length of intestine that has to be colonized before symptoms are produced. The problem is further complicated by the suggestion, mentioned earlier, that malnutrition might produce changes in the flora (Gorbach *et al.*, 1970). Whether the malabsorption produced by the bacteria gave rise to the malnutrition, or the malnutrition changed the flora requires more study.

IV. Whipples disease

Bacteria are thought to be responsible for the malabsorbtive condition called Whipples Disease. The disease responds to antibiotic therapy and "bacillary bodies" can be demonstrated in sections of intestinal mucosa (England *et al.*, 1960; Davis *et al.*, 1963; Philips and Finlay, 1967). Attempts to cultivate a specific pathogen have, however, not been successful (Sherris *et al.*, 1965).

V. The influence of malabsorption not caused by bacteria on the intestinal flora

From a bacteriological viewpoint the most significant aspect of malabsorption syndromes whether congenital or acquired is the increase in nutrients available for bacterial metabolism in the colon. Faecal fats reflect the results of bacterial action upon the dietary fat, hydroxylation and other reactions can occur (Webb *et al.*, 1963; Wiggins *et al.*, 1969; Thomas, 1972). Utilization of protein by the flora may lead to an increase in the protein degradation products (phenols, indoles, amines) and an increase in these substances in the stool. The significance of this colonic putrefaction has been discussed with respect to theories of auto-intoxication (e.g. Hale White *et al.*, 1913) but has been little studied except with respect to hepatic encephalopathy (Chapter 16).

The effects of carbohydrate malabsorption are best illustrated by the consideration of disaccharidase deficiencies. Congenital deficiencies of

lactase, sucrase-iso maltase and other disaccharidases (Neale, 1971) are well
known; deficiency of Trehalase has also been described. Secondary
deficiencies may also occur in coeliac disease and after an attack of acute
gastroenteritis. Lactase deficiency is acquired on weaning by a large
proportion of the world's population; this deficiency is related to
ethnic/cultural groupings and may be related to the historical development
of milk drinking (Neale, 1971). Disaccharide malabsorption leads to
fermentative diarrhoea, the pH of the stool is lowered and the amount of
lactic acid vastly increased (Fraser, 1968; Neale, 1971).

CHAPTER 14

Acute Diarrhoeal Disease

Diarrhoea is an important if somewhat ill-defined symptom of many diseases. Indeed diarrhoeal diseases, most usually caused by bacteria but assisted by malnutrition, are among the common causes of infant mortality in under-developed countries (Gordon and Scrimshaw, 1970). Among adults acute diarrhoeal disease remains an important public health problem. On the basis of animal experimentation the intestinal flora is thought to contribute to the pathogenesis of diarrhoeal disease due to enteric bacterial pathogens. The intestinal flora may also be involved in the pathogenesis of some diarrhoeal diseases of uncertain aetiology. Even known protozoal pathogens such as *Entamoeba histolytica* do not produce disease in the absence of an intestinal flora (Phillips and Wolfe, 1959).

Before proceeding to discuss the causes of diarrhoeal disease it is perhaps necessary to consider some technical points. Intestinal pathogens are often said to produce "enterotoxin"; this does not imply the existence of one substance called enterotoxin. The response of test systems, most commonly the rabbit ileal loop, to culture filtrates and growing cultures is used to ascribe enterotoxicity to strains of bacteria. The description of enterotoxin rests on various functional parameters. Enterotoxin induces a temporary, reversible functional defect in the mucosal cells; transport of water and electrolytes are affected, without causing any structural damage. Various test systems are described by Moon and Whip (1971).

The ability of bacteria to invade the intestinal mucosa is important in the pathogenesis of some intestinal diseases.

The ability of strains to penetrate the conjunctiva of guinea-pig (Sereny Test) or to invade He-La cell monolayers correlates well with the ability to invade the lamina propia of guinea-pigs (Dupont *et al.*, 1971). One or more of these tests is used to indicate the ability of bacteria to invade the intestinal mucosa. Invasiveness of salmonella has been examined in the ileum of rats and monkeys (Takeuchi, 1967).

Gastroenteritis may also be caused by a wide variety of infectious agents. Two varieties of gastroenteritis can be distinguished: intoxifications caused by the ingestion of preformed toxin produced by bacteria growing in foods and infections resulting from the establishment of pathogens in the intestine.

Initiation of infection may be prevented by the destruction of the pathogen by the stomach acid, its removal from the small intestine by clearance mechanisms or its exclusion from the intestine by the normal flora.

I. Protective function of the flora

Animal experiments suggest that the intestinal flora has an important protective function in preventing the initiation of infection by intestinal pathogens. Thus the pre-treatment of mice with streptomycin increases their susceptibility to oral challenge with salmonellae (Miller and Bohnhoff, 1962; Bohnhoff and Miller, 1962; Bohnhoff et al., 1964; Meynell, 1963; Abrams and Bishop, 1966). In man the prolonged carriage of salmonellae by patients given neomycin probably reflects an analogous mechanism (Association for the study of Infectious Diseases, 1970).

Treatment of mice and guinea-pigs with antibiotics increases their susceptibility to infection by shigellae and in the case of guinea-pigs also to Vibrio cholerae (Freter, 1956). Germ-free guinea-pigs are susceptible to Vibrio cholerae infection and susceptible to shigellae (Formol et al., 1961) while conventional animals are not.

The mechanisms of microbial interference are not understood. However, the production of volatile fatty acids is important in the inhibition of Salmonella typhimurium in the mouse gut. Savage (1972) suggested that the spatial arrangement of micro-organisms were important especially at the mucosal surface. Thus, organisms such as shigellae might be excluded from the mucosa by the indigenous microbes adherent to the wall of the colon.

II. The agents of diarrhoeal disease

1. Bacillus cereus

The consumption of fried rice containing large numbers (more than 10^6/gram) of Bacillus cereus has been associated with outbreaks of food poisoning (B.M.J. 1972a). Examination of strains isolated from outbreaks of food poisoning demonstrated that many strains produced enterotoxin (Spira and Goepfert, 1972). The disease is thought to result from the ingestion of preformed toxin.

2. Clostridium botulinum

Botulism is the pre-eminent example of a disease caused by a preformed toxin. The neurotoxins of Clostridium botulinum are the most toxic substances known. After ingestion the toxins are absorbed and attach to the motor nerve terminals. It is of interest in the context of the present discussion that diarrhoea occurs only as an early symptom of the disease and is followed by obstinate constipation (Hobbs, 1968). This might result from a disruption of the relationship between the segmental contractions of the small bowel, which ensure adequate contact of contents with the absorptive surfaces and the propulsive peristaltic movements. Such dis-association might allow the very rapid emptying of the small bowel with resultant diarrhoea. The cessation of all movement would produce constipation.

3. *Clostridium perfrigens (welchii)*

Clostridium perfringens is responsible for two diseases of the intestine. Type A strains are a major cause of food poisoning. Both heat-resistant and heat-sensitive strains have been implicated although heat-resistant strains have been more prominent, perhaps because of their ability to survive cooking (Sutton and Hobbs, 1965). The disease may result from growth of clostridia in the gut and the *in situ* liberation of toxin, though the ingestion of preformed toxin may be important. Studies in the rabbit ileal loop have demonstrated the production of enterotoxin (Duncan *et al.*, 1968) and this ability to influence mucosal physiology may account for the enteropatho-genicity of particular strains.

Type C *Clostridium perfringens* causes necrotizing jejunitis (enteritis necroticans), a severe and often fatal disease. Cases of the disease have been reported in Germany (Darmbrand), New Guinea (pig-bel), and Uganda. The disease is characterized by necrosis and inflammation of the small bowel and may represent an intestinal form of gas gangrene (Murrell *et al.*, 1966a, b; Willis, 1969).

4. *Escherichia coli*

Escherichia coli causes diarrhoea in infants and adults. The *E. coli* enteropathogenic in infants have long been considered to be restricted to certain O groups. Recent studies on the episomal control of enterotoxin production casts doubt on the significance of these specific reactions.

Animal studies have demonstrated that strains of enteropathogenic *Escherichia coli* can produce disease in ways analogous to those discussed for *Vibrio cholerae*, *Shigella* and *Salmonella* (Savage, 1972).

The ability to penetrate epithelial cells can be transferred from *Shigella flexneri* to *Escherichia coli* (Formol *et al.*, 1965). The ability of *Escherichia coli* to produce enterotoxin is controlled by an episome (Smith and Halls, 1968). Thus any particular strain might acquire either or both abilities.

In pigs which suffer a natural infection similar to that seen in infants, the organisms adhere to the mucosa of the small intestine (Arbuckle, 1971). Some enteropathogenic strains of *Escherichia coli* produce an enterotoxin which can be demonstrated by its effect on isolated loops of intestine (e.g. Smith and Gyles, 1970; Smith and Halls, 1967); such enterotoxin does not give rise to any mucosal damage (Craig, 1972). Other *Escherichia coli* enteropathogenic for neonatal swine are able to invade the colonic mucosa (Staley *et al.*, 1970). Enterotoxin is produced by strains isolated from infants (Taylor *et al.*, 1958). It seems likely that in children at least, the gastroenteritis produced by *Escherichia coli* results from the growth of, and production of enterotoxin by the organisms in the small intestine. The resultant exsorption of fluid produces the diarrhoea.

Outbreaks of diarrhoea in adults due to *Escherichia coli* were studied by Rowe *et al.* (1970) and Gorbach *et al.* (1971). Only one of the strains isolated belonged to a recognized enteropathogenic serological group, however, enterotoxin production was demonstrated. The strain isolated by Rowe *et al.*, 014 K? H-28, was later shown to reproduce the disease on administration to volunteers (Formol *et al.*, 1971).

Outbreaks of enteric disease in adults similar to dysentery have been observed. Studies on strains of *E. coli* isolated from these outbreaks showed that they were invasive in test systems and reproduced the disease when fed to volunteers (DuPont *et al.*, 1971).

5. *Salmonella*

Salmonella are transported through the intestinal mucosa into the subepitheleal tissues; penetration occurs in the small intestine (Takeuchi and Sprinz, 1967; Sprinz *et al.*, 1966). The exact location of infection is however, uncertain; some animal models suggest a large intestinal involvement with an ileocaecal lesion (Powell *et al.*, 1971). In man the finding that organisms can often be isolated from vomit suggests small intestinal involvement. Probably the whole intestine is involved. Studies of *Salmonella typhimurium* in the rabbit ileum suggests that invasiveness alone is not enough to produce diarrhoea. Some other factors are necessary to produce the exsorption of fluid but these factors do not seem to be analogous to the enterotoxin produced by other intestinal pathogens (Gianella *et al.*, 1973).

The disease produced by most Salmonellae is entirely distinct from the fever produced by organisms such as *Salmonella typhi*. In such organisms invasiveness is very highly developed enabling bacteria to pass through the mucosa into the lymphatic system. Growth of *Salmonella typhi* occurs intracellularly in phagocytes and the clinical manifestations occur as the bacteria re-enter the blood stream from intracellular sites.

6. *Shigella*

In dysentery, due to the various shigella species, the pathogen invades the superficial layers of the mucosa producing some cell damage but not followed by systemic spread (Sprinz, 1969). Ulceration of the colon and in some cases, of the terminal ileum, occurs. The bacteria invade the colonic epithelial cells and then multiply within them passing into adjacent cells. The death of these patches of infected cells produces the ulceration and bloody diarrhoea (LaBrec *et al.*, 1964; Ogawa *et al.*, 1966; Takeuchi *et al.*, 1968). Some strains of *Shigella dysenteriae* produce an "enterotoxin" similar in action to that of *Vibrio cholerae*. This toxin may be responsible for some of the manifestations of the disease (Van Heynigen, 1971; Craig, 1972).

In view of the recent studies on salmonella (Gianella *et al.*, 1973) indicating that invasion alone does not produce fluid exsorption, other factors may be produced by strains lacking enterotoxin.

The role of the intestinal flora in preventing infection by Shigella species may well be the occupation of mucosal space since, even in man, bacteria are demonstrable adherent to the colonic mucosa (Savage, 1972; Nelson and Mata, 1970).

7. *Staphylococcus aureus*

Some staphylococci elaborate enterotoxin. Staphylococcal enterotoxin is a neurotoxin acting on the central nervous system and is not known to act on the intestinal mucosa; it should therefore be distinguished from the other enterotoxins discussed in this chapter. The enterotoxin is formed by staphylococci growing in food and on ingestion produces violent diarrhoea and vomiting.

Staphylococci can also cause a severe enterocolitis in patients undergoing treatment with broad spectrum antibiotics (Altemeier *et al.*, 1963; Asar and Drapanas, 1968).

Ulceration of the colonic mucosa and necrosis occur. The mechanism of this disease is obscure; it may be that removal of the normal flora from the mucosal surface allows colonization of the mucosa with the staphylococci.

8. *Vibrio cholerae* and *Vibrio cholerae,* biotype El Tor

The disease produced by El Tor vibrios is not distinguishable from that produced by classical cholera vibrios although a higher proportion of asymptomatic infections may occur (Bart *et al.*, 1970).

The diarrhoea in cholera is caused by toxic factors, "enterotoxin", released by the *Vibrio cholerae* growing in the small intestine. There is no structural damage to the intestinal mucosa; the main defect seems to be a functional disarrangement of water balance. The vibrios grow either in the lumen of, or adherent to the mucosa of the small intestine, so no invasion of the mucosa occurs (Sprintz *et al.*, 1962; Savage, 1972).

Although animal experiments suggest that the normal flora protects against *Vibrio cholerae* infection it is difficult to visualize by what mechanism since the small intestinal flora of man seems too sparse to be significant. Savage (1972) suggests that indigenous bacteria, by occupying space on the mucosa, prevent mucosal adherence and hence initiation of infection. The importance of adherence is underlined by the work of Freter (1969) who suggested that protective antibody may prevent adhesion or promote shedding. However, more recent work shows that IgA antibody may also prevent production of enterotoxin (Fubara and Freter, 1972).

9. *Vibrio parahaemolyticus*

A food-borne infection caused by *Vibrio parahaemolyticus* has been described in various parts of the world including the United Kingdom (Brit. M.J. 1972b; Barrow and Miller, 1972). These organisms produce enterotoxin (Bhattacharya *et al.*, 1971) and may thus produce a disease similar to that of other enterotoxic bacteria.

Vibrio fetus has also been described as a cause of diarrhoea mainly in infants (Mandel and Ellison, 1963).

10. *Viruses*

No bacterial pathogen can be isolated from many cases of diarrhoea, and this disease has been ascribed to the activity of viruses. Evidence in support of this hypothesis is difficult to find. In a study of infantile diarrhoea by Cramblett *et al.* (1971) an exhaustive search for viruses yielded similar numbers of isolates from patients and controls (Table 14.1). While there is a suggestion that ECHO viruses and adenoviruses may be implicated the evidence is not very convincing.

TABLE 14.1

Isolation of viruses in diarrhoeal disease (Data of Cramblett *et al.*, 1971)

			No. of patients yielding virus				
	No. of subjects yielding viruses	No. of subjects studied	Poliovirus	ECHO virus	Coxsackie virus	Adenovirus	Herpes simplex
Children with diarrhoea	271	46	12	19	2	12	1
Controls	180	33	17	9	2	4	1

11. *Other diarrhoeal agents*

Many other bacteria have been reported to cause diarrhoea (Table 14.2), *Pseudomonas aeruginosa,* produces an enterotoxin (Kubota and Lin, 1971). The status of these organisms as infective agents is unclear, though they may be important following antibiotic treatment. *Streptococcus faecalis* var *liquifaciens* has been described as a cause of food poisoning (Hobbs, 1968).

TABLE 14.2

Bacteria suggested as causes of diarrhoea

Streptococcus faecalis var *liquifaciens*
Pseudomonas aeruginosa
Proteus mirabilis
Yersinia enterocolytica
Pleisiomonas shigelloides
Aeromonas spp.

III. Diarrhoeas thought to be infective

A. WEANLING DIARRHOEA

Gastroenteritis is a major cause of death among infants and young children in many developing countries. Indeed, gastroenteritis of infancy is still common in Great Britain. Estimates suggest that 100,000 cases occur in a year of which about 10% are admitted to hospital (Wheatly, 1968).

Not all of these cases of disease can be accounted for; "acknowledged" bacterial pathogens are rarely found in more than 20% of these infants. Virus infections has been invoked to account for other cases but attempts to demonstrate viruses have proved disappointing and the aetiology of at least 65% of cases remains unexplained.

Studies of jejunal specimens obtained at necropsy (Dammin, 1964) showed large numbers of bacteria in the jejunum of children who died from "weanling diarrhoea" and Dammin postulated that this non-specific bacterial multiplication might occur because malnutrition had impaired the health of the mucosa and this combination of insults produced the disease. However, more recent studies (James *et al.*, 1972) showed that bacterial over-growth can sometimes be demonstrated in malnourished children both with and without diarrhoea, and in well nourished children who had recovered from diarrhoea. Similarly Mata *et al.* (1972) demonstrated high counts of bacteria in the small intestine of both normal children and those with malnutrition. Gracey *et al.* (1969) demonstrated an abnormal flora in children with diarrhoea due to sugar intolerance. As discussed below re-distribution of the small intestinal flora often occurs during diarrhoea.

The relative resistance of breast-fed infants to gastroenteritis was demonstrated by Ross and Dawes (1954); although this resistance has long been suspected, the reason is not known. Studies in Guatemala showed that most cases of gastroenteritis occur shortly after cessation of breast feeding (Gordon, 1971). To explain these observations three aspects of the problem have been considered: the role of protective antibody from breast milk, the nutritional status of the breast-fed infant and changes in the intestinal flora, due to the changed diet, reducing the protective effect of the flora.

Maternal antibody to *Escherichia coli* may occasionally be transferred in the milk and this would presumably contribute to immunity since placental transfer does not occur (Sussman, 1961). However, the role of maternal antibody in the 65% of cases whose aetiology is unexplained cannot be assessed. Maternal antibody may contribute to the control of the flora by its action in the intestinal lumen; IgA is the main immunoglobulin in both colostrum and intestinal secretions.

Malnutrition increases susceptibility to intestinal and many other infections (Scrimshaw *et al.*, 1968). The inadequacy of the Guatamalan diet as compared to breast milk may explain the peak of intestinal infection following weaning (Gordon, 1971).

Earlier work summarized by Rosebury (1961) suggested that the colonic flora of breast-fed infants is dominated by *Bifidobacterium bifidus* and that these bacteria prevented colonization by *Escherichia coli*. There is, however, some doubt as to the significance of these findings since a recent study revealed little difference in the degree of colonization by *Escherichia coli* in bottle or breast-fed infants (Bullen and Willis, 1971). Nevertheless, there is evidence that breast feeding may affect the type of Bifidobacterium isolated from the feaces (Braun *et al.*, 1964). Our few observations suggest that on weaning bacteroides and fusobacteria become more common in the faeces and these bacteria and their interaction with the colonic mucosa might repay further studies. This finding would support those of Mata *et al.* (1972) who showed a decrease in the number of bifidobacteria on weaning. Study of the problem in the United Kingdom is complicated by the slow stabilization of the flora under hospital conditions and the difficulty of obtaining specimens from infants whose diet of breast milk is not supplemented.

B. TRAVELLERS DIARRHOEA

Visitors are liable to suffer attacks of diarrhoea within a short time of arriving in a new country. Few cases, probably not more than 5%, are due to shigellas or salmonellas (Varela *et al.*, 1959; Rowe *et al.* 1970). Adeno- and enteroviruses have not been implicated (Bell and Grist, 1967). Attack rates of 33% and higher have been reported for travellers between the United States and Mexico (Kean, 1963) and in the Middle East. The attack rate in temperate areas may be lower but it is not negligible (Kean, 1963; Dandoy, 1966). Visitors to the Lebanon and Iran (Hanveld, 1960; Kean, 1969) from temperate areas had a higher attack rate than those from the tropics. Some evidence suggests that the incidence is higher among young adults than among old adults, but this may result from differences in life style.

Changes in the intestinal flora due to acquisition of local strains of bacteria have been postulated as the principal cause of travellers' diarrhoea. The only direct evidence was obtained by Rowe *et al.* (1970) who studied a group of British troops transferred to Aden. A previously undescribed serotype of *Escherichia coli* (0148K? H-28) was isolated from 19 of 35 patients during the acute phase of the disease but not from any healthy man. This strain was later shown to produce enterotoxin and was able to produce gastro-intestinal infections in volunteers (Formol *et al.*, 1971).

IV. Alterations in the flora

In diarrhoea caused by known pathogens the most obvious change in the flora is the appearance of the pathogen. Each of the pathogenic bacteria producing intestinal disease tends to locate in a particular region of the intestine (Table 14.3). The ecology of the small intestine is disturbed in acute diarrhoea. Some pathogens, for example *Vibrio cholerae*, colonize the small bowel but an abnormal distribution within the small gut of bacteria included in the normal flora is found in many patients with diarrhoea. Enterobacteria were isolated from the jejunum of more than 25% of the patients with acute diarrhoeal disease studied by Cohen *et al.* (1967). Bacteria, in addition to *Vibrio cholerae*, including enterobacteria and other intestinal organisms can be isolated from jejunal specimens obtained from patients with cholera (Gorbach *et al.*, 1970). A similar redistribution of bacteria occurs in patients with diarrhoea induced by the infusion of saline into the colon (Gorbach *et al.*, 1970a).

TABLE 14.3

Location of intestinal pathogens

Organism	Location of infection
Clostridium perfringens	Small intestine
Escherichia coli	Small *or* large intestine
Salmonella spp.	Small and large intestine
Shigella spp.	Large intestine
Vibrio cholerae	Small intestine

The most obvious change in the faecal flora, when the diarrhoea is caused by a pathogen, is the finding of large number ($10^7 - 10^8$ per gram) of the pathogen, (Thompson 1955; Gorbach *et al.*, 1970b). A reduction in the number of anaerobes and an increase in the numbers of various enterobacteria is often demonstrable in liquid and semi-liquid faeces, no matter what caused the diarrhoea (Gorbach, 1971).

V. General considerations

Acute diarrhoea may result from the ingestion of a preformed toxin or from the establishment of a pathogenic micro-organism in the intestine followed by the production of toxic factors. Toxins may act locally on the mucosa or systemically on the nervous system. Bacteria may maintain themselves in the intestine by invasion of or adherence to the mucosa (Table 14.4).

Enterotoxin acting on the mucosa produces diarrhoea by stimulating the exsorption of fluid. The exact mechanism is uncertain. Toxins acting on the nervous systems may produce diarrhoea by altering the propulsion of intestinal contents. The osmotic effects of un-absorbed intestinal contents entering the colon as a result of small intestinal hurry may also be

TABLE 14.4

Factors influencing fluid exsorption and maintenance of infection of some
intestinal pathogens

Organism	"Factor" influencing fluid exsorption	Mechanism maintaining infection of intestine
Clostridium perfringens	Enterotoxin	?
Escherichia coli	Enterotoxin	K antigen "adhesion" to mucosa
	?	Mucosal invasion
Salmonella spp.	?	Mucosal invasion
Shigella spp.	?	Mucosal invasion
Staphylococcus aureus	Staph enterotoxin (a neurotoxin)	Not applicable
Vibrio cholerae	Enterotoxin	"Adhesion" to mucosa

significant, such effects being aggravated by the fermentation of undigested substances by the large intestinal flora. The destruction of the colonic mucosa by invasive organisms would decrease the colonic absorption of water and this together with the exudation of body fluids would produce diarrhoea.

CHAPTER 15

Role of Bacteria in the Aetiology of Cancer

It has been estimated that 80%-90% of human cancer is of environmental aetiology and is, therefore, potentially preventable. The carcinogens responsible may be preformed in the environment or may be ingested in the form of a precarcinogen and metabolized to the carcinogen in the body. In the latter context the role of bacteria in the production of carcinogens merits considerable investigation. In this section we discuss some of the ways in which bacteria might be involved in human carcinogenesis. These include the production of nitrosamines, the possible production of carcinogenic metabolites of the biliary steroids, and of amino acids.

In any situation where the bacteria produce carcinogens from dietary components or from secretions produced as a response to dietary components, there will be a link between diet and cancer. We will also, therefore, discuss the epidemiological evidence in favour of a dietary factor in the aetiology of certain cancers.

I. Bacterial production of carcinogens

A. FROM STEROIDS

A number of steroids have been shown to be carcinogenic in animal studies, and these include deoxycholic acid (Badger *et al.*, 1940; Cook *et al.*, 1940; von Ghiron, 1939), bis-nor-Δ^5-cholenic acid (Lacassagne *et al.*, 1961), apocholic acid (Lacassagne *et al.*, 1966), and oestradiol (Lacassagne, 1932; Cutts, 1965; McMahon and Cole, 1969); three of these have been shown to be products, or possible products, of bacterial metabolism of the biliary steroids in the human gut. Deoxycholic acid is, of course, a major biliary bile acid and is produced by the bacterial dehydroxylation of the primary bile acid cholic acid. It is present in large amounts in the human large bowel, and the rate of excretion in faeces of deoxycholic acid correlates well with the incidence of colon cancer when national populations are considered (Fig. 15.1). Is deoxycholic acid genuinely carcinogenic? The animal studies are equivocal since there have been studies showing no carcinogenicity. The average Englishman excretes 1.5 kg of deoxycholate

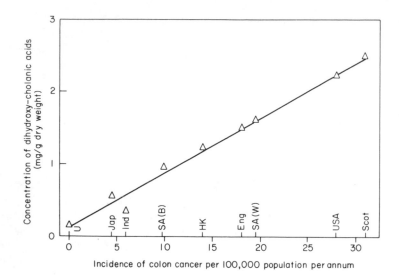

Fig. 15.1. The relation between the faecal concentration of dihydroxy-cholanic acids (mainly deoxycholic acid) and the incidence of colon cancer in 9 populations. These are: U = Uganda; Jap = Japan; Ind = India; S SA(B) = the black population of Johannesburg; HK = Hong Kong; Eng = England (London); SA(W) = the white population of Johannesburg; USA = United States, and Scot = Scotland.

per 50 years of life and with an incidence of colon cancer of 18 per 100,000; this does not indicate to us .that it need be a very potent carcinogen to be responsible for the incidence of colon cancer.

Bis-nor-Δ^5-cholenic acid, which was shown by Lacassagne *et al.* (1961) to be carcinogenic, is closely related to the product of cholesterol side chain cleavage by bacteria as demonstrated by Sih *et al.* (1968a, b); the cholesterol metabolite differs in that it retains the 3-hydroxyl group (Fig. 15.2). There is little evidence concerning the production of this metabolite *in vivo* in the gut and it will not be available until we have more information on the host of minor acid steroids in the faecal bile acid fraction.

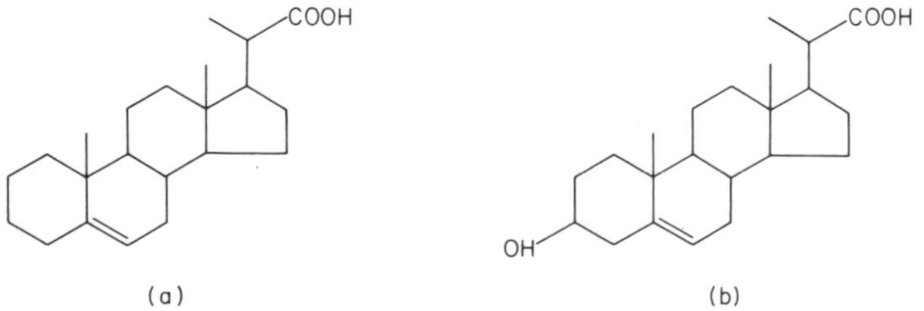

(a)   (b)

Fig. 15.2. Bis-nor-5-cholenic acid (a) and its 3β-hydroxy derivative (b) formed by bacterial degradation of cholesterol.

Oestradiol has been shown to be carcinogenic in rats, giving rise to breast tumours (Lacassagne, 1932; Cutts, 1965). In addition, many breast tumours (human as well as animal) are oestrogen dependent and their growth is curtailed by ovariectomy, adrenalectomy and hypophysectomy (Huggins, 1967). Bacteria produce oestrone and 17-methoxy-oestradiol from 4-androstene-3, 17-dione,3-oxo-cholestenone and 3-oxo 4-cholen-24-oic acid (see Chapter 9) *in vitro*. We have no evidence concerning the production of phenolic steroids *in vivo*.

In addition to these known carcinogens, it is possible that bacteria might produce a polycyclic aromatic hydrocarbon from steroids. The mechanisms by which bacteria can introduce nuclear double bonds into the steroid nucleus have been discussed earlier (Chapter 9.) and they include (a) nuclear desaturation in conjugation with an oxo group; (b) removal of the 10-methyl group; (c) dehydration reactions; (d) nuclear desaturation in conjugation with other nuclear double bonds. Using these four types of reaction the bile acid nucleus can be fully aromatized to a substituted cyclopentaphenanthrene (Fig. 15.3). Reaction 1 is a 3α-hydroxydehydro-

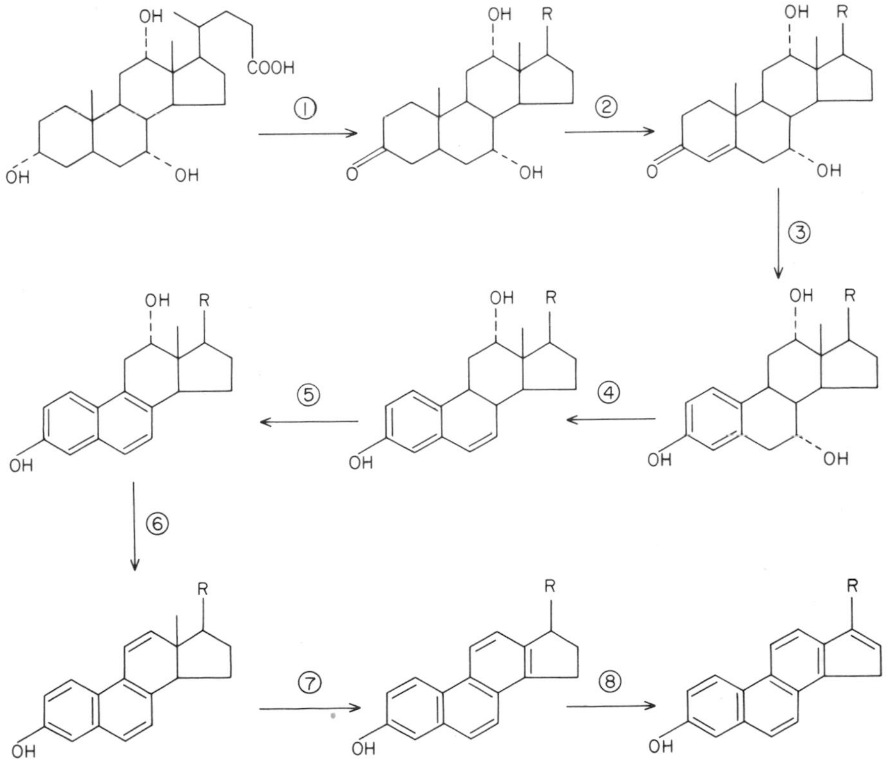

Fig. 15.3. A possible pathway for the aromatization of the bile acid nucleus.

genation, carried out by most species of gut bacteria (see Table 7.6). Reaction 2 is the dehydrogenation of the C4-5 bond to give a conjugated 4-en-3-one structure; this reaction has been demonstrated in a range of opalescent-negative clostridia. Reaction 3 is the aromatization of ring A with the removal or transfer of the C—19 methyl group; this reaction has been demonstrated with clostridia. Reaction 4 is the 7-dehydration yielding a C6-7 double bond stabilized by conjugation with ring A; the 7-dehydration reaction is carried out by a wide range of bacterial genera including bacteroides, bifidobacteria, clostridia, veillonellae and *Strep. faecalis*. Reaction 5, which completes the aromatization of rings A and B is a nuclear dehydrogenation which we have demonstrated using clostridia. Reaction 6, is a 12-dehydration reaction yielding a C11-12 double bond conjugated to rings A and B; this reaction is discussed in Chapter 7 and has been detected in some strains of human intestinal non-sporing anaerobic bacteria. Reaction 7, the removal of the methyl group at C-13, has not been reported for gut bacteria, although it has been demonstrated with a soil organism. It is assumed that this demethylation will be accompanied by, or followed by, a nuclear dehydrogenation to aromatize ring C, yielding a 17-substituted cyclopentaphenanthrene.

The substituted cyclopentaphenanthrenes have been studied extensively by Coombs and Croft (1969). They showed that the 17-methyl-Δ-16 series (Fig. 15.4) were carcinogenic, the unsubstituted homologue having weak activity, the 11-methoxy and 12-methyl derivatives being somewhat more active, and the 11-methyl and 11,12-dimethyl derivatives having the highest activity. Where ring D was saturated the carcinogenic activity was lower; the unsubstituted 3-methoxy, 11-methoxy and 12-methyl derivatives were inactive but some carcinogenic activity was demonstrated with the 11β-methyl and the 11,12-dimethyl derivatives. A high level of carcinogenic activity was also obtained in the 17-oxo series with the 11-methyl and 11-methoxy derivatives. Thus it is possible to extend the postulated series of reactions shown in Fig. 15.3 in two ways to obtain the known carcinogens, 3-methoxy-17-methylcyclopenta-(a)-phenanthrene, (1) and 17-methylcyclopenta-(a)-phenanthrene. In addition, the 11α-hydroxylation of steroids has been demonstrated with a wide range of soil organisms (Capek *et al.,* 1966); if this reaction is also performed on the dehydrogenated product by gut bacteria, it opens the way for 11-methoxy formation, possibly by a similar pathway to that observed in 17-methoxy oestradiol formation (Chapter 9).

Thus gut bacteria produce substances known to be carcinogenic from endogenous steroids (bile acids and cholesterol in particular), and it can reasonably be postulated that bacteria might be capable of producing a polycyclic aromatic molecule from the steroid skeleton. Is this relevant to human cancer? We believe that it may be relevant in the aetiology of cancer

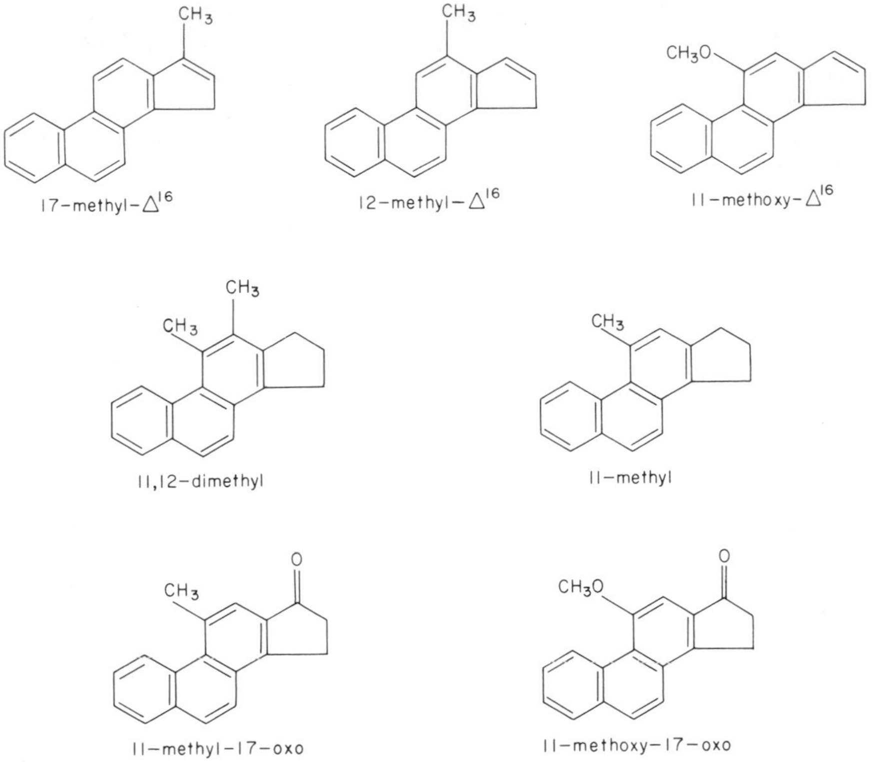

Fig. 15.4. The structures of some carcinogenic cyclopentaphenanthrenes.

of the colon and of cancer of the breast, and this is discussed later in this chapter.

B. Production of Phenols and their Possible Significance

The metabolism of tyrosine to yield phenolic metabolites was described in Chapter 6, Section VII; the major phenols produced are phenol, p-cresol and p-ethylphenol together with a range of phenolic acids.

Boutwell and Bosch (1959) demonstrated that local application of some phenols promotes the development of skin tumours in mice if it follows a single initiating dose of the potent carcinogen dimethyl benzanthracene. This indicates that phenols have a co-carcinogenic effect; the phenols tested and found to be active, included phenol, p-cresol and 2-ethylphenol. Similar evidence of tumour promoting activity in phenols was obtained by Wynder and Hoffmann (1968).

There is further evidence that is compatible with the hypothesis that the co-carcinogenic effect of phenols may play a role in cancer. Tannenbaum and Silverstone (1949) found that feeding a low protein diet to C3H mice reduced the incidence of spontaneous hepatomas, suggesting that protein or protein metabolites may be involved in the formation of these tumours. Similarly, animals fed a low protein diet were more resistant to the spontaneous formation of mammary tumours (White and White, 1944). It is known that a low protein diet results in an alteration in the activity of intestinal mucosal enzymes (Deo *et al.*, 1965; Solimano *et al.*, 1967; Platt *et al.*, 1964) and of hepatic enzymes (Novikoff, 1959) and this may provide the explanation of the effects of changes in dietary protein, but it is also known that such a diet results in a decreased rate of urinary excretion of phenols (Bakke, 1969d). Similarly, Grant and Roe (1969) showed that germ-free status significantly protected male C3H mice from the early development of liver-cell tumours in response to dimethyl benzanthracene given shortly after birth, and significantly protected mice of both sexes, to the development of malignant lymphoma, mammary, ovarian and uterine tumours following the same treatment. Thus the gut flora produces a known co-carcinogen from protein in the diet, and the removal of the gut flora or reduction in the dietary protein protects animals from carcinogenic activity. In the light of this a role for these phenols in the aetiology of cancer should not be ignored and may be relevant in cancer of the colon, where there is a good correlation between the incidence of colon cancer and the amount of protein in the diet.

C. Bacterial Metabolism of Tryptophan and its Relation to Cancer

It has been suggested (Price, 1966; Bryan, 1969; Yoshida *et al.*, 1971; Bryan, 1971) that an increased rate of excretion of tryptophan metabolites may result in an increased risk of bladder cancer. This suggestion stems from the work of Dunning *et al.* (1950) who showed that a high incidence of bladder cancer resulted when rats were fed 2-acetylaminofluorene combined with DL-tryptophan or indole. No such tumours were produced by 2-acetylaminofluorene alone. These results were confirmed by Boyland *et al.*, (1954) who further showed that tryptophan could be replaced by indoleacetic acid or indole; in contrast, 2-acetylaminofluorene could not be replaced by benzidine or by β-napthylamine. It was later shown by Dyer and Morris (1961) that 2-acetylaminofluorene stimulates tryptophan metabolism and that pyridoxine reverses this effect; they suggested that it is the disturbed metabolism of tryptophan which results in the carcinogenesis with 2-acetylaminofluorene merely causing the disturbance.

The metabolism of tryptophan by gut bacteria has been discussed in Chapter 6. Many of the products are aromatic amines (Fig. 15.5), and there is a considerable body of evidence to implicate aromatic amines in the

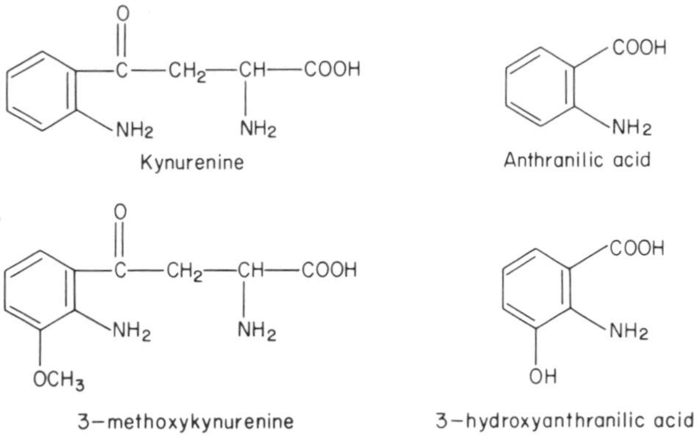

Fig. 15.5. Some aromatic amino metabolites of tryptophan.

aetiology of bladder cancer. A number of studies have shown that in patients with bladder cancer there is an increased rate of urinary excretion of the aromatic amines anthranilic acid, 3-hydroxy-anthranilic acid, kynurenine and 3-hydroxy-kynurenine compared with normal controls (Boyland and Williams, 1956; Brown et al., 1960; Quagliarello et al., 1961). Price and Brown (1962) investigated patients with industrial bladder cancer and found that the tryptophan metabolite concentration was normal showing that a raised concentration was not due to the presence of a bladder tumour per se. Urinary tryptophan metabolite concentration, in addition to being related to the incidence of bladder cancer, is also used as an indicator for breast cancer, since approximately half of such patients excrete elevated urinary concentrations of tryptophan metabolites (Rose, 1967; Rose et al., 1971). Hepatic tryptophan metabolism is controlled by steroid hormones, and this increase in metabolism could be due either to an absolute rise in oestrogen level or an impairment in androgen production; it has been demonstrated that in patients with elevated urinary concentrations of tryptophan metabolites the urinary level of an androgen (aetiocholanolone) is significantly reduced (Davis et al., 1970) supporting the latter explanation.

There have been a number of investigations into the carcinogenicity of tryptophan metabolites in addition to those of Dunning et al. and Boyland et al. referred to earlier. The structural similarity between some tryptophan metabolites and some known bladder carcinogens is illustrated in Fig. 15.6. A number of tryptophan metabolites have been tested for carcinogenicity by the bladder implantation technique. For these studies, the test compound is mixed with a suitable substance (such as cholesterol) and inserted as a small pellet into the bladder lumen. The test compound is then leached out slowly by urine over a prolonged period of time and so comes

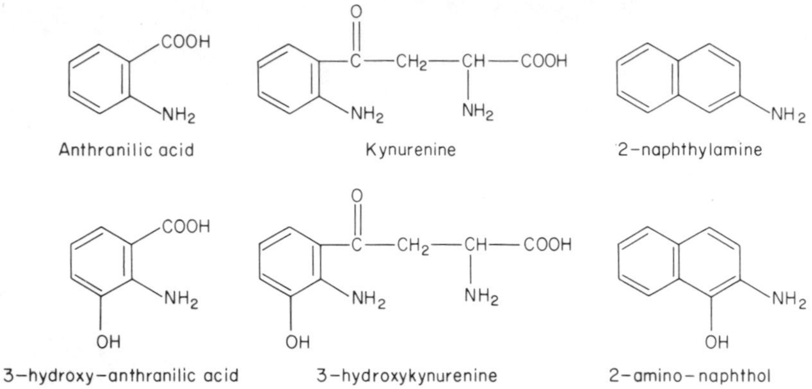

Fig. 15.6. The relationship between some tryptophan metabolites and some known bladder carcinogens (Rose, 1972).

into contact with the bladder mucosal surface. Using this technique Allen *et al.* (1957) obtained a 27% incidence of tumours in the bladders of mice exposed to 3-hydroxy-kynurenine and 3-hydroxy-anthranilic acid. The method has been refined by Bryan and his colleagues (for example, Bryan and Springberg, 1966; Bryan, 1969) and they have concluded that, as judged by this technique, 8-hydroxy-quinaldic acid, and xanthenuric acid and its 8-methylether, 3-hydroxy-kynurenine and 3-hydroxy-anthranilic acid are carcinogenic and, in addition, kynurenine, quinaldic acid and acetyl-kynurenine might also be active. Of these, quinaldic acid and 8-hydroxy-quinaldic acid are produced only by the gut flora, whilst the others are produced by mammalian and bacterial enzymes. 3-hydroxy-anthranilic acid, given in the absence of a foreign body, produces both leukaemias and lymphorecticular tumours (Bryan, 1968) although none of the tryptophan metabolites tested was able to give rise to bladder tumours under these conditions. However, Bryan and Springberg (1966) showed that although the 8-methylether of xanthenuric acid injected subcutaneously gave no tumours; tumours appeared if a pellet of pure cholesterol had previously been inserted into the mouse bladder. In addition 3-hydroxy-kynurenine and 3-hydroxy-anthranilic acid are mutagenic to cultured mammalian tissue cells (Kuznetsova, 1969).

There is little data on the contribution of the bacterial flora to the urinary tryptophan metabolite concentration. Of the metabolites known to be present in urine, indole, quinaldic and 8-hydroxy-quinaldic acid are due soley to the gut bacteria, but the flora will also make a contribution to the level of the other metabolites as well. Studies of germ-free as compared to conventional animals would add considerably to our knowledge of this subject, as would a study of the urine of patients undergoing bowel sterilization prior to colonic surgery.

D. BACTERIAL PRODUCTION OF N-NITROSAMINES

The production of N-nitrosamines by bacteria from nitrate or nitrite and secondary amines has been discussed in Chapter 6. The relevance of nitrosamine formation to human cancer is dealt with later in this chapter.

E. MISCELLANEOUS BACTERIAL REACTIONS YIELDING CARCINOGENS

1. *Ethionine production*
Ethionine is the S-ethyl analogue of methionine and was first discovered as a synthetic carcinogen (Farber, 1963) who showed that in the rat it is incorporated into protein in several tissues *in vivo*. This presumably requires activation of the carboxyl group with ATP, but Farber showed that in the rat liver the S-atom was also activated by ATP and the resulting S-adenosyl-ethionine appeared to ethylate some of the hepatic nucleic acid.

Studies of bacterial cultures grown in mineral salts-glucose medium supplemented with sulphate or methionine have shown that ethionine is produced by a number of species, including *Esch. coli* (Fisher and Mallette, 1961); the ethionine was in the free amino acid form within the cells and in the culture supernatant, and was not incorporated into bacterial protein. Thus any ethionine produced *in vivo* in the human gut would be available for carcinogenic action against the host. As yet, the production of ethionine in the gut has not been extensively studied.

2. *Hydrolysis of conjugated carcinogens*
The bacterial hydrolysis of cycasin to yield the carcinogen methylazoxy-methanol has been discussed in Chapter 5, Section III. To what extent this hydrolysis of plant glycoside to yield a carcinogenic aglycone in the gut as a general reaction is not known. A number of polycyclic aromatic hydrocarbons are known to undergo entero-hepatic circulation (Smith, 1966) and presumably the gut flora contributes to this by hydrolysing glucuronide conjugates produced in the liver prior to biliary secretion. Again, this is a subject that has not been extensively studied and would appear to warrant further attention.

II. Production of nitrosamines by bacteria, and its relation to human cancer

The nitrosamines probably consitute the group of carcinogens most intensively studied. This is because they are extremely potent carcinogens and are organ specific, the target organ depending on the test animal, the nitrosamine and the dosage used.

Thus, dimethylnitrosamine given in repeated small doses gives rise to liver tumours in rats, but if given in a single large dose produces kidney tumours in the same animal. Dibutyl-nitrosamine and N-nitrosopiperidine, also when administered to the rat, give rise to bladder and oesophageal tumours respectively. Table 15.1 gives some examples of the types of tumours that can be produced with nitrosamines.

TABLE 15.1

Some examples of the types of tumours that can be obtained using nitrosamines (for details see Magee and Barnes, 1967)

Tumour site	Nitrosamine used	Test animal	Conditions used
Liver	DMN	Rat	In food
Kidney	DMN	Rat	Single large dose i.p.
Lung	N-nitrose piperidine	Hamster	s.c. twice weekly
Oesophagus	N-nitroso-N-methyl-aniline	Rat	In food or drinking water
Bladder	Dibutylnitrosamine	Rat	i.p.

The possible role of nitrosamines in human cancer has excited much interest since nitrate is widely used by the food industry as a preservative, and is in any case naturally present in many food-stuffs and in many supplies of drinking water. Secondary amines are also present in many food-stuffs (Table 15.2), although the documentation for this is somewhat

TABLE 15.2

Secondary amines present in human foodstuffs

Secondary amine	Food item
Dimethylamine	Fish, cooked meats, tea
Diethylamine	Fish, cooked meats, tea
Piperidine	Spices, bread flavours, tobacco smoke, cooked meat
Pyrrolidine	Wine, bread flavours, tobacco smoke, cooked meat
Sarcosine	Toothpaste
Piperazine	Drugs (e.g. treatment of worm infestations)
Others	Drugs, wines and fermented foods, tobacco smoke, etc.

scarce. The investigation of nitrosamines as an environmental hazard has centred on two main lines:

(a) The pre-formation of nitrosamines in food-stuffs (by the reaction of secondary amines with nitrite, the latter being produced by the bacterial reduction of nitrate) and in cigarette smoke. These studies have revealed reassuringly few examples of nitrosamines present in foods at levels greater than 5 μg/kg; some examples are given in Table 15.3.

TABLE 15.3

Levels of some nitrosamines found in foods

Food item	Nitrosamine reported	Concentration
Fish - salmon	DMN	about 10 ppb
- shad	DMN	about 10 ppb
- sable	DMN	about 10 ppb
Cooked meats		
- salami	DMN	10-20 ppb
- hams	DMN	about 10 ppb
- sausages	DMN	10-20 ppb
Cooked bacon	DMN, DEN N-nitro-sopyrrolidine	1-40 ppb
Spirits	DMN	< 10 ppb
	N-nitrosopyrrolidine	trace
	N-nitrosopiperidine	trace

(b) The formation of nitrosamines *in vivo* in the stomach via the acid catalysed reaction between secondary amines present in food and nitrite presumably added as a preservative. The amounts likely to be formed by this mechanism are small because normal food-stuffs contain only small amounts of secondary amine, and because nitrite is destroyed by acid conditions so that little is left for nitrosation. Although there is a wealth of information indicating that the stomach conditions in the rat are suitable for the formation of N-nitrosamines, there is little information on the amount of amines likely to be ingested, on which amines are present in which food items, and on the level of nitrate likely to be ingested.

The bacterial catalysis of the N-nitrosation reaction has been discussed previously, (Chapter 6); since bacteria are able to promote this reaction at physiological pH values, the sites in which nitrosamines might be formed *in vivo* must be extended to include all those in which nitrate, secondary amine and bacteria might coexist. Since bacteria are able to reduce nitrate to nitrite, the important factor is no longer the amount of ingested nitrite, which is likely to be small, but the amount of ingested nitrate, which will be considerably larger. Nitrate is present in high concentrations in many root vegetables (Table 15.4) as well as being present as a food additive in processed meat products and in drinking water. Although it is likely that

TABLE 15.4

Concentration of nitrate reported in some vegetable
sources (from Ashton, 1970)

Vegetable item	Nitrate concentration (mg/kg)
Radish (raw)	500-3000
Turnip (cooked)	1500
Carrots (raw)	100-200
Cabbage (raw)	200
Lettuce (raw)	about 1000
Kale (air dried)	37000
Broccoli (raw)	about 1000
Spinach (raw)	1000-2000
Beetroot (cooked)	2500
Celery (raw)	about 1000
Peas (raw)	10
Potato (raw)	10-100

only small amounts of secondary amines are ingested with food, quite large amounts of dimethylamine, piperidine and pyrrolidine are produced in the large bowel and excreted in the urine. This secondary amine level is independent of the day to day diet and is relatively constant. Thus, secondary amine will be present in the stomach and small intestine in small amounts dependent on the nature of the food consumed recently, and in the large intestine and urine in relatively large amounts independent of the diet.

A. THE FATE OF INGESTED NITRATE

The fate of ingested nitrate in rats has been studied by Hawksworth and Hill (1971). The rats were fed 120 μmoles of nitrate by stomach tube and the urine collected for 48 hours after feeding. In two of the rats 90% of the nitrate was recovered in the urine within 8 hours of feeding whilst the other two rats excreted 63% and 42% respectively in the same period of time. Thus most of the nitrate is excreted very rapidly and must be absorbed very rapidly from the upper small intestine, it is very unlikely that much nitrate could reach the large intestine if taken as an aqueous solution. Similar studies using guinea pigs have produced similar results. The higher daily volume of urine permitted hourly assays of urine nitrate (Fig. 15.7) which showed even more clearly how rapidly the ingested nitrate reached the

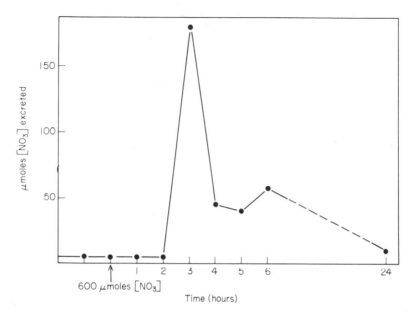

Fig. 15.7. The excretion of nitrate in guinea-pig urine after the administration of 600 μmoles nitrate by gastric intubation.

urine. In neither the rat nor the guinea pig was nitrite detected in the urine, indicating that any nitrite formed in the gut was either destroyed *in situ* by reaction for example with primary amines to yield nitrogen via the formation of an unstable diazonium salt,

$$R . NH_2 + HNO_2 \rightarrow [[R . N_2{}^+] \ {}^-OH] \rightarrow R . OH + N_2$$

or was destroyed by the nitrite oxidase enzymes present in erythrocytes during transport from the gut to the kidneys.

We know of no similar studies in humans, but comparison of normal urinary nitrate levels in people living in Worksop with those of people living in Paddington have been made. In Paddington the public water supply contains about 18 ppm of nitrate compared with 90 ppm in the drinking water of Worksop at that time. It has been estimated (Ashton, 1970) that the average weekly intake of nitrate is about 450 mg of which 72% is from vegetables and processed meat products, the remaining 28% being from the drinking water (Table 15.5). These average weekly intake figures apply to Paddington, but in Worksop, the high nitrate content of the drinking water resulted in a weekly nitrate intake more than double that of people living in Paddington; only 35% of this total was from food and 67% was from the drinking water (Hill *et al.*, 1973). Of 72 urine specimens from Paddington, 34 (47%) had no detectable nitrate, and the mean concentration was

TABLE 15.5

Estimated weekly nitrate intake in areas where the public water supply
contains 18 ppm and 90 ppm nitrate (based on data by Ashton, 1970)

Dietary nitrate source	Amount consumed per week	Mean nitrate content	mg nitrate consumed per week	
			Low nitrate area	High nitrate area
Processed meats	420 g	500 μg/g	210	210
Vegetables*	600 g	200 μg/g	120	120
Water	7 litres		126	630
			Totals 456	960

* Not including potatoes

1.0 mM. Only 2/72 had more than 5 mM nitrate (Fig. 15.8a). In contrast of 50 urine samples from Worksop only 8 (16%) had no detectable nitrate, the mean concentration was 2.6 mM, and 5/50 had more than 5 mM (Fig. 15.8b). Assuming that the normal volume of urine per day is about 1000 ml the daily excretion of nitrate in Paddington is about 60mg and in Worksop about 170 mg; these figures are very similar to those for the mean daily intake, indicating that in man, as in the rat and guinea pig, nitrate is excreted virtually quantitatively in the urine, and that very little, if any, nitrate reaches the large bowel (where it would be reduced and destroyed by the gut flora) and is therefore unavailable for nitrosation reactions at that site.

Thus in normal people, bacteria will be absent from the stomach and upper small intestine and the bladder, but will be present in large numbers in the large bowel. Nitrate will be present in the stomach, upper small intestine and the bladder, but absent from the large bowel, whilst secondary amines will be present in large amounts in the large bowel and the bladder, and in small amounts in the stomach and upper small intestine; there is no site at which all three reactants will co-exist.

However, there are a number of disease states that are relatively common and which will allow the reactants to coexist. Bladder infections are extremely common, and it has been shown by Sinclair and Tuxford (1971) that in a rural general practice in England the incidence of bladder infection was 186 per thousand patients per year. Urinary tract infections are much more common in women than in men, and more than 80% of these infections are due to *Esch. coli,* which is the organism which most effectively catalyses the N-nitrosation reaction. In the bladder there will be large amounts of secondary amine and nitrates; the bacterial counts are normally 10^9 organisms/ml (Savage *et al.,* 1967) and these organisms will

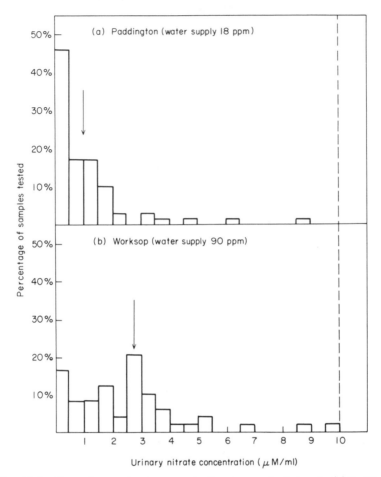

Fig. 15.8. The urinary nitrate concentration in people living in (a) Paddington; (b) Worksop. The vertical arrow indicates the mean value.

have plenty of time to act on the reactants, since in assymptomatic bladder infection the incubation time will optimally be overnight. Thus, the conditions for nitrosamine production—high reactant concentration, large numbers of organisms and long incubation time—are as nearly ideal as could be expected (apart from those in the colon where there would be many more bacteria and the transit time of 70 hours would allow much more time for nitrosation).

In order to demonstrate that nitrosamines produced in the bladder are a potential hazard it is necessary to demonstrate first that nitrosamines are, in fact, produced *in vivo*, and secondly, that nitrosamines produced in the bladder can get into general circulation and so reach the target organ.

We have demonstrated the *in vivo* production of nitrosamines in rats with experimental bladder infection (Hill and Hawksworth, 1972). Rats were anaesthetized, the bladder was exposed and a stitch inserted, followed by the injection of 0.5 ml containing 10^7 *Esch. coli.* The stitch acts as a foreign body and consequently a chronic bladder infection is set up. These rats were fed nitrate and piperidine or pyrrolidine, and the urine collected for 48 hours; the urine was shown to contain N-nitrosopiperidine or N-nitrosopyrrolidine depending on the amine fed to them. Thus the nitrosation is catalysed by bacteria *in vivo* when large amounts of amine and nitrate are fed to the rats; no nitrosamine was detected in the urine of uninfected rats or in infected rats fed only nitrate or only secondary amine. Unfortunately, these experiments cannot readily be performed using low levels of amine or nitrate since nitrosamine can only be confirmed using mass spectroscopy which requires relatively large amounts of nitrosamine. In agreement with these *in vivo* results in the rat, Brooks *et al.* (1972) have produced evidence which indicates the presence of dimethyl nitrosamine in the urine of a person with a bladder infection. The methods used were not definitive and were developed for the detection of nanogram levels of nitrosamine, but they suggest that a search for nitrosamines in the urine of people with bladder infections and ingesting large amounts of nitrate would be fruitful.

The next question is whether nitrosamines produced in the bladder can enter the blood system and so reach the target organ, despite the widely held belief that the bladder is an inert organ. It has been demonstrated that a number of tryptophan metabolites, glycine and glucose are absorbed from the urinary bladder (Bryan and Morris, 1966; Morris and Bryan, 1966; Bryan *et al.,* 1965). In our experiments C^{14} labelled dimethyl-nitrosamine or H^3 labelled nitrosopiperidine were introduced into the bladder via a bladder catheter (the ureters were first ligated to prevent reflux) and blood was collected via a carotid canula at intervals. C^{14} was detected in the blood within 5 minutes of introducing nitrosamine into the bladder, the level reaching a maximum value at approximately 30-60 minutes (Fig. 15.9). After various times such rats were sacrificed and the organs removed to see whether the C^{14} was bound by a "target". As expected the label concentrated in the liver and kidney (the major target organs for this nitrosamine in the rat). Similar studies with H^3-labelled N-nitrosopiperidine in the rat showed that the H^3 label is concentrated in the liver and the oesophagus (Table 15.6). In the hamster, N-nitrosopiperidine causes tumours of the lung, and when introduced into the bladder (in the H^3 labelled form) the label accumulated in the liver and the lung.

In addition to the infected bladder, the stomach of people with achlorhydria or anacidity will also be heavily colonized with bacteria and will be a site where bacteria, nitrate and secondary amine may be present

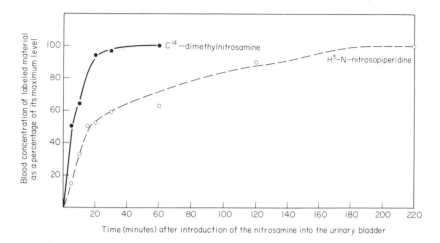

Fig. 15.9. Blood levels of labelled material at various times after the introduction into the rat urinary bladder of C^{14}-dimethylnitrosamine and H^3-nitrosopiperidine. The blood levels are expressed as the percentage of the maximum level reached.

TABLE 15.6

Distribution of ^{14}C and ^3H in the organs of rats 3 hours after the administration via a bladder catheter of ^{14}C-dimethylnitrosamine and ^3H-N-nitrosopiperidine respectively

Organ	% of counts following ^{14}C-dimethylnitrosamine	% of counts following ^3H-N-nitrosopiperidine
Blood	50	20
Liver	32	43
Kidney	6	25
Spleen	1	<1
Stomach	7	10
Oesophagus	<1	<1
Lung	2	0

together. Here, both the nitrate and secondary amines will be of dietary origin. The total gastric juice in achlorhydrics contains 10^5-10^7 organisms per ml of mixed flora (Drasar *et al.*, 1969) which is much lower than the numbers present in infected urine. The secondary amine concentration will also be lower than that in urine (since only dietary amine will be involved) and the incubation will be less than in the bladder (since the gastric emptying time is usually short). Production of nitrosamine from piperidine and nitrate in the isolated rat stomach by bacteria has been demonstrated by Alam *et al.* (1971). Because of its poor gastric acidity, the conditions in the normal rat stomach are similar to those in achlorhydric man. Solutions of the reactants were instilled into the isolated stomach and incubated *in vivo* for 40 minutes. The nitrosamine produced would be readily absorbed from the stomach or from the upper small intestine and so enter the general circulation.

There is, of course, no definitive data on the "target" sites of nitrosamines in humans, but epidemiological studies can, we believe, give some strong leads already; these should become very strong in the near future. The nitrosamines that might be produced *in vivo* are dimethyl-nitrosamine (in the stomach by acid or bacterially catalysed reactions, and in the urinary bladder) N-nitrosopiperidine and N-nitrosopyrrolidine (both in the urinary bladder) and there are a number of situations which are amenable to epidemiological study.

In Worksop the high nitrate content of the drinking water supply results in a greatly increased intake of nitrate per day (Table 15.5) and consequently a high gastric and urinary concentration of nitrate. Assuming that the incidence of urinary tract infection and of gastric achlorhydria in Worksop is not markedly different from that in the rest of the country this should result in an increased incidence of nitrosamine-induced cancer and this should be detectable epidemiologically. The cancer deaths for the years 1958-1971 were analysed by site, age and sex and compared with the expected numbers (derived from the data from the Sheffield cancer registry). This analysis showed that, whilst the numbers of deaths from cancer of the bladder, breast, lung and colon were similar to those expected, there was an increased number of deaths from cancer of the stomach, liver, kidney and oesophagus in both men and women (Table 15.7). Although the most spectacular increase was in the deaths

TABLE 15.7

Number of cancer deaths in Worksop during the period 1958-1971 compared with the numbers expected from the age structure of the population and the death rates for the Sheffield registry area

Site of tumour	Male deaths		Female deaths	
	Expected	Found	Expected	Found
Stomach	70	93(+33)	43	83(+93)
Liver	1.8	10(+456)	1.4	8(+472)
Oesophagus	10.4	14(+34)	8.0	10(+25)
Kidney	6.6	13(+97)	3.4	5(+47)
Bladder	39	37(−5)	12	12(0)
Breast			133	119(−10)

(Figures in brackets indicate the percentage difference)

from primary hepatic carcinoma (563%), it must be noted that the numbers were small and that diagnosis of primary hepatic carcinoma is not easy and not absolutely reliable. However, the increased number of deaths from stomach cancer was very significant because of the large numbers involved, the age distribution of the increase (mainly in the oldest age groups) and the sex difference (a much greater increase in female than in male deaths). This encourages us to investigate cancer of the stomach further. The increased deaths from cancer of the oesophagus was noted but was not investigated further because of the numbers involved.

The death rate from stomach cancer varies with social class (Stocks, 1960), rainfall, longitude and latitude (Gardner *et al.*, 1969) within the U.K. A number of control towns whose water supplies contained less than 10 ppm nitrate were selected where the population had the same social class structure (obtained from the 1961 census) and which were close to Worksop (to take account of the other relevant variables) and the deaths from stomach cancer for a recent ten year period obtained. From this data, and from the age structure of the population, the death rates per 100,000 per annum were calculated and compared with those for Worksop. The results showed that after the known important factors had been taken into account, the number of deaths from stomach cancer in a population consuming large amounts of nitrate were very much higher than those in populations consuming much smaller amounts of nitrate (Table 15.8). The nitrosamine most likely to be produced in the stomach from dietary sources is dimethylnitrosamine, and the evidence of Brooks *et al.* (1972) would indicate that it is also the most likely to be formed in the bladder. The data from Worksop are compatible with the hypothesis that bacteria in the stomach or bladder produce dimethylnitrosamine which then gives rise

TABLE 15.8

Death rates from gastric cancer in Worksop and in some control (low-nitrate) areas

	Death rates per 10,000 per annum							
	Males				Females			
	35-44	45-64	65-74	>75	35-44	45-64	65-74	>75
Sheffield	0.3	6.2	21.4	31.0	0.3	2.3	8.8	22.8
Wakefield	0.3	4.5	17.7	23.0	0.3	2.6	11.5	15.7
Chesterfield	0.5	3.2	18.9	28.8	0.4	3.2	9.8	22.5
Doncaster	0.3	4.4	18.7	31.6	0.1	0.6	8.5	21.6
Matlock	0.5	2.2	11.2	9.8	0	1.6	3.5	13.6
Total controls	0.3	5.3	20.2	29.2	0.3	2.3	8.9	21.7
Worksop	0.8	5.3	22.2	49.0	0.6	2.5	15.2	42.0

to gastric carcinoma. It is now necessary to look for supporting evidence for this hypothesis. Correa *et al.* (1970) have noted that in Narino, a southern province of Colombia, the incidence of gastric cancer is much higher than in the rest of Colombia. Further investigations of this area has revealed towns where the nitrate content of the drinking water is very high and where the death rate from stomach cancer is also alarmingly high (Gordillo, private communication). A study of this area should throw light on the questions (a) how much nitrosamine is formed under these conditions in the infected bladder, and (b) is dimethylnitrosamine the only nitrosamine formed or are the N-nitroso derivatives of piperidine and pyrrolidine also formed?

It has been noted by Stahlsberg and Taksdal (1971) that patients who have undergone gastric surgery for the removal of benign lesions more than 15 years before death have a higher incidence of gastric cancer than do normal control patients. In contrast, those dying within 15 years of such surgery have no increased incidence of gastric cancer and in fact appear to be at slightly less risk than the normal population. Most of the surgical procedures cited results in gastric achlorhydria and colonization of the stomach by bacteria (Drasar and Shiner, 1969). It is generally accepted that patients with pernicious anaemia (and, therefore, gastric achlorhydria) have an increased death rate from gastric cancer. These are conditions which would permit bacteria to produce nitrosamines in the stomach from dietary material. The nitrosamine most likely to be produced would be dimethyl-nitrosamine. The long latent period before cancer is manifest, observed by Stahlsberg and Taksdal, is in agreement with the Worksop data (which also implies lengthy latent period).

Thus there is a body of circumstantial evidence compatible with the hypothesis that bacteria can produce nitrosamines *in vitro*, that these are relevant to human cancer, and that the target organ of dimethylnitrosamine is the stomach.

III. Bacteria, steroids and cancer of the colon

A. EPIDEMIOLOGICAL CONSIDERATIONS

Cancer of the large bowel is much more common in North-West Europe and in North America than in Africa, Asia and in South America (Doll, 1967, 1969). The areas with a low incidence of the disease, with the exception of Japan, have a low standard of living and the high incidence areas have a high standard. The geographical differences do not appear to be explicable on a racial basis, since the Japanese who migrate to California retain their low incidence while they retain their original cultural habits; but subsequent "westernized" generations have a higher, more "Californian" incidence of colon cancer (Buell and Dunn, 1965). Similarly, increasing "westernization" of Japanese in Japan is associated with an increased incidence of colon cancer (Wynder *et al.*, 1969). Nor can geography explain the difference since, in addition to the data on "westernized" Japanese, the three racial groups in South Africa and in Hawaii differ in their incidence in colon cancer (Doll, 1969) despite the fact that they live in the same external environment.

Several studies have indicated a possible relation between colon cancer and diet, although there is a singular lack of unanimity about the responsible dietary component (as is illustrated in Table 15.9) with all major components being incriminated. We have analysed the FAO statistics

TABLE 15.9

The dietary items implicated by various authors in the aetiology of colon cancer

Dietary component	Reference
Fat	Wynder and Shigematsu (1967)
	Wynder *et al.* (1969)
Protein	Gregor *et al.* (1969)
Refined sugar	Burkitt (1969)
Roughage (lack of)	Walker *et al.* (1970)
	Burkitt (1971)

on food consumption, the U.N. data on *per capita* income, and various measures of standard of living (Drasar and Irving, 1973). Dietary protein and fat correlate much more closely with the incidence of colon cancer than do either the other diet components or the measures of living standards (Table 15.10) with animal protein and combined fat (i.e. that which is present in meat and vegetables, and excluding cooking fats and oils, butter etc.) giving the best correlations (Fig. 15.10). In addition, from the same statistics, we have calculated the roughage intake assuming that (a) vegetables contain an average 3% roughage, and (b), the cereal used in Western countries is highly milled and contains no roughage whereas that used in Africa, Asia etc. is unmilled and contains 3% fibre, and the correlation between this derived figure and the incidence of colon cancer is included in Table 15.10.

Studies of the correlation between the intake of individual food items and the incidence of colon cancer have not proved fruitful, but a study by Berg *et al.* (1972) of Japanese people living in Hawaii showed a correlation with the intake of meat.

TABLE 15.10

The relation between various measures of standard of living and the
incidence of colon cancer (from Drasar and Irving, 1973)

		Correlation coefficient with colon cancer incidence
Diet		
Total fat		0.81
Animal fat		0.84
Bound fat		0.88
Total protein		0.70
Animal protein		0.87
Refined sugar		0.32
	cereals	−0.31
Fibre containing foods	potatoes and starchy foods	−0.10
	nuts	0.10
	vegetables	0.05
	fruit	0.22
Other measures		
Income		0.70
Vehicles		0.76
T.V. sets		0.24

B. HYPOTHESES

There are two major hypotheses concerning the role of diet in the aetiology
of colon cancer. These place prime importance on dietary fibre and dietary
fat and protein respectively; there is a considerable overlap between the
approach of these two groups. Both groups accept that the carcinogen is
not ingested as such but that it is produced *in situ* in the colon. Our
hypothesis is that:

(a) bacteria can produce carcinogens or co-carcinogens from dietary
components or from intestinal secretions produced in response to the diet;

(b) the nature of the diet affects the composition of the intestinal
bacterial flora;

(c) since diet controls the amount of substrate for carcinogen formation,
the nature of the flora acting on it, and to some extent the conditions
under which the reactions take place, this would explain the correlation
between diet and the incidence of colon cancer.

To a considerable extent this is common ground, and it is at this point
that the two groups diverge.

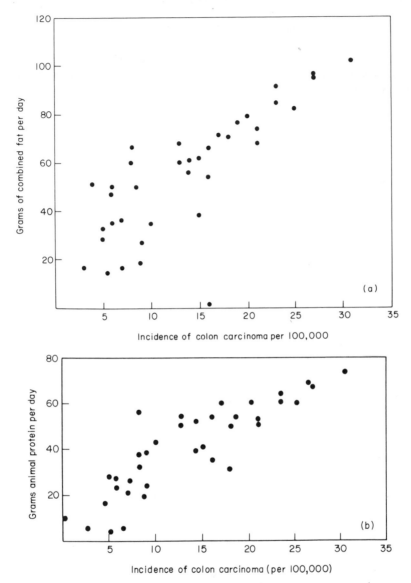

Fig. 15.10. The correlation between the incidence of colon cancer and (a) bound fat; (b) total animal protein.

The role of fibre in the aetiology of colon cancer has been strongly advocated by Burkitt (1971) and by Walker (1970); it has received a wide measure of support. The argument put forward by Burkitt is that diseases which have a common cause will be associated in geographical distribution

HIF–8*

and also in individuals. "Conversely, when two or more diseases are recognized as associated in geographical distribution or in individuals, they may be suspected of having common or related causes". He then points out the association between diverticular disease, appendicitis, peptic ulcer, coronary disease and colon cancer, and supports Cleave's hypothesis (1956) that these are all related to refined carbohydrate leading to a deficiency in dietary fibre. He suggests, in agreement with Walker *et al.* (1970) that the low fibre content of a western diet results in faecal arrest which leads to modification of the gut flora, degradation of bile salts to produce carcinogens and then carcinogenesis.

Burkitt *et al.* (1973) have demonstrated that the intestinal transit time in Africans living on a high fibre diet is short compared with that of western man living on a low fibre diet. Thus, in the generalized hypothesis set out above, they would place most importance in (c) on the conditions in the gut, the rapid transit in Africans making (a) and (b) unimportant.

The relation between colon cancer and dietary fat was suggested by Wynder and Shigematsu (1967) and by Wynder *et al.* (1969) and we have extended this (Aries *et al.*, 1969; Hill *et al.*, 1971; Drasar and Hill, 1972). Our main stress is on points (a) and (b) with less stress on the intestinal conditions. As has been shown (in Section I of this chapter) a number of steroids are known to be carcinogens, and it is possible that bacteria might be able to produce a substituted cyclopentaphenanthrene structure from the steroid nucleus. The amount of bile acid in the faeces is very dependent on the amount of fat in the diet (Hill, 1971) as illustrated in Fig. 15.11, so that our working study was to investigate:

(a) the bacterial flora in faeces of people living in areas with high and low risks of colon cancer;
(b) the faecal steroids of people living in high and low risk areas;
(c) the ability of bacteria to modify the bile acid molecule;

The countries studied were England, Scotland and the United States (all high risk countries) and Uganda, India and Japan (as low risk countries).

The effect of diet on the gut flora has been discussed in Chapter 3. In summary, the flora of the low risk countries contained fewer bacteroides, more streptococci and a lower ratio

$$\frac{\text{anaerobic bacteria}}{\text{aerobic bacteria}}$$

(Table 15.11). Within the enterococci, people from low risk countries had a higher proportion of *Strep. faecium* and a lower proportion of *Strep. faecalis* so that, although Ugandans had 20 times as many enterococci per gram as did English people, the difference in the numbers of *Strep. faecium* was 60 fold (Table 15.12). The Gram-positive non-sporing anaerobes

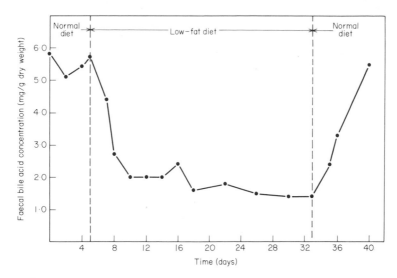

Fig. 15.11. The effect of dietary fat on the faecal bile acid concentration. The low fat diet contained less than 30 g fat per day compared with the normal diet which contained 100-120 g fat per day.

TABLE 15.11

The faecal bacterial flora of people living in areas where the incidence of colon cancer is high (England, Scotland, United States) or low (Uganda, India, Japan); taken from Hill *et al.* (1971)

	Mean $\log_{10}$ colonies per g wet weight					
	England	Scotland	U.S.A. (white)	Uganda	India	Japan
Anaerobes						
Bacteroides	9.8	9.8	9.8	8.2	9.2	9.4
Bifidobacteria	9.8	9.9	10.1	9.3	9.6	9.7
Clostridia—op$^+$ve	4.2	4.2	3.4	4.0	4.2	4.6
op$^-$ve	5.7	5.6	5.5	5.1	5.7	5.5
Veillonella	4.2	3.8	3.4	5.3	5.8	5.7
Aerobic						
Enterobacteria	7.9	7.6	7.4	8.0	7.9	9.3
Enterococci	5.8	5.3	5.9	7.0	7.3	8.1
Bacillus spp.	3.7	3.3	3.6	4.5	4.9	4.4
Lactobacillus spp.	6.5	7.7	6.5	7.2	7.6	7.4
Streptococcus	7.1	6.8	7.0	7.8	7.9	8.5
$\log_{10} \dfrac{\text{anaerobes}}{\text{aerobes}}$	2.1	2.5	2.7	1.1	1.5	0.5

TABLE 15.12

Enterococci of people living in India and England

	England	India	Indian English
Total enterococci	6.3×10^5	2.0×10^7	31.5
No. of *Strep. faecalis*	4.1×10^5	4.4×10^6	10.7
No. of *Strep. faecium*	2.0×10^5	1.3×10^7	65.0
No. of *Strep. bovis/equinus*	0.2×10^5	2.7×10^6	135.0

TABLE 15.13

Faecal steroids of people living in various countries

Population studied		Acid steroids				Neutral steroids		
		% tri-subst.	% di-subst.	% mono + unsubst.	Total	% Cholesterol	% Coprostanol	Total
England	(71)	11	43	46	5.56	29	63	10.83
Scotland	(18)	5	46	49	6.18	29	66	10.10
U.S.A.								
white	(42)	10	44	46	6.12	32	61	11.19
black	(12)	–	–	–	6.27	28	66	10.37
S. Africa								
white	(13)	12	54	34	5.56	40	52	.8.51
black	(23)	15	52	33	·2.60	56	32	4.47
Uganda	(11)	12	56	32	0.45	45	49	1.82
India	(18)	10	69	21	0.51	38	55	1.51
Japan	(36)	34	51	15	1.23	60	36	4.47

isolated from the low incidence countries included many more Eubacteria than did those of the high incidence countries (Drasar *et al.*, 1973; Peach *et al.*, 1973).

The faecal steroid analysis (Table 15.13) showed that:

(a) the concentration of total acid steroids and total neutral steroids was much higher in faeces from people living in the high risk areas;

(b) the degree of dehydroxylation of acid steroids was much higher in people from high risk countries. Thus, 45-50% of the acid steroids of people living in high risk areas were mono or unsubstituted compared with 32%, 21% and 13% for Ugandans, Indians and Japanese respectively;

(c) similarly, the proportion of neutral steroid in the form of the products of microbial degradation of cholesterol were much higher in faeces of people from the high risk countries than in faeces of people from low risk areas.

Thus, if bacteria can make a carcinogenic compound from biliary steroids, then the faecal steroids from the high risk countries have been more extensively metabolized and are more likely to contain the relevant metabolite, and since the substrate concentration is also much higher the chances of significant amounts of the relevant compound being produced are greater.

Study of isolated pure strains indicated that a much greater proportion of the anaerobes from high risk countries were able to dehydroxylate cholic acid *in vitro* (Table 15.14); this is in accord with the more extensive dehydroxylation *in vivo* by these organisms.

TABLE 15.14

The ability of bacteria from various populations to 7α-dehydroxylate cholic acid

Organism	England	Scotland	U.S.A.	India	Uganda
Enterobacteria	0/87	0/30	—	0/32	0/180
Enterococci	10/90	12/30	—	0/24	5/162
Clostridia	24/70	17/38	6/10	0/14	4/60
Bacteroides	22/50	14/24	5/10	1/20	14/42
Bifidobacteria	23/57	13/24	5/10	1/20	5/137

In addition to the six countries listed, faecal steroid analyses have also been carried out on black and white South Africans living in Johannesburg, and on people living in Hong Kong, giving a total of 9 population groups. The relation between faecal steroid concentration and the incidence of colon cancer of these 9 groups (Fig. 15.12) shows a good correlation for total neutral steroid and total acid steriod and an extremely close correlation for dihydroxycholanic acids (mainly deoxycholic acid). Deoxycholic acid is one of the steroids which has been shown to be carcinogenic.

A further study has been undertaken of faeces from people living in Hong Kong. Here, the people were divided into three groups depending on their income. It is known that in Japan the higher income groups have a higher incidence of colon cancer, and this is thought to be related to the westernization of their diet. Our analysis (Table 15.15) showed that the concentration of faecal steroids in the three groups were different, the highest income group having more total neutral steroid, total acid steroid and dihydroxycholanic acid. From the dihydroxycholanic acid assays, we would predict that the high income group (more than £200 per month) would have a greater incidence of colon cancer than the low income group (approximately £40 per month) by a factor of 1.4-1.5. The data needed to check this is not, at present, available.

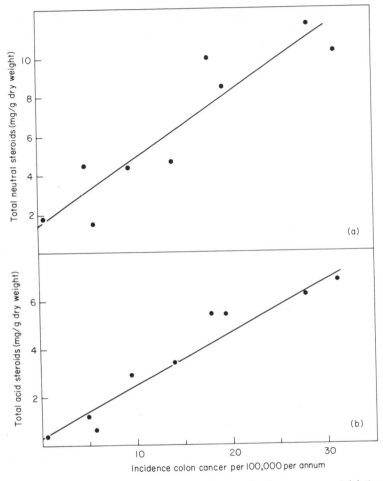

Fig. 15.12. The relation between the incidence of colon cancer and (a) the faecal neutral steroid concentration; (b) the faecal total acid steroid concentration.

In addition to the steroid metabolites, a number of products of protein metabolism have been shown to be co-carcinogenic; these include the phenolic products of tyrosine metabolism and the tryptophan metabolites. The incidence of colon cancer is closely correlated with the amount of dietary animal protein and it is very probable that the products of protein metabolism play a major part in the aetiology of colon cancer.

C. CONCLUSIONS

We have placed our stress on the substrate concentration for carcinogen formation, although we recognize the importance of the physiological

TABLE 15.15

Faecal steroids and bacteria in 3 income groups living in Hong Kong

	Population group		
	A	B	C
Acid steroids (mg/g dry weight)			
total	4.63	3.01	2.18
dihydroxy	1.47	1.16	1.10
Bacteria (Log counts/g wet weight)			
Bacteroides	9.7	9.6	9.3
Enterococci	4.7	5.4	6.0

A = income greater than £200 per month; B = between £80 and £120 per month; C = approximately £40 per month.

conditions within the gut. For example, in Chapter 7 the effect of E_h and pH on the dehydroxylase reaction is discussed and these varied with the population groups studied. The acid stool pH of the Africans and Indians studied is more likely to be due to disaccharidase deficiency than to the diet *per se,* and the mild fermentive diarrhoea induced by this must have some effect on transit times. If transit time is of supreme importance, as is suggested by those who favour fibre as the crucial dietary component in the aetiology of colon cancer, then lactase deficiency is probably of major importance. In studies of cancer patients Wynder *et al.* (1967) showed that neither constipation, nor the use of purgatives was associated with cancer of the colon. Further, there is little evidence that transit time as such, grossly affects the composition of the gut flora or their ability to degrade steroids. Our studies of obese patients and volunteer medical students living on a liquid diet containing no fibre showed that, though the transit time was so long that the interval between stool samples was often 14 days, the degradation of faecal steroids by the gut bacteria was the least found by us in any population (Crowther *et al.,* 1973). Even with the transit times found with Africans there is plenty of time for metabolism to proceed. However, the fibre content of the diet may well be of importance in determining the faecal carcinogen concentration. In the local production of a carcinogen in the gut, it is not the total daily production of carcinogen that is important but the concentration of carcinogen in contact with the gut wall. Thus the bulking effect of fibre might effectively dilute the carcinogen.

Knowledge of the aetiology of colon cancer might help us to virtually eliminate this, numerically, the second most important form of cancer. This could be achieved either by removing from the diet the substrates for carcinogen formation or by adding to the diet inhibitors which prevent carcinogen formation, or by adding bulking agents to the diet to dilute the carcinogen to an inactive concentration.

IV. Bacteria, steroids and cancer of the breast

Endocrine factors can undoubtedly be of major significance in the aetiology of breast cancer, and this is amply demonstrated by the beneficial effect of ovariectomy, adrenalectomy and hypophysectomy in curtailing the growth of some tumours (Huggins, 1967). These surgical treatments remove the oestrogen synthesizing sites from the body and there is a very strong evidence for a direct role for oestrogens in the aetiology of breast cancer either as a direct carcinogen or synergistically together with some other factor.

The evidence that oestrogens are carcinogenic has been described earlier in this chapter. In addition to the data showing that oestrogens are able to induce tumours in the breast (Lacassagne, 1932; Cutts, 1965) and in the kidney (Kirkman, 1959), many oestrogen dependent tumours have been described. In one of these the production of anti-oestrogen antibodies in the prospective host both delayed the onset of tumour growth and prolonged the survival of the animals. Thus, although the ability of oestrogen to induce primary tumours has been questioned it is undoubtedly true that they can stimulate the development of tumours once these have been induced (King, 1971) and removal of the oestrogen source results in regression of the tumour.

In addition to these endocrine factors, there is a wealth of data, both experimental and epidemiological, implicating diet in the aetiology of breast cancer. Carroll and Khor (1970) have investigated the effect of dietary fat on mammary tumour production in rats treated with 7,12-dimethyl-benzanthracene. Rats fed on a diet containing 20% corn oil developed more tumours than did control rats fed a low fat diet. The type of diet fed after treatment with the carcinogen had a greater influence on the production of mammary tumours than did the type fed before the carcinogen was given, indicating that the effect is excreted mainly at the promotional stage of mammary carcinogenesis, rather than at the induction stage. There is a lot of epidemiological data implicating diet in the aetiology of breast cancer, and many of the arguments run parallel to those already described for cancer of the colon. Thus, the incidence of breast cancer is high in North-West Europe and in North America, and is low in Africa, Asia and South America (Doll, et al., 1970). Within a country it is highest in the higher social economic classes. Japanese living in Hawaii have a higher incidence than those in Japan, although first generation migrants to

California retain their low incidence experience. This striking similarity between the epidemiology of colon cancer and cancer of the breast has led Wynder (1968) to postulate a role of dietary fat in the aetiology of breast cancer. He suggested that the dietary fat might lead to alterations in the mammary adipose tissue which result in increased hormone retention. We have postulated an alternative mechanism (Hill, *et al.*, 1971b) implicating the production of oestrogens by gut bacteria, described previously in Chapter 9. We know that bacteria are able to aromatize ring A of the steroid nucleus, and that people living in high incidence countries have a higher faecal concentration of acid and neutral steroids. Our hypothesis is, therefore, that

(a) bacteria can produce oestrogenic steroids in the gut from biliary steroids; oestrogens undoubtedly have a role in the development of mammary tumours;

(b) the amount of biliary steroid substrate is dependent on the amount of dietary fat;

(c) this rationalizes the observed relationship between dietary fat and breast cancer.

As with colon cancer, a number of measures of living standards are correlated with the incidence of breast cancer, but the best correlations are with dietary bound fat and animal protein (Fig. 15.13; Table 15.16). It is likely that, as with colon cancer, the products of protein metabolism which are known to be carcinogenic or co-carcinogenic, have an important role in the aetiology of breast cancer.

TABLE 15.16

The relation between various measures of standard
of living and the incidence of breast cancer (Drasar and
Irving, 1973)

	Correlation coefficient with breast cancer
Diet	
Total fat	0.80
Animal fat	0.80
Bound fat	0.78
Total protein	0.59
Animal protein	0.79
Refined sugar	0.50
Other measures	
Income	0.68
Vehicles	0.70
T.V. sets	0.31

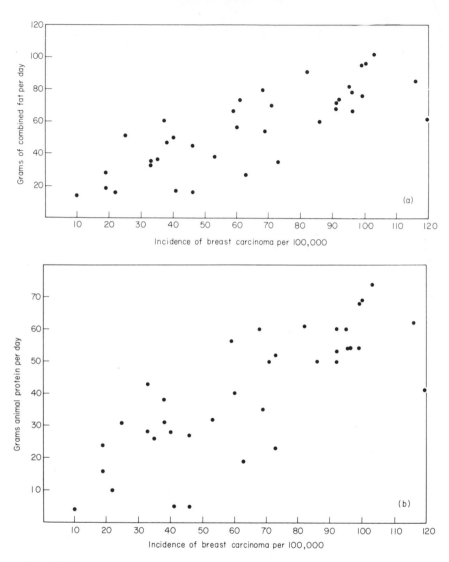

Fig. 15.13. The relation between the incidence of breast cancer and (a) dietary fat; (b) dietary animal protein.

If our hypothesis is true, then people living on a high fat diet should have higher levels of circulating oestrogenic steroid and also higher urinary levels. The normal production rate of oestradiol is 0.5 mg/day by the body (Hellman *et al.*, 1970); *in vitro*, pure cultures of clostridia achieve a 10% conversion to oestrogen steroids, and the daily excretion rate of faecal steroid is approximately 700 mg/day. Potentially, therefore, the gut flora

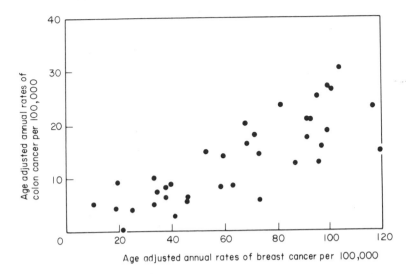

Fig. 15.14. The relation between the incidence of colon cancer and the incidence of breast cancer.

could make a very significant contribution to the body oestrogen pool. In a proportion of patients treated surgically there is a failure to prevent oestrogen synthesis, and, therefore, no improvement in the patient. In some of these the surgical failure may be due to poor technique, but in some it may be due to bacterial production of oestrogens preventing any significant fall in plasma oestrogen levels and a continuous supply to the tumour.

Since we have postulated that breast cancer and colon cancer have virtually the same aetiology (although that of breast cancer is complicated by a wide range of other factors) there should be a close correlation between the two, and this is illustrated in Fig. 15.14. The hypothesis is, at least, worthy of consideration and can give rise to a wealth of experimental studies which may prove to be wrong but will undoubtedly help to illuminate a rather hazy subject.

CHAPTER 16

Gut Bacteria and Hepatic Disease

Many of the products of bacterial metabolism in the gut are potentially toxic, including ammonia, pharmacologically active amines, phenols and phenolic acids and ethanol, all of which are produced by meat digestion. All of these are absorbed from the gut and travel to the liver via the portal blood system, where they are detoxified before excretion in the urine. The concentration of these potential toxins is high in the portal blood and low in the systemic venous blood. In any situation where the portal blood can by-pass the liver their concentration increases in the systemic blood and can reach toxic levels; this is the generally accepted aetiology of hepatic coma associated with cirrhosis or with porto-systemic anastamosis.

Cirrhotic patients often enter coma following a high protein meal or intestinal bleeding (see review by Sherlock, 1958) and it was concluded that the coma was the result of protein digestion. Different proteins have different abilities to trigger off hepatic coma, blood being the worst source of protein from the patient's point of view (Bessman et al., 1958) and milk and cheese diets being somewhat better than others (Fenton et al., 1966). Coma could also be induced by feeding urea, ammonium chloride and methionine. This has led to the conclusion that ammonia produced in the gut is the principal cause of hepatic coma, although the pharmacologically active amines and phenols may also be of importance.

I. Hyperammonemia

Intestinal bacteria produce ammonia via a variety of pathways (which have been discussed in Chapter 6), the principal of which is urea hydrolysis. Urea undergoes an enterohepatic circulation, being produced in the liver and then entering the colon by passive diffusion, where it is hydrolysed to ammonia and CO_2. The ammonia then re-enters the portal blood, again by diffusion, and returns to the liver to be converted back to urea. Approximately 15-30% of the total urea pool (i.e. about 7 g) is hydrolysed each day (Walser and Bodenlos, 1959; Jones et al., 1969).

The evidence for the existence of a mucosal urease is equivocal, but the major source of colonic urease is the gut bacteria. Faecal homogenates hydrolyse urea readily and urease is produced by a range of gut bacterial genera, including Klebsiella, Proteus, Bacteroides etc. Treatment of patients with neomycin or other antibiotics reduces the faecal urease activity (Evans *et al.*, 1966); in addition, germ-free animals fail to catabolize urea to any significant extent (Levenson *et al.*, 1959). In a recent publication, Wolpert *et al.* (1971), reported experiments indicating that urea is hydrolysed by bacteria in close association with the gut mucosa and not by those in the colonic lumen.

This conclusion was reached because urea delivered to the gut bacteria systemically was much more efficiently hydrolysed than that administered intraluminally. Hardly any urea is detectable in faeces, so that virtually all of the urea entering the gut is hydrolysed to ammonia.

In the normal healthy person, the ammonia generated in the gut is restricted to the portal blood system, but in hepatic disease the liver fails to detoxify the ammonia and it enters the general circulation (White *et al.*, 1955) and this results in the chronic or recurrent neuropsychiatric disorder related to protein intolerance. Ultimately the result is hepatic coma due to the direct cerebrotoxic effect of ammonia which has a direct toxic action on intermediary oxidative metabolism in the brain (Schenker *et al.*, 1967). Similar symptoms arise, for the same reasons, in protein intolerance due to portal-systemic anastamosis (Ridwell, 1955). Hyperammonemia has been reviewed by Summerskill (1969).

The major course of therapy of hepatic coma is the control of the intestinal ammonia production and nitrogen metabolism. This has been attempted by either (a) reducing the supply of nitrogen compounds to the gut, (b) reducing the number of ammonia-producing bacteria, (c) reducing the amount of time available for bacteria to produce ammonia, and (d) preventing the escape of ammonia from the gut. Reduction in the amount of protein in the diet reduces the amount of substrate available for ammonia production; different proteins also result in different blood ammonia levels. For example, blood protein is the best source of ammonia, results in the highest levels of ammonia in the circulating blood and stimulates hepatic coma very readily (Bessman *et al.*, 1958); this may explain the frequency with which hepatic coma is associated with intestinal bleeding. Milk and cheese diets have been recommended by Fenton *et al.* (1966) since the resultant blood ammonia level is lower than that resulting from a meat diet. It has been suggested that the reduced ammonia production may be due not only to an altered substrate but also to an altered gut flora, since milk is said to favour the growth of bifidobacteria and lactobacilli in the gut (both thought to be non-producers of urease). A direct reduction in the protein intake is often very difficult since the patients with neuropsychiatric symptoms are usually very protein sensitive and thus are close to nitrogen imbalance. Thus the treatment designed to remove one set of symptoms inevitably results in the acquisition of a new set.

Attempts to reduce the numbers of ammonia producing organisms has taken two forms, antibiotic therapy and replacement therapy. A number of antibiotics have been shown to reduce ammonia production in the colon for a short time; these include a range of broad spectrum antibiotics including neomycin (Wolpert *et al.*, 1969; Dawson *et al.*, 1957) and chlortetracycline (Sherlock *et al.*, 1956), but these antibiotics have the usual side effects of diarrhoea and steatorrhoea which often accompany disturbance of the gut flora, and staphylococcal enterocolitis (Walker *et al.*, 1965). Replacement therapy is based on the concept that, since many organisms fail to hydrolyse urea, replacement of the usual (ureolytic) flora with one that is non-ureolytic will solve the problem. Lactobacilli are non-urease producing organisms and these are fed to the patient in milk (usually 1-2 litres per day) with little sucess. Alternatively the bacteria may be administered as a powder (with no more success). The response of the gut flora to such therapy emphasizes once again its remarkable stability and, in the light of current knowledge on the factors controlling the gut flora, widespread success for such therapy would be very surprising.

The amount of ammonia produced should be reduced if the time available for its production is reduced, and this is the rationale behind the use of enemas and purgatives in the treatment of hepatic coma. Dawson *et al.* (1957) pointed out that their patients treated with neomycin produced three stools per day and suggested that their success with this treatment might be due to the purgative action of neomycin rather than its antibiotic activity. Bowel cleansing is a common treatment for hepatic coma associated with intestinal bleeding as a means of removing the blood from the bowel as rapidly as possible before it can be converted to toxic products (Bessman *et al.*, 1958). There is still some question regarding the amount of agent to be used and ultimate effectiveness of this treatment. Inevitably it would appear to be a short-term measure.

The fourth course of treatment is also, to us, the most intellectually attractive; this involves reducing the absorption of ammonia from the gut rather than trying to reduce the amount produced. Ammonia, in its non-ionized form, is readily absorbed from the colon by passive diffusion because the normal colonic pH is approximately equal to, or even somewhat higher than, that of the circulating blood. When the colonic pH is reduced, as for example, in fermentative diarrhoea, much of the ammonia is in the form of the ammonium ion and the ammonia will be on a pH gradient. In these conditions ammonia will move from the blood to the colon on the pH gradient rather than in the reverse direction on the concentration gradient and the blood ammonia level will be reduced without altering the amount produced in the gut. This is the rationalization for the lactulose therapy.

Lactulose (β 1-4 galactosylfructose) is the oxo-isomer of lactose differing only in the aglycone; nevertheless this is not a substrate for the β-galactosidase produced by the human small intestinal mucosa (Dahlquist and Gryboski, 1965). It is readily fermented, however, by the gut bacteria (Hoffmann *et al.*, 1964) and in particular by the enterococci, bifidobacteria and lactobacilli (but not by *Esch. coli*, the best producers of β-galactosidase) to fatty acids thereby reducing the colonic pH. The dose used is adjusted so as to induce two soft stools per day and under these conditions the faecal pH reaches 4-5 without causing undue discomfort (Bircher *et al.*, 1966; Elkington *et al.*, 1969). The virtue of this regime is that it allows the patient to increase his protein intake to 70 g per day without mental or neurological deterioration (Bircher *et al.*, 1966). The treatment will fail when either the colonic pH is not sufficently reduced or the symptoms are due to some protein breakdown other than ammonia.

Hepatic coma associated with cirrhosis and protein intolerance is a major clinical problem, because the condition of the patient by the time he reaches hospital is usually dire. Consequently no method of treatment is likely to produce good results in a high proportion of patients. The results, such as these, of hepatic failure are a measure of the efficiency with which the liver normally detoxifies intestinal ammonia.

II. Production of toxic amines and phenols

In addition to ammonia, bacteria produce a range of amines from protein by decarboxylation of the constituent amino acids; the failure to detoxify these may also contribute to the hepatic coma associated with cirrhosis. The mean blood ammonia level in hepatic coma patients is much higher than that in cirrhotics without coma, but many individuals with hepatic coma have normal blood ammonia levels. This suggests that although hyperammonemia is the main contributor to hepatic coma it is not the major factor in all cases. It is known that coma can be induced by the addition of methioine to the diet and the toxic effects are probably not entirely due to the ammonia produced (Phear and Ruebner, 1956). Bacteria produce a range of amines including tyramine, histamine, cadaverine, agmatine together with a number of unidentified amines (Melnykowycz and Johansson, 1955; Phear and Ruebner, 1956). The administration of oxytetracycline abolishes these amines from the blood. Perry *et al.* (1966) showed that there were a number of amines produced in the gut and excreted in the urine; these included histamine, tyramine, octopamine and piperidine. In two patients treated with monoamine oxidase inhibitors there were at least four additional amines present in the urine in addition to the normal amines, the concentration of these latter normal amines was much higher than in the control people. Thus it is evident that in normal circumstances the hepatic amine oxidase very efficiently detoxifies the amines produced in the gut. In cirrhosis the hepatic monoamine oxidase may be inactive or by-passed, so allowing the amines to freely circulate.

Many of the amines have pharmacological activity and are potentially toxic. Young rats have low levels of amine oxidase and so are unable to cope with large amounts of tyramine; consequently excess tyrosine in the diet is toxic and in sufficient quantities is lethal to young rats (Martin, 1942).

Tyramine, like the diamines cadaverine and putrescine, is a depressor substance whilst histamine and the mono-amines are pressor substances. In addition, agmatine has an insulin-like activity and histamine is known to stimulate the secretion of stomach acid, as well as having a general inflammatory activity increasing vascular permeability, leucotaxis etc. It has been suggested that histamine produced in the intestine may play a role in the aetiology of peptic ulcer associated with cirrhosis. The concentration of histamine in portal blood is much higher than that in the circulating blood (Anrep *et al.*, 1953). The excretion of histamine is increased by feeding meat (Irvine *et al.*, 1959a) the histidine released on meat hydrolysis being decarboxylated by the gut bacteria. It was further shown that histamine released in the gut can effect stomach acid secretion. (Irvine *et al.*, 1959a, b). He introduced histamine into the jejunum and, while small amounts had little effect, the stomach acid secretion was increased progressively as the amount of histamine increased. In a review of the influence of the liver on gastric secretion Clarke (1960) concluded that a humoral excitant of gastric secretion is released into the portal system from the enteric tract and is normally destroyed in the liver; it originates principally from the small bowel and colon and its production is stimulated by feeding meat. One such excitant is histamine although there may be others; the excitant becomes quantitatively of importance when the portal blood by-passes the liver via a shunt or due to cirrhosis.

III. Steatorrhoea and gallstones associated with hepatic disease

Cirrhotic patients have a reduced bile acid pool due to impairment of the bile synthesizing systems. The ratio of chenodeoxycholate to cholate in the pool is increased, as is the ratio of taurine/glycine conjugates.

Bacteria metabolize bile salts via hydrolysis of the amide bond to release free bile acids, then dehydroxylation of these free acids to produce the secondary bile acids. The secondary bile acids deoxycholate and lithocholate are toxic to mammalian cells and it might therefore be suspected that the products of bacterial metabolism would play a role in the side effects of hepatic disease. Such a role has proved difficult to establish.

The product of dehydroxylation of chenodeoxycholic acid, lithocholic acid, has a wide spectrum of toxic activities, summarized by Palmer (1970).

Experimental hepatic necrosis can be established in a wide range of laboratory animals by feeding lithocholate (Holsti 1960; Hunt, 1963, 1964, 1965). Cirrhosis is characterized by a high serum concentration of bile acids, and in particular a disproportionate increase in the concentration of serum chenodeoxycholate (Vlahcevic *et al.*, 1970). The level of lithocholate in serum tends to increase with the serum chenodeoxycholate level (Carey and Williams, 1965) and so it might be expected that relatively large amounts of lithocholate reach the liver. Studies of biliary bile acids in cirrhotics, however, reveal a very low level of secondary bile acids compared with levels in normal people. This low level of secondary bile acids in the bile cirrhotics must therefore (Vlahcevic *et al.*, 1970) be due to:

(a) A failure of the gut bacteria in cirrhotic patients to dehydroxylate chenodeoxycholic acid. Then, although in general the serum lithocholate level follows that of chenodeoxycholate, in these patients this relationship falls down;

or (b) a failure of the absorption of secondary bile acids from the colon of cirrhotics resulting in, once again, a failure of the relation between serum lithocholate and serum chenodeoxycholate to hold good;

or (c) a failure of the liver to deal with secondary bile acids via conjugation and re-secretion in the bile.

Thus, explanations (a) and (b) imply that the more toxic secondary bile acids never reach the liver and, therefore, can have no role in the perpetuation of human cirrhosis, whilst explanation (c) implies the opposite, that secondary bile acids reach the liver and are not detoxified and are, therefore, free to manifest their toxic activities. As yet there is no clear data available which would clarify this situation. However, (c) would fit best the animal studies.

The low concentration of biliary bile acids, both primary and secondary, results in a low luminal concentration of bile acids. When the concentration falls below the critical micellar concentration fat absorption is impaired resulting in the steathorrhea associated with cirrhosis. The role of the bile acids in fat absorption and the significance of the critical micellar concentration have been discussed already in Chapter 14.

Cholesterol is only poorly soluble in water and one of the functions of the bile salts is to be a component of the ternary mixture which keeps biliary cholesterol in solution. The physical chemistry of this ternary mixture has been reviewed by Small (1970); basically, for a given amount of cholesterol there are minimum amounts of bile salt and lecithin needed to maintain the cholesterol in solution. When the amount of bile salt falls below its critical concentration then some of the cholesterol precipitates, probably as microcrystals. If this process is prolonged then there is an agglomeration of these small crystals into macroscopic gallstones. Vlahcevic *et al.* (1972) have shown that, in non-cirrhotic people, the bile pool size of gallstone patients is much lower than that in control people. In both patients and controls the rate of synthesis of bile acids by the liver was 350 mg/day; the rate of turnover and faecal loss was much greater in the gallstone patients. The faecal loss of bile acids is dependent on the rate of microbial degradation (Kellog and Wostmann, 1969) so that here the gut bacteria may play a major role in the aetiology of gallstone formation. In cirrhotic patients this is compounded by impaired synthesis of bile acids on the liver, resulting in a further decrease in the acid pool and a further increase in the tendency of cholesterol to precipitate on the bile. In cirrhotic patients the degree of microbial responsibility for the reduced bile acid pool is probably small whereas in the non-cirrhotics the role of the gut flora can be crucial.

CHAPTER 17

The Significance of Gut Bacteria in Normal People

I. Ageing and survival

All diseases, not caused by specific pathogens, have been ascribed to alimentary toxaemia due to the activity of the intestinal bacteria (Hale White *et al.,* 1913). Metchnikoff (1907) considered that the life span was limited and senility caused by the auto-intoxication produced by intestinal putrefaction. In order to limit putrefaction he advocated the replacement or suppression of the putrefactive flora by a lactic flora and stated that this could be achieved by fermented milk products containing large numbers of lactobacilli. A vogue developed for the use of Lactobacillus milk and other means of transforming the flora (Rettger and Cheplin, 1921; Dugeon, 1926). The effectiveness of such treatments in the implantation of *Lactobacillus acidophilus* was not proved, only the numbers of lactobacilli poured into the gut assisting their persistence (Rettger *et al.,* 1935). Indeed although the contention that the toxic wastes of the intestinal flora cause disease is a plausible one, it rests largely on unproven assumptions (Topley and Wilson, 1936). Interest in auto-intoxication lapsed because of the lack of any firm data until re-awakened by studies on liver disease (Philips *et al.,* 1952).

Recent studies of gnotobiotic animals have shown the need to re-examine this problem. In a study of cholesterol metabolism the cholesterol content of the aorta in old germ-free rats was found to be significantly lower than that in control animals, (Wostmann and Wiech, 1961). This observation parallels the finding of Gordon *et al.* (1966) that germ-free mice lived approximately 100 days longer than conventional animals. At death the ages of the genetically similar mice were, in days (mean and standard errors); germ-free males 723 ± 19; females 681 ± 12; conventional males 480 ± 10; females 516 ± 10. The increased survival of males, relative to females, in the germ-free group as compared with the conventional animals may be related to the females' greater resistance to infection (Wheater and Hurst, 1962).

Although these studies seem to demonstrate the involvement of the intestinal flora in ageing the component of the flora involved has not been identified, and much more work is necessary before concepts formulated by Metchnikoff (1907) could be seriously revived.

II. Nutrition and digestion

The existence of germ-free animals that have bred for generations in the absence of bacteria indicates that the intestinal flora is not essential for life. Indeed the addition of antibiotics to animal feeds leads to increased growth that may be attributable to a reduction of the intestinal bacteria of the host. Mice raised in a clean environment have a simplified flora and utilize food more efficiently (Dubos, 1965). Ruminants are dependent on bacterial action for the utilization of their normal diet (Hungate, 1966) and non-ruminants may obtain as much as 20% of their energy requirements by the caecal absorption of bacterial products (McBee, 1970). Bacterial products are absorbed from the human colon but the extent of their contribution to nutrition is uncertain (Hotzel and Barnes, 1966).

A. VITAMINS

Intestinal bacteria are able to synthesize vitamins and may require them for growth (Table 17.1). The degree to which these benefit man is a matter of debate and colonic absorption occurs only slowly (Wiseman, 1964). This latter difficulty is overcome in some animals by the practice of coprophagy

TABLE 17.1

Vitamin requirements of selected intestinal bacteria

Selected intestinal bacteria	Minimal vitamin requirement for growth*			Utilization of vitamin B_{12}
	Growth in vitamin-free mineral salts media	Growth in media of known composition (may include vitamins)	Complex growth requirements several vitamins needed	
Escherichia coli	+	+	−	+
Bacteroides fragilis	−	+	+	+
Streptococcus faecalis	−	+	+	±
Bifidobacterium bifidus	−	+	+	+

* Although many bacteria are able to synthesize vitamins if these are available in the culture medium the preformed vitamins are usually utilized.

but this habit is not widespread in man. In the rat, for example, vitamin K (Black *et al.,* 1942), biotin and folic acid (Nielsen and Evenhjen, 1942), the B complex, vitamin E (Daft and Sebrell, 1942) and possibly certain essential amino-acids (Martin, 1942) are synthesized by the flora and utilized by the host.

A similar utilization of intestinally synthesized thiamine (Najjar and Holt, 1943), riboflavin (Najjar *et al.,* 1944) and nicotinic acid (Ellenger *et al.,* 1944) in man has been postulated. The presence of a few small intestinal bacteria and the ability of the salivary bacteria to synthesize vitamins (Disraly *et al.,* 1959) makes a small bacterial contribution feasible, since intestinal bacteria are capable of synthesizing numerous vitamins including B_1, B_2, B_6, B_{12}, K, folic acid and biotin (Dyke *et al.,* 1950; Mickelsen, 1956; Rerat, 1964).

B. Intestinal Structure and Function

The most obvious morphological difference between germ-free and normal rodents is the vastly enlarged caecum in the former (Luckey, 1963). Although the relevance of this observation to man is unclear it does point to the potential magnitude of the influence of the flora on intestinal structure. The small intestine of germ-free animals is less on both weight and surface area compared to controls (Gordon and Pesti, 1971). This seems to be associated with a smaller amount of lamina propria tissue but not with any less intestinal function. Mucosal and luminal enzymes concerned in the digestion of carbohydrate, protein, and fat are present in comparable amounts under both conditions (Coates, 1968). As judged by the absorption of xylose, absorption from the germ-free intestine is enhanced (Heneghan, 1963). The villus architecture of germ-free pigs and guinea pigs is much more regular than in those with a normal bacterial load. Cell turnover in the intestine of germ-free animals is lower than in conventional animals; similarly, the mitotic indices are lower, and cellular migration from crypt to villus tip takes longer in germ-free animals (Gordon, 1960; Gordon and Kardos, 1961; Williams *et al.,* 1971; Abrams, 1967; Abrams *et al.,* 1963; Lesher *et al.,* 1964).

Associated with the problem of caecal enlargement caecal water absorption is impaired in germ-free animals. The mechanism of this impairment is not entirely clear but an inhibitory substance secreted in the saliva and destroyed by the intestinal flora has been demonstrated (Csakey, 1968). The accumulation of mucus in the germ-free intestine may also play a role.

III. Body defence mechanism

The intestinal flora constitutes one of the main defences against intestinal infection, bacterial interactions preventing the establishment of pathogens in the intestine. However, important though this function of the flora is it represents a property of the flora rather than a property of the body and is, therefore, discussed elsewhere (Chapter 14). This section is concerned with the influence of intestinal bacteria on the humoral and cellular defence system of the body.

A. HUMORAL DEFENCE SYSTEMS

Antibodies to components of the intestinal flora and to many other organisms are widespread in man, and the assumption is made that these antibodies are formed in response to antigens absorbed through the gut. Blood Group (ABO) antibodies probably also arise as a result of stimulation by absorbed bacterial antigens (Springer *et al.*, 1962). The ability of oral cholera and typhoid vaccines to produce a response underlines the importance of intestinal absorption of antigens.

The exposure of germ-free animals to antigenic stimuli is much less than that of normal animals and as a consequence the levels of serum gamma globulin is much less than in control animals (e.g. Wostmann, 1968). However, the half-life of the globulins is similar (Wostmann and Olsen, 1964; Snell, 1964), and the association with bacteria leads to an antibody response (Wostmann, 1961). Although germ-free animals are capable of producing an immune response this differs from that in conventional animals. The primary response is reduced in magnitude (Olsen and Wostmann, 1966) probably because of the reduction in Reticuloendothelial system in the germ-free state, and lasts for a longer time (Wostmann, 1968). Peritoneal macrophages from germ-free animals digest foreign antigens more slowly than those from normal animals (Bauer *et al.*, 1964) and this may be of great significance in the transmission of antigenic information for antibody synthesis. Complement levels also seem to be low in germ-free animals (Newton *et al.*, 1960).

B. CELLULAR DEFENCE SYSTEMS

The lymphatic tissues are much less in the germ-free than in the normal state, especially in areas normally in contact with a profuse flora (Bauer, 1968). These differences may be to some extent due to sub-clinical infections since when control animals are housed and fed under the same conditions as the germ-free animals there are no significant differences in the size and weight of the lymphatic organs; further, the distribution and number of small lymphocytes is similar in both groups (Bauer *et al.*, 1964). However, when control animals are housed and fed under open laboratory conditions lymph nodes and spleens are larger than those in the germ-free state (Luckey, 1963).

As mentioned previously, the macrophages from germ-free animals are less efficient in the digestion of bacteria and other antigens than those from normal animals (Luckey, 1963; Bauer, 1968). This may be attributable to the relative paucity of lysosomal enzymes in cells from germ-free animals, however, the phagocytic ability of cells in germ-free animals is apparently unimpaired (Thorbeche and Benaceraff, 1959; Heisse and Myrvik, 1966; Bauer, 1968).

Large lymphocytes although present in germ-free animals presumably resulting from dietary antigenic stimulation, occur in smaller numbers than in conventional animals. Response to particulate and soluble antigens is qualitatively similar to that in normal animals but the response is delayed (Bauer, 1968).

Bacteria are the main source of antigenic materials in healthy animals and the level of immunological activity in lymphatic tissue parallels the intensity of its exposure to the micro flora (Bauer, 1968). The intestinal flora is the most important stimulant of the body defence mechanism. On exposure to living or dead pathogens and non-pathogens, the normal animal is at an advantage for mustering its defences compared to its germ-free counterpart (Gordon and Pesti, 1971).

IV. Ulcerative colitis

Ulcerative colitis is said to be primarily a disease of developed countries (Burkitt, 1971). Dietary relationships similar to those suggested for cancer of the colon have been inferred. While many explanations of the aetiology of this disease have been advanced we are concerned here only with the role of the bacterial flora.

Taylor (1972) has suggested two ways that intestinal bacteria might be implicated in the aetiology of non-specific ulcerative colitis:

(i) Damage to the colonic mucosa by bacterial pathogens or other agents might be followed by the invasion of the mucosa by the normal flora with resultant immune sensitization directed against some mucosal component sharing antigenic determinants with an intestinal bacterium.

(ii) The normal flora could react with the damaged mucosa to form antigenic complexes that stimulate the production of anti-colonic antibodies.

Foetal and germ-free colonic mucosa possesses antigens that cross-react with *E. coli* 014; antibodies to these antigens are demonstrable in the sera of about 30% of ulcerative colitis patients (Perleman and Broberger, 1969). *Clostridium dificile* can stimulate the production of anti-colon antibodies in gnotobiotic rats (Hammarstrom *et al.,* 1969). Antibody to various anaerobic bacteria was demonstrated in the colonic mucosa of ulcerative

TABLE 17.2

Occurrence of selected bacterial groups in faeces from patients with Ulcerative colitis

Patients with	Log_{10} bacteria/gram faeces. Mean (Range)					
	Entero-bacteriaceae	Bactero-ides	Strept-ococcus	Lacto-bacillus	Gram+ non-sporing anaerobes	References
Ulcerative colitis	7.2(5.2-8.2)	5.8(N-10.1)	4.4(N-9.2)	5.0(N-7.7)	D	Cook (1967)
Moderate Ulcerative colitis	6.4	9.1	5.7	5.8	6.8	Gorbach et al. (1968)
Severe Ulcerative colitis	8.6	9.3	6.0	4.9	7.2	Gorbach et al. (1968)
Crohn's Disease	7.7	9.7	6.1	5.2	6.1	Gorbach et al. (1968)

N = Not detected; D = Less than 100 bacteria

colitis patients by Monterio et al. (1971); however, these findings may only indicate that during colonic inflammation an immune response to the intestinal flora occurs.

The faecal flora of patients with ulcerative colitis has not been examined in great detail, but recent studies suggest that it does not differ markedly from that of normal people (Table 17.2) although the faeces of more severely affected patients contain more enterobacteria (Cooke, 1967; Gorbach et al., 1968; Seneca and Henderson, 1950).

No firm conclusions can be drawn until more data is available.

References

Abrams, G. D. (1967). *Proc. Soc. exp. Biol. (N.Y.)*126, 301.

Abrams, G. D., Bauer, H. and Sprinz, H. (1963). *Lab. Invest.* 12, 355.

Abrams, G. D. and Bishop, J. E. (1966). *J. Bact.* 92, 1604.

Ackerman, D. (1910). *Z. Biol.* 57, 104.

Adinolfi, M., Glynn, A. A., Lindsay, M. and Milne, C. M. (1966). *Immunology* 10, 517.

Alam, S. Q., Boctor, A. M., Rogers, Q. R. and Harper, A. E. (1967). *J. Nutr.* 93, 317.

Alam, B. S., Saporoschetz, I. B. and Epstein, S. S. (1971). *Nature, Lond.* 232, 199.

Allen, M. J., Boyland, E., Dukes, C. E., Horning, E. S. and Watson, J. G. (1957). *Brit. J. Cancer* 11, 212.

Altemeir, W. A., Hummel, R. P. and Hill, E. O. (1963). *Ann. Surg.* 157, 847.

Anaerobe Laboratory. (1970). "Outline in Clinical Methods in Anaerobic Bacteriology." Cato, E. P., Cummings, C. S., Holdeman, L. V., Johnson, J. L., Moore, W. E. C., Smibert, R. M. and Smith, L. D. S. Published by Anaerobe Laboratory., Blacksburg, Virginia, U.S.A.

Anaerobe Laboratory. "Anaerobe Laboratory Manual" (1972). Holdeman, L. V. and Moore, W. E. C. Published by Anaerobe Laboratory, Blacksburg, Virginia, U.S.A.

Anapara, J., Perry, T. L., Hanly, C. and Peck, E. (1964). *Clin. Chim. Acta* 10, 286.

Anchel, M. and Schoenheimer, R. (1938). *J. biol. Chem.* 125, 23.

Anderson, C. M. and Langford, R. F. (1958). *Brit. med. J.* 1, 803.

Anderson, E. S. (1968). *Ann. Rev. Microbiol.* 22, 131.

Anderson, E. S. and Smith, H. R. (1972). *Brit med. J.*.iii, 329.

Angel, A. and Rogers, K. J. (1968). *Nature, Lond.* 217, 84.

Anrep. G. V., Barsoum, G. S. and Talaat, M. (1953). *J. Physiol. (Lond.)* 120, 419.

Aranki, A., Syed, S. A., Kenney, E. B. and Freter, R. (1969). *Appl. Microbiol.* 17, 568.

Arbuckle, J. B. R. (1971). *J. Path.* 104, 93.

Aries, V. C., Crowther, J. S., Drasar, B. S. and Hill, M. J. (1969a). *Gut* 10, 575.

Aries, V. C., Crowther, J. S., Drasar, B. S., Hill, M. J. and Ellis, F. R. (1971). *J. Path.*103,54.

Aries, V. C. and Hill, M. J. (1970a). *Biochim. biophys. Acta (Amst.)* 202, 526.

Aries, V. C. and Hill, M. J. (1970b). *Biochim. biophys. Acta (Amst.)* 202, 535.

Arnold, A., Edgren, D. C. and Palladino, V. S. (1953). *J. Neuro. Ment. Dis.* 117, 135.

Asatoor, A. M. (1965). *Biochim. biophys. Acta (Amst.)* 100, 290.

Asatoor, A. M. (1968). *Clin. Chim. Acta* 22, 223.

Asatoor, A. M. and Simenhoff, M. L. (1965). *Biochim. biophys. Acta (Amst.)* 111, 384.

Ashton, M. R. (1970). *B.F.M.I.R.A.* Lit. Survey No. 7.

Association for the Study of Infectious Disease. Joint project by Members. (1970). *Lancet ii*, 1159.

Avery-Jones, F., Gummer, J. W. P. and Lennard-Jones, J. E. (1968). "Clinical Gastroenterology", 2nd Edn. Blackwell, Oxford.

Azar, H. and Drapanas, T. (1968). *Amer. J. Surg.* 115, 209.

Bach-Nielsen, P. and Amdrap, E. (1965). *Acta chir. scand.* **129**, 521.

Badenoch, J. (1960). *Proc. roy. Soc. Med.* **53**, 657.

Badger, G. M., Cook, J. W., Hewett, C. L., Kennaway, E. L., Kennaway, N. M., Martin, R. H. and Robinson, A. M. (1940). *Proc. roy. Soc. B.* **129**, 439.

Baker, S. J. and Mathan, V. I. (1968). *Amer. J. clin. Nutr.* **21**, 984.

Bakke, O. M. (1969a). *Scand. J. Gastroenterology* **4**, 603.

Bakke, O. M. (1969b). *Scand. J. Gastroenterology* **4**, 419.

Bakke, O. M. (1969c). *J. Nutr.* **98**, 209.

Bakke, O. M. (1969d). *J. Nutr.* **98**, 217.

Bakke, O. M. (1970). *Acta pharmacol. (Kbh.)* **28**, 28.

Bakke, O. M. (1971). *Acta pharmacol. (Kbh.)* **29**, 107.

Barber, M. and Franklin, R. H. (1946). *Brit. med. J. i*, 951.

Barnes, E. and Goldberg, H. S. (1968). *J. gen. Microbiol.* **51**, 313.

Barrow, G. I. and Miller, D. C. (1972) *Lancet i*, 485.

Bart, J. K., Huq, Z., Khan, M. and Mosley, W. H. (1970) *J. infect. Dis.* **121**, Suppl. 17-24.

Bartle, H. J. and Harkins, M. J. (1925). *Amer. J. med. Sci.* **169**, 373.

Batchelor, F. R., Chain, E. B., Richards, M. and Rolinson, G. N. (1961). *Proc. roy. Soc. B.* **154**, 522.

Bauer, H. (1968). In "The Germ-free Animal in Research" (Ed., Coates, M. E.). Academic Press, N.Y. and London, p. 210.

Bauer, H., Horowitz, R. F., Levenson, S. M. and Popper, H. (1963). *Amer. J. Path.* **42**, 471.

Bauer, H., Horowitz, R. E., Watkins, K. C. and Popper, H. (1964). *J. Amer. med. Ass.* **187**, 713.

Baumann, E. (1879). *Ber. dtsch. chem. Ges.* **12**, 1450.

Bayes, B. J. and Hamilton, J. R. (1969). *Arch. Dis. Childh.* **44**, 76.

Beaver, M. H. and Wostmann, B. S. (1962). *Brit. J. Pharmacol.* **19**, 385.

Beerens, H., Castel, M. M. and Abraham, R. (1960). *Ann. Inst. Pasteur* **99**, 454.

Bell, E. J. and Grist, N. R. (1967). *Brit. med. J. ii*, 741.

Benveniste, R. and Davies, J. (1971). *Biochem. J.* **10**, 1787.

Bernhardt, F. W. and Zilliken, A. (1959). *Arch. Biochem.* **82**, 462.

Bernheimer, A. W. and Schwartz, L. L. (1965). *J. bact.* **89**, 1387.

Berthelot, R. (1911). *C. r. hebd. seanc. Acad. Sci. (Paris)* **156**, 641.

Berthelot, R. (1918). *Ann. Inst. Pasteur* **32**, 17.

Berthelot, A. and Bertrand, D. M. (1910). *C. r. hebd. Seanc. Acad. Sci. (Paris)* **154**, 1643.

Bessman, A. N., Mirick, G. S. and Hawkins, R. (1958). *J. clin. Invest.* **37**, 990.

Bhat, P., Shantakumari, S., Rajan, D., Mathan, V. I., Kapadia, C. R., Swarnabi, C. and Baker, S. J. (1972). *Gastroenterology* **62**, 11.

Bhattacharya, S., Bose, A. D., and Ghosh, A. D. (1971). *Appl. Microbiol.* **22**, 1159.

Bircher, J., Muller, J., Guggenheim, P. and Haemmerli, U. P. (1966). *Lancet i*, 890.

Bishop, R. F. (1963). *Brit. J. exp. Path.* **44**, 189.

Bishop, R. (1965). *Ernährungsforschung* **10**, 417.

Bishop, R. F. and Allcock, E. A. (1960). *Brit. med. J. i*, 766.

Bisset, K. A. and Davis, G. H. G. (1960). "The Microbial Flora of the Mouth". Heywood and Co., London.

Black, S., Overman, R. S., Elvehjem, C. A. and Link, K. P. (1942). *J. biol. Chem.* **45**, 137.

Bohnhoff, M. and Miller, C. P. (1962). *J. infect. Dis.* **111**, 117.

Bohnhoff, M., Miller, C. P. and Martin, W. R. (1964). *J. exp. Med.* **120**, 805.

Bolin, T. D., Crane, G. G. and Davis, A. E. (1968). *Aust. Ann. Med.* **17**, 300.

Bolin, T. D. and Davis, A. E. (1969). *Nature, (Lond.)* **222**, 382.

Boni, P. (1967). *Riv. Ist. sieroter. ital.* **42**, 261.

Booth, A. N., Emerson, O. H., Jones, F. J. and Deeds, F. (1957). *J. biol. Chem.* **229**, 51.

Booth, A. N. and Williams, R. T. (1963a). *Nature, Lond.* **198**, 684.

Booth, A. N. and Williams, R. T. (1963b). *Biochem. J.* **88**, 66.

Booth, C. C. and Heath, J. (1962). *Gut* **3**, 70.

Borgstrom, B. (1964). *J. Lipid Res.* **5**, 222.

Bornside, G. H. and Cohn, I. (1965). *Amer. J. dig. Dis.* **10**, 844.

Boutwell, R. K. (1967). *In* "Phenolic Compounds and Metabolic Regulation" (Eds., Finkle, B. J. and Runeckles, V. C.). Appleton-Century-Crofts, N.Y.

Boutwell, R. K. and Bosch, D. K. (1959). *Cancer Res.* **19**, 413.

Bouwman, R. J. (1923). *Pharm. Weekbl.* **60**, 845.

Boyland, E., Harris, J. and Horning, E. S. (1954). *Brit. J. Cancer* **8**, 647.

Boyland, E. and Williams, D. C. (1956). *Biochem. J.* **64**, 578.

Branche, W. C., Young, V. M., Robinet, H. G. and Massey, E. D. (1963). *Proc. Soc. exp. Biol.* (N.Y.) **114**, 198.

Braun, O. H., Dehnert, J., Hoffman, K., Kienetiz, M., Mayer, J. B., Reploh, H., Reuter, G. Seeliger, H. D. R. and Werner, H. (1964). *Dtsch. med. Wschr.* **89**, 1647.

Breed, R. S., Murray, E. G. D. and Smith, N. R. (1957). "Bergey's Manual of Determinative Bacteriology". 7th Edn. Baillière, Tindall and Cox, London.

British Medical Journal (1972a). *i*, 189.

British Medical Journal (1972b). *i*, 701.

Brooks, J. B., Cherry, W. B., Thacker, L. and Alley, C. C. (1972). *J. infect. Dis.* **126**, 143.

Brot, N., Smit, Z. and Weissbach, H. (1965). *Arch. Biochem.* **112**, 1.

Brown, C. L., Hill, M. J. and Richards, P. (1971). *Lancet ii*, 406.

Brown, R. R., Price, J. M., Satter, E. J. and Wear, J. B. (1960). *Acta Unio Intern. Contra Cancrum* **16**, 299.

Brown, W. R., Savage, D. C., Dubois, R. S., Alp, M. H., Mallory, A. and Kern, F. (1972). *Gastroenterology* **62**, 1143.

Brunser, O., Eidelman, S. and Klipstein, F. A. (1970). *Gastroenterology* **58**, 655.

Bryan, G. T. (1968). *Cancer Res.* **24**, 582.

Bryan, G. T. (1969a). *Amer. industr. Hyg. Ass. J.* **30**, 27.

Bryan, G. T. (1969b). *J. nat. Cancer Inst.* **43**, 255.

Bryan, G. T. (1971). *Amer. J. clin. Nutr.* **24**, 841.

Bryan, G. T., Morris, C. R. and Brown, R. R. (1965). *Cancer Res.* **25**, 1432.

Bryan, G. T. and Morris, C. R. (1966). *Nature, Lond.* **210**, 857.

Bryan, G. T, and Springberg, P. D. (1966). *Cancer Res.* **26**, 105.

Bryant, M. P. and Burkey, L. A. (1953). *J. Dairy Sci.* **36**, 205.

Buchanan, R. E., Holt, J. G. and Lessel, E. F. (1966). "Index Bergeyana". Livingstone, Edinburgh and London.

Buck, A. C. and Cook, E. M. (1969). *J. med. Microbiol.* **2**, 521.

Buehler, H. J., Katzman, P. A. and Doisy, A. D. (1951). *Proc. Soc. exp. Biol. (N.Y.)* **76**, 672.

Buell, P. and Dunn, J. E. (1965). *Cancer* **18**, 656.

Bullen, C. L. and Willis, A. T. (1971). *Brit. med. J. iii*, 338.

Burke, V. and Anderson, C. M. (1966). *Aust. J. Pediat.* **1**, 147.

Burkitt, D. P. (1971a). *J. nat. Cancer Inst.* **47**, 913.

Burkitt, D. P. (1971b). *Cancer* **28**, 3.

Burnett, G. W. and Sherp, H. W. (1962). "Oral Microbiology and Infectious Disease", 2nd Edn. Williams and Wilkins, Baltimore.

Burrows, A. C. (1968). *Ann Rev. Microbiol.* **22**, 254.

Burrows, W., Elliot, M. E. and Havens, I. (1947). *J. infect. Dis.* **81**, 261.

Burrows, W. and Havens, I. (1948). *J. infect. Dis.* **82**, 231.

Capek, A., Hanc, O. and Tadra, M. (1966). "Microbial Transformation of Steroids". Academia, Prague.

Carey, J. B. and Williams. (1965). *Science,, N.Y.* **150**, 620.

Carey, J. B., Zaki, F. G., Hoffbauer, F. W. and Nwokolo, C. (1967). *J. Lab. clin. Med.* **69**, 737.

Carey, J. B., Wilson, I. D., Zaki, F. G. and Hanson, R. F. (1966). *Medicine (Baltimore)* **45**, 461.

Carroll, K. K. and Khor, H. T. (1970). *Cancer Res.* **30**, 2260.

Chuttani, K. H. and Kaethuri, D. (1968). *J. trop. Med. Hyg.* **71**, 96.

Clarke, M. L. (1960). *Amer. J. Med.* **29**, 740.

Clarke, M. L., Lanz, H. C. and Senior, J. R. (1969). *J. clin. Invest.* **48**, 1587.

Cleave, T. L. (1956). *J. roy. nav. med. Serv.* **42**, 55.

Closon, J., Salvatore, G., Michel, R. and Roche, J. (1959). *C. r. Soc. Biol.* **153**, 1120.

Cohen, G. N., Nisman, B. and Raynaud, M. (1946). *C. r. hebd. Seance. Acad. Sci. (Paris)* **225**, 647.

Cohen, G. N., Nisman, S. and Raynaud, M. (1946). *Amer. J. dig. Dis.* **10**, 892.

Cohn, I. Jnr., (1970). *Surg. Gynec. Obstet.* **130**, 1006.

Cohn, R., Kalser, M. H., Arteaga, I., Yawn, E., Frazier, D., Leite, C. A., Ahearn, D. G. and Roth, F. (1967). *J. Amer. med. Ass.* **201**, 835.

Coleman, D. L. and Baumann, C. A. (1957). *Arch. Biochem.* **72**, 219.

Colman, G. C. (1969). *J. gen. Microbiol.* **50**, 149.

Collee, J. G., Rutter, J. M. and Watt, B. (1971). *J. med. Microbiol.* **4**, 271.

Connor, W. E., Witick, D. T., Stone, D. B. and Armstrong, M. L. (1969). *J. clin Invest.* **48**, 1363.

Cooke, E. M. (1967). *J. Path. Bact.* **94**, 439.

Cooke, E. M., Ewins, M. and Shooter, S. (1969). *Brit. med. J. iv*, 593.

Cooke, E. M., Shooter, R. A., Kumen, P. J., Rousseau, S. A. and Foulkes, A. L. (1970). *Lancet i*, 436.

Cook, G. C. and Kajubi, S. K. (1966). *Lancet i*, 725.

Cook, J. W., Kennaway, E. L. and Kennaway, N. M. (1940). *Nature, Lond.* **145**, 627.

Coombs, M. M. and Croft, C. J. (1969). *Progr. exp. Tumor Res. (Basel)* **11**, 69.

Cordaro, J. T., Sellers, W. M., Ball, R. J. and Schmidt, J. P. (1966). *Aerospace Med.* **37**, 594.

Correa, P., Cuello, C. and Duque, E. (1970). *J. nat. Cancer Inst.* **44**, 297.

Cotran, R., Kendrick, M. I. and Kass, E. H. (1960). *Proc. Soc. exp. Biol. (N.Y.)* **104**, 424.

Craig, J. P. (1971). "Microbial Toxins". Academic Press, London and N.Y.

Craig, J. P. (1972). "Microbial Pathogenicity in Man and Animals". Soc. Gen. Microbiol. Symposium Series.

Cramblett, H. G., Azimi, P. and Haynes, R. E. (1971). *Ann. N.Y. Acad. Sci.* **176**, 80.

Cregan, J. and Hayward, N. J. (1953). *Brit. med. J. i*, 1356.

Cregan, J., Dunlop, E. E. and Hayward, N. (1953). *Brit. med. J. ii*, 1248.

Crowther, J. S. (1971). *J. appl. Bact.* **34**, 477.

Crowther, J. S. (1971b). *J. med. Microbiol.* **4**, 343.

Crowther, J. S., Drasar, B. S., Goddard, P., Hill, M. J. and Johnson, K., (1973). *Gut* **14**, 790.

Csáky, T. Z. (1968). "The Germ-free Animal in Research" (Ed., Coates, M. E.). Academic Press, N.Y. and London.

Cutts, J. H. (1965). *Canad. Cancer Conf.* **6**, 50.

Cvjetanović, B., Mel, D. M. and Felsenfeld, O. (1970). *Bull. Wld. Hlth. Org.* **42**, 499.

Dack, G. M. and Petran, E. (1934). *J. infect. Dis.* 54, 204.

Dacre, J. C. and Williams, R. T. (1968). *J. Pharm. Pharmacol.* 20, 610.

Dacre, J. C., Scheling, R. R. and Williams, R. T. (1968). *J. Pharm. Pharmacol.* 20, 619.

Daft, F. S. and Sebrell, W. H. (1942). *Publ. Hlth. Rep. (Wash.)* 58, 1542.

Dahlquist, A. and Gryboski, J. D. (1965). *Biochim. biophys. Acta (Amst.)* 110, 635.

Dahlquist, A., Bull, B. and Gustafsson, B. E. (1965). *Arch. Biochem.* 109, 150.

Dammin, G. J. (1964). *Bull. Wld. Hlth. Org.* 31, 29.

Dandoy, S. (1966). *Calif. Med.* 104, 458.

Danielsson, H. (1960). *Acta physiol. scand.* 48, 364.

Davidson, L. S. P. (1928). *J. Path. Bact.* 31, 557.

Davidson, S. J. and Talalay, P. (1966). *J. biol. Chem.* 241, 906.

Davies, A. (1922). *Lancet i,* 1009.

Davies, T. D., McBee, J. W., Borland, J. L., Kurtz, S. M. and Ruffin, J. M. (1963). *Gastroenterology* 44, 112.

Davis, H. L., Leklem, J. E., Carlson, I. and Brown, R. R. (1970). *Proc. Amer. Ass. Cancer Res.* 11, 19.

Dawson, A. M. (1971). *J. clin. Path.* 24, Suppl. 5.

Dawson, A. M., McLaren, J. and Sherlock, S. (1957). *Lancet ii,* 1263.

Dawson, A. M. and Isselbacher, K. J. (1960). *J. clin. Invest.* 39, 730.

Deeds, F., Booth, A. N. and Jones, F. T. (1957). *J. biol. Chem.* 225, 615.

Dellipiani, A. W. and Girdwood, R. H. (1964). *Clin. Sci.* 26, 359.

Deo, M. G., Sood, S. K. and Ramalingaswami, V. (1965). *Arch. Path.* 80, 141.

Dick, G. F. (1941). *Amer. J. Digest. Dis.* 8, 255.

Dietschy, J. M. (1969). *Gastroenterology* 57, 461.

Distaso, A. and Sugden, J. H. (1919). *Biochem. J.* 13, 153.

Dixon, J. M. S. (1960). *J. Path. Bact.* 79, 131.

Dixon, J. M. S. and Paully, J. W. (1963). *Gut* 4, 169.

Dodgson, K. S., Spencer, B. and Thomas, J. (1953). *Biochem. J.* 53, 452.

Dodgson, K. S., Spencer, B. and Wynn, C. H. (1956). *Biochem. J.* 62, 500.

Doig, A. and Girdwood, R. H. (1960). *Quart. J. Med.* 115, 333.

Doll, R. (1967). *Nat. Cancer Inst. Monogr.* 25, 173.

Doll, R. (1969). *Brit. J. Cancer* 23, 1.

Doll, R., Muir, P. and Waterhouse, J. (Eds.) (1970). "Cancer in Five Continents", Vol. II. Springer, Berlin.

Donaldson, R. M. (1962). *Gastroenterology* 4, 271.

Donaldson, R. M. Jr. (1964). *New Engl. J. Med.* 270, 938, 994, 1050.

Donaldson, R. M. (1965). *J. clin. Invest.* 44, 1815.

Donaldson, R. M. (1968). "Handbook of Physiology (Section 6)", Vol. 5. American Physiological Soc., Washington, p. 2807.

Donaldson, R. M. (1970). *Advance. intern. Med.* 16, 191.

Donaldson, R. M., Corrigan, H. and Natsios, G. (1962). *Gastroenterology* 43, 282.

Drasar, B. S. (1967). *J. Path. Bact.* 94, 417.

Drasar, B. S., Hill, M. J. and Shiner, M. (1966). *Lancet i,* 1237.

Drasar, B. S. and Shiner, M. (1969). *Gut* 10, 812.

Drasar, B. S., Shiner, M. and McLeod, G. M. (1969). *Gastroenterology* 56, 71.

Drasar, B. S., Hill, M. J. and Williams, R. E. O. (1970). *In* "The Safety Testing of Food Additives". Blackwell, Oxford.

Drasar, B. S. and Hill, M. J. (1972). *Amer. J. clin. Nutr.* 25, 1399.

Drasar, B. S., Renwick, A. G. and Williams, R. T. (1972). *Biochem. J.* 129, 881.

Drasar, B. S., Crowther, J. S., Goddard, P., Hawksworth, G., Hill, M. J., Peach, S., Williams, R. E. O. and Renwick, A. (1973). *Proc. Nutr. Soc.* 32, 49.

Drasar, B. S. and Irving, D. (1973). *Brit. J. Cancer* 27, 167.

Druckrey, H., Preussman, R., Ivankovic, S. and Schmahl, D. (1967). *Z. Krebsforsch.* **69**, 103.

Dubos, R. (1965). "Man Adapting". Yale University Press, New Haven and London.

Dubos, R. and Shaedler, R. W. (1962). *Amer. J. med. Sci.* **244**, 265.

Dubos, R., Schaedler, R. W., Costello, R. and Hoet, P. (1965). *J. exp. Med.* **122**, 67.

Dugeon, L. S. (1926). *J. Hyg.* **25**, 119.

Duncan, I. B. R., Goudie, J. G., Mackie, L. M. and Howie, J. W. (1954). *J. Path. Bact.* **67**, 282.

Duncan, C. L., Sugijama, H. and Strong, D. H. (1968). *J. Bact.* **95**, 1560.

Dunning, W. F., Curtis, M. R. and Maun, M. E. (1950). *Cancer Res.* **10**, 454.

Dunstan, W. R. and Henry, T. R. (1903). *Proc. roy. Soc. B.* **72**, 85.

DuPont, H. L., Formol, S. B., Hornick, R. B., Snyder, M. J., Libonati, J. P., Sheahan, D. G., LaBrec, E. H. and Kalas, J. P. (1971). *New Eng. J. Med.* **285**, 1.

DuPont, H. L., Hornick, R. B., Snyder, M. J., Libonati, J. P., Formal, S. B. and Gangarosa, E. J. (1972). *J. Infect. Dis.* **125**, 5.

Dyer, N. H. and Hawkins, C. (1972). *In* "Recent Advances in Gastroenterology" (Eds., Badenoch, J. and Brooke, B. N.) Churchill-Livingstone, London.

Dyer, N. H. and Morris, H. P. (1961). *J. nat. Cancer Inst.* **26**, 315.

Editorial (1972). *Brit. med. J.* i, 2.

Edwards, P. R. and Ewing, W. H. (1972). "Identification of the Enterobacteriaceae". Burgess, Minneapolis.

Eggerth, A. H. (1935). *J. Bact.* **30**, 277.

Eggerth, A. H. and Gagnon, B. H. (1933). *J. Bact.* **25**, 389.

Elder, H. H. A. (1947). *J. trop. Med. Hyg.* **50**, 212.

Elkington, S. G., Floch, M. H. and Conn, H. O. (1969). *New Engl. J. Med.* **281**, 408.

Ellenger, P., Coulson, R. A. and Benesch, R. (1944). *Nature, Lond.* **154**, 270.

Elliot, R. B., Maxwell, G. M. and Vawser, N. (1967). *Med. J. Aust.* **1**, 46.

Engel, A. (1929). *Acta med. scand.* **20**, 150.

England, M. T., French, J. M. and Rawson, A. B. (1960). *Gastroenterology* **39**, 219.

England, N. W. J. (1968). *Amer. J. clin. Nutr.* **21**, 962.

Engler, R., Holtz, P. and Raudonat, H. W. (1958). *Arch. exp. Pathol. Pharmacol.* **233**, 393.

Evans, W. B., Royagi, T. and Summerskill, W. H. (1966). *Gut* **7**, 635.

Everett, M. T., Brogan, T. D. and Nettleton, J. (1969). *Brit. J. Surg.* **56**, 679.

Falanje, J. M. (1970). *J. trop. Med. Hyg.* **73**, 119.

Faloon, W. W. and Fisher, C. J. (1958). *Ann. N.Y. Acad. Sci.* **76**, 196.

Farber, E. (1963). *Advanc. Cancer Res.* **7**, 383.

Farmer, E. D. and Lawton, F. E. (1966). "Stone's Oral and Dental Disease", 5th Edn. Livingstone, Edinburgh and London.

Fenton, J. C. B., Knight, E. J. and Humpherson, P. L. (1966). *Lancet* i, 164.

Finegold, S. M. (1970). *Amer. J. clin. Nutr.* **23**, 1466.

Finegold, S. M., Posnich, D. J., Miller, L. G. and Hewitt, W. L. (1965). *Ernährungsforschung* **10**, 316.

Finegold, S. M., Sutter, V. L., Boyle, J. D. and Shimada, K. (1970). *J. infect. Dis.* **122**, 376.

Finegold, S. M., Atteberry, H. R. and Sutter, V. L. (1972). *Amer. J. clin. Nutr.* **25**, 1391.

Fingl, E. (1965). *In* "The Pharmacological Basis of Therapeutics" (Eds., Goodman, L. S. and Gilman, A.). Macmillan, N.Y., p. 1009.

Fisher, C. J. and Faloon, W. W. (1957). *New Engl. J. Med.* **256**, 1030.

Fisher, J. F. and Malletter M. F. (1961). *J. gen. Physiol.* **45**, 1.

Flatz, G., Saenguidom, C. H. and Sanguanbhokhai, T. (1969). *Nature, Lond.* 221, 758.

Floch, M. H., Gershengoren, W., Diamond, S. and Hersh, T. (1970). *Amer. J. clin. Nutr.* 23, 8.

Florey, H. W. (1933). *J. Path. Bact.* 37, 282.

Folin, O. and Denis, W. (1915). *J. biol. Chem.* 22, 309.

Fore, H., Walker, R. and Goldberg, L. (1967). *Food Cosm. Toxicol.* 5, 459.

Formal, S. B., Dammin, G., Sprinz, H., Schneider, H., Horowitz, R. E. and Forbes, M. (1961). *J. Bact.* 82, 284.

Formal, S. B., LaBrec, E. H., Kent, T. H. and Falkow, S. (1965). *J. Bact.* 89, 1374.

Formal, S. B., DuPont, H. L., Hornick, R., Snyder, M. J., Libonati, J. and LaBrec, E. H. (1971). *Ann. N.Y. Acad. Sci.* 176, 190.

Frazer, A. C. (1968). "Malabsorption Syndromes". Heinemann, London.

French, J. M. (1961). *Postgrad. med. J.* 37, 259.

French, J. M., Gaddie, R. and Smith, W. M. (1956). *Quart. J. Med.* 25, 333.

Freter, R. (1956). *J. exp. Med.* 104, 411.

Freter, R. (1962). *J. infect. Dis.* 111, 37.

Freter, R. (1969). *Tex. Rep. Biol. Med.* 27, 299.

Freter, R. (1970). *Infect. and Immunity* 2, 556.

Freter, R., De, S. P., Mondal, A., Shrivasta, D. L. and Sunderman, F. W. (1965). *J. infect. Dis.* 115, 83.

Freter, R. and Fabara, E. S. (1972). *Amer. J. clin. Nutr.* 25, 1357.

Fritz, P. J. and Melius, P. (1963). *Canad. J. Biochem.* 41, 719.

Fung, C. K. and Proulx, P. (1969). *Canad. J. Biochem.* 47, 371.

Gale, E. F. (1940). *Biochem. J.* 34, 392 and 846.

Gale, E. F. (1941). *Biochem. J.* 35, 66.

Gale, E. F. (1952). "The Chemical Activities of Bacteria". University Tutorial Press, London.

Gall, L. S. (1965). Special communication from Aerospace Medical Center.

Garber, N., Zohar, D. and Michlin, H. (1968). *Nature, Lond.* 219, 407.

Garton, G. A. (1963). *J. Lipid Res.* 4, 237.

Garton, G. A. and Williams, R. T. (1949). *Biochem. J.* 45, 158.

Gaylor, D. W., Clarke, J. S., Kudinoff, Z. and Finegold, S. M. (1960). *Antimicrob. Ag. Ann.* 392.

Gerson, C. D., Kent, T. H., Saha, J. R., Siddiqui, N. and Lindenbaum, J. (1971). *Ann. intern. Med.* 75, 41.

Ghiron, V. (1939). Summary of Communications 3rd. Int. Cancer Congress.

Giannella, R. A., Briotman, S. A. and Zamcheck, N. (1971). *Amer. J. dig. Dis.* 16, 1007.

Giannella, R. A., Selwyn, A., Broitman, A. and Zamcheck, N. (1971). *Amer. J. dig. Dis.* 16, 1000.

Giannella, R. A., Formal, S. B., Dammin, G. J. and Collins, H. (1973). *J. clin. Invest.* 52, 441.

Gibbons, R. J., Socransky, S. S., Sawyer, S., Kapsimalis, B. and Macdonald, J. B. (1963). *Arch. oral Biol.* 8, 281.

Gibbons, R. J., Kapsimalis, B. and Socransky, S. S. (1964). *Arch. oral Biol.* 9, 101.

Gibbons, R. J. and Kapsimalis, B. (1967). *J. Bact.* 93, 510.

Girard, J. P. and Kalbernatten, A. (1970). *Europ. J. clin. Invest.* 1, 188.

Glazko, A. J., Dill, W. A. and Rebstock, M. C. (1950). *J. biol. Chem.* 183, 679.

Glazko, A. J., Dill, W. A. and Wolf, L. M. (1952). *J. Pharmacol. exp. Ther.* 104, 452.

Glazko, A. J., Wolf, L. M., Dill, W. A. and Bratton, A. E. (1949). *J. Pharmacol. exp. Ther.* 96, 445.

Glazko, A. J., Carnes, H. E., Kazenko, A., Wolf, L. M. and Reutner, T. F. (1958). *In* "Antibiotics Annual 1958" (Eds., Welch, H. and Marti-Ibanez, F.). Med. Encyclopedia Inc., New York, p. 792.

Goddard, P. and Hill, M. J. (1971). *Biochem. J.* 124, 73p.

Goddard, P. and Hill, M. J. (1972). *Biochem. biophys. Acta (Amst.)* 280, 336.

Goldstein, F. (1971). *Gastroenterology* 61, 780.

Gold stein, F., Wirts, C. W. and Kramer, S. (1961). *Gastroenterology* 40, 47.

Goldstein, F., Wirts, G. W. and Kowlessar, O. D. (1970). *Arch. intern. Med.* 72, 215.

Goldsworthy, N. E. and Florey, H. W. (1930). *Brit. J. exp. Path.* 11, 192.

Goodman, L. S. and Gilman, A. (1965). "The Pharmacological Basis of Therapeutics". Macmillan, New York, p. 1158.

Gorbach, S. L. (1967). *Gut* 8, 530.

Gorbach, S. L. (1971a). *Gastroenterology* 60, 1110.

Gorbach, S. L. (1971b). *J. clin. Invest.* 50, 881.

Gorbach, S. L., Plant, A. G., Nahas, L., Weinstein, L., Spanknebel, G. and Levitan, R. (1967). *Gastroenterology* 53, 856.

Gorbach, S. L., Nahas, L., Lerner, P. I. and Weinstein, L. (1967). *Gastroenterology* 53, 845.

Gorbach, S. L., Nahas, L., Plant, A. G., Weinstein, L., Levitan, R. and Patterson, J. F. *Gastroenterology* 54, 874.

Gorbach, S. L. and Tabaqchali, S. (1969). *Gut* 10, 963.

Gorbach, S. L., Banwell, J. G., Mitra, R., Chatterjee, B. D., Jacob, B. and Mazumder, D. N. (1969). *Lancet i*, 74.

Gorbach, S. L., Banwell, J. G., Jacobs, B., Chatterjee, B. D., Mitra, R., Brigham, K. L. and Neogy, K. N. (1970). *J. infect. Dis.* 121, 38.

Gorbach, S. L., Neale, G., Levitan, R. and Hepner, G. W. (1970). *Gut* 11, 1.

Gorbach, S. L., Banwell, J. G., Jacobs, B., Chatterjee, B. D., Mitra, R., Sen, N. N. and Mazumder, D. N. (1970). *Amer. J. clin. Nutr.* 23, 1545.

Gorbach, S. L., Banwell, J. G., Chatterjee, B. D., Jacobs, B. and Sack, R. B. (1971).*J. clin. Invest.* 50, 881.

Gordon, H. A. (1960). *Amer. J. dig. Dis.* 5, 841.

Gordon, H. A. and Bruckner-Kardoss, E. (1961). *Amer. J. Physiol.* 201, 175.

Gordon, H. A., Bruckner-Kardoss, E. and Wostmann, B. S. (1966). *J. Gerontol.* 21, 380.

Gordon, H. A. and Pesti, L. (1971). *Bact. Rev.* 35, 390.

Gordon, J. E. (1971). *Ann. N.Y. Acad. Sci.* 176, 9.

Gordon, J. E. and Scrimshaw, N. S. (1970). *Med. Clin. N. Amer.* 54, 1495.

Gracey, N., Burke, V. and Anderson, C. M. (1969). *Lancet ii*, 384.

Grant, G. A. and Roe, F. J. C. (1969). *Nature, Lond.* 222, 1282.

Grundy, S. M., Ahrens, E. H. and Salen, G. (1968). *J. Lip. Res.* 9, 374.

Grundy, S. M. and Ahrens, E. H. (1969). *J. Lip. Res.* 10, 91.

Guerra, R., Wheby, M. S. and Bayless, T. M. (1965). *Ann. intern. Med.* 63, 619.

Gustaffson, B. E., Bergstrom, S., Lindstedt, S. and Norman, A. (1957). *Proc. Soc. exp. Biol. (N.Y.)* 94, 467.

Gustaffson, B. E. and Fitzgerald, R. J. (1960). *Proc. Soc. exp. Biol. (N.Y.)* 104, 319.

Gustaffson, B. E. and Lanke, L. S. (1960). *J. exp. Med.* 112, 975.

Gustaffson, B. E., Midtvedt, T. and Norman, A. (1968). *Acta Path. Mic. Scand.* 72, 433.

Haenel, H. (1961). *J. appl. Bact.* 24, 242.

Haenel, H. (1963). *Zbl. Bakt. I. Abt. Orig.* 188, 219.

Haenel, H., Müller-Beuthow, W. and Scheunert, A. (1957). *Zbl. Bakt. I. Abt. Orig.* 168, 37.

Haenel, H., Feldheim, W., Müller—Beuthow, W. and Ruttloff, H. (1958). *Zbl. Bakt., I. Abt. Orig.* 173, 76.

Haenel, H., Gassman, B., Grutte, F. K. and Müller-Beuthow, W. (1964). *Zbl. Bakt. I. Abt. Orig.* 192, 491.

Hale White, W., Andrewes, F. W., Harley, V., Saundby, R., Arbuthnot Lane, W. and Colyer, J. F. (1913). *Proc. roy. Soc. Med.* 6, 1.

Hall, W. T. and McGavin, M. D. (1968). *Pathologia veterinaria* 5, 26.

Hamilton, J. D., Dyer, N., Dawson, A. M., O'Grady, F. W., Vince, A., Fenton, J. C. B. and Mollin, D. L. (1970). *Quart. J. Med.* XXXIX 265.

Hamilton-Miller, J. M. T. (1966). *Bact. Rev.* 30, 761.

Hammarström, S., Perlmann, P., Gustafsson, B. E. and Lagercrante, R. (1969). *J. exp. Med.* 129, 747.

Hampton, J. C. and Rosario, B. (1965). *Lab. Invest.* 14, 1464.

Hanahan, D. J. and Everett, N. B. (1950). *J. biol Chem.* 185, 919.

Handelman, S. L. and Mills, J. R. (1965). *J. dent. Res.* 44, 1343.

Haneveld, G. T. (1960). *Trop. Geogr. Med.* 12, 339.

Hanke, M. T. and Koessler, K. K. (1924). *J. biol. Chem.* 59, 867.

Hansen, I. L. and Crawford, M. A. (1968). *Biochem. Pharmacol.* 17, 338.

Hansson, K., Lundh, G., Stenrau, U. and Wallerstrom, A. (1963). *Acta chir. scand.* 126, 338.

Hardcastle, J. D. and Wilkins, J. L. (1970). *Gut* 11, 1038.

Haughton, B. G. and King, H. K. (1961). *Biochem. J.* 80, 268.

Hawksworth, G. M. (1970). *J. Med. Microbiol.* 3, 9.

Hawksworth, G. M. (1973). "Ph.D. Thesis, London University."

Hawksworth, G. M., Drasar, B. S. and Hill, M. J. (1971). *J. Med. Microbiol.* 4, 451.

Hawksworth, G. M. and Hill, M. J. (1971a). *Biochem. J.* 122, 28.

Hawksworth, G. M. and Hill, M. J. (1971b). *Brit. J. Cancer* 25, 520.

Hayaishi, O., Taniuchi, II., Tashiro, M. and Kuno, S. (1961). *J. Biol. Chem.* 236, 2492.

Hayakawa, S., Saburi, Y. and Tamaki, K. (1958). *J. Biochem. (Tokyo)* 45, 419.

Hayakawa, S., Kanematsu, Y. and Fujiwara, T. (1969). *Biochem. J.* 115, 249.

Hayakawa, S. and Hattori, T. (1970). *Fed. Eur. Biochem. Soc. Lett.* 6, 131.

Heneghan, J. B. (1963). *Amer. J. Physiol.* 205, 417.

Heuise, E. R. and Myrvik, Q. N. (1966). *Fed. Proc.* 25, 439.

Hellman, L., Bradlow, H. L. and Zumoff, B. (1970). *Advanc. clin. Chem.* 13, 1.

Henning, N., Zeitler, G., and Neugebauer, I. (1958). *Münsch. med. Wschr.* 100, 1858.

Hentges, D. J. (1969). *J. Bact.* 97, 513.

Hentges, D. J. (1970). *Amer. J. clin. Nutr.* 23, 1451.

Hersh, T., Flock, M. H., Binder, H. J., Conn, H. O., Prizont, R. and Spiro, H. M. (1970). *Amer. J. clin. Nutr.* 23, 1595.

Hess, A. F., (1912). *J. inf. Dis.* 11, 71.

Hewetson, J. T. (1904). *B. M. J.,* 2, 1457.

Heynigen, W. E. Van. (1971). "Microbial Toxins", Vol 2A. Academic Press, London and N.Y., p. 69.

Hill, M. J. (1971a). "Some Implications of Steroid Hormones in Cancer" (Eds., Williams, D. C. and Briggs, M. H.). Heinemann, London, p. 84.

Hill, M. J. (1971b). *J. Pathol.* 104, 129.

Hill, M. J. and Drasar, B. S. (1968). *Gut* 9, 222.

Hill, M. J. and Aries, V. C. (1971). *J. Pathol.* 104, 129.

Hill, M. J., Drasar, B. S., Aries, V. C., Crowther, J. S., Hawksworth, G. M. and Williams, R. E. O. (1971). *Lancet i,* 95.

Hill, M. J., Goddard, P. and Williams, R. E. O. (1971b). *Lancet ii,* 472.

Hill, M. J. and Hawksworth, G. M. (1972). *In* "N-Nitroso Compounds: Analysis and Formation" (Eds., Bogovski, P., Preussman, R. and Walker, E. A.). International Agency for Research on Cancer (Lyon) p. 116.

Hill, M. J., Hawksworth, G. M. and Tattersall, G. (1973). *Brit J. Cancer* 28, 572.

Hirai, K. (1921). *Biochem. Z.* 114, 71.

Hirtzmann, M. and Reuter, G. (1963). *Med. Klin.* 58, 1408.

Hobbs, B. C. (1968). "Food Poisoning and Food Hygiene". Arnold, London.

Hobbs, J. R. (1971). *J. clin. Path.* 24, suppl. 5, 146.

Hoehn, W. M., Schmidt, L. H. and Hughes, H. B. (1944). *J. biol. Chem.* 152, 59.

Hofmann, A. F. (1965). *Gastroenterology* 48, 484.

Hofmann, A. F. (1969). "Bile Salt Metabolism" (Eds., Schiff, L., Carey, J. B. and Dietschy, J. M.) Thomas, Springfield, p. 160.

Hofmann, A. F. and Small, D. M. (1967). *Ann. Rev. Med.* 18, 333.

Hoffman, K. (1964). *Zbl. Bakt. I. Abt. Orig.* 192, 500.

Hoffmann, K., Mossel, D. A. R., Korus, W. and Van der Kamer, J. H. (1964). *Klin. Wschr.* 42, 126.

Holsti, P. (1960). *Nature, Lond.* 186, 250.

Holsti, P. (1962). *Acta path. microbiol. scand.* 54, 479.

Holt, R. (1967). *Lancet i,* 1259.

Holtz, P. (1958). *Klin. Wschr.* 36, 238.

Hooker, J. D. (1896). (Ed.) *"Journal of the Rt. Hon. Sir John Banks* during Captain Cook's first voyage in H.M.S. Endeavour in 1768-71". Macmillan, London and New York, p. 466.

Hopper, A. F., Wannemacher, R. W. and McGovern, P. A. (1968). *Proc. Soc. exp. Biol. Med. N.Y.* 128, 695.

Hoskins, L. C. (1968). *Gastroenterology* 54, 218.

Hoskins, L. C. and Zamcheck, N. (1968). *Gastroenterology* 54, 210.

Hötzel, D. and Barnes, R. H. (1966). *Vitam. and Horm.* 24, 115.

Houte van J. and Gibbons, R. J. (1966). *Antonie v. Leeuwenhoek* 32, 212.

Huggins, C. (1967). *Science, N.Y.* 156, 1050.

Hulsman, W. C. and van Eps, L. W. S. (1967). *Clin. chim. Acta.* 15, 233.

Hungate, R. E. (1950). *Bact. Rev.* 14, 1.

Hungate, R. E. (1966). "The Rumen and its Microbes". Academic Press, N.Y. and Lond.

Hunt, J. N. (1959). *Physiol. Rev.* 39, 491.

Hunt, R. D. (1963). *Proc. Soc. exp. Biol. (N.Y.)* 113, 139.

Hunt, R. D. (1964). *Proc. Soc. exp. Biol. (N.Y.)* 115, 277.

Hunt, R. D. (1965). *Fed. Proc.* 24, 431.

Ichihara, K., Yoshimatsu, H. and Sakamoto, Y. (1965). *J. Biochem. (Tokyo)* 43, 803.

Indahl, S. R. and Scheline, R. R. (1968). *Appl. Microbiol.* 16, 667.

Irvine, W. T., Duthie, H. L. and Waton, N. G. (1959a). *Lancet i,* 1061.

Irvine, W. T., Duthie, H. L., Ritchie, H. D. and Waton, N. G. (1959b). *Lancet i,* 1064.

Iveson, P., Parke, D. V. and Williams, R. T. (1966). *Biochem. J.* 100, 28.

James, W. P. T., Drasar, B. S. and Miller, C. (1972). *Amer. J. clin. Nutr.* 25, 564.

Jeejeebhoy, K. N., Desai, H. G., Borkar, A. V., Despande, V. and Pathare, S. M. (1968). *Amer. J. clin. Nutr.* 21, 994.

Jersky, J. and Kinsley, R. H. (1967). *S. Afr. med. J.* 41, 1194.

Joncs, E. A., Smallwood, R. A., Craigie, A. and Rosenoer, V. M. (1969). *Clin. Sci.* 37, 825.

Kaiharo, M. and Price, J. M. (1961). *J. biol. Chem.* 236, 508.

Kalser, M. H., Cohen, R., Arteaga, I., Yawn, E., Mayoral. L., Hoffert, W. R. and Frazier, D. (1966). *New Engl. J. Med.* 274, 500 and 558.

Kauffmann, F. (1969). "The Bacteriology of Enterobacteriaceae". Munksgaarde, Copenhagen.

Kean, B. H. (1963). *Ann. intern. Med.* 59, 605.

Kean, B. H. (1969). *Lancet ii*, 583.

Kellog, T. F. and Wostmann, B. S. (1969). *J. Lipid Res.* 10, 495.

Kemp, P. and White, R. W. (1968). *Biochem. J.* 106, 55.

Kendall, A. I., Day, A. A., Walker, A. W. and Haner, R. C. (1927). *J. infect. Dis.* 40, 677.

Kenworthy, R. and Allen, W. D. (1966a). *J. comp. Path.* 76, 31.

Kenworthy, R. and Allen, W. D. (1966b). *J. comp. Path.* 76, 291.

Kelper, C. R. and Tove, S. B. (1967). *J. biol. Chem.* 242, 5686.

Kern, F. and Meiroff, W. E. (1970). "Bile Salt Metabolism" (Eds., Schiff, L., Carey, J. B. and Dietschy, J. M.). Thomas, Springfield, p. 284

Ketyi, I. and Barna, K. (1964). *Acta microbiol. Acad. Sci. Hung.* 11, 173.

Khoury, K. A., Floch, M. H. and Hersh, T. (1969). *J. exp. Med.* 130, 659.

Kim, Y. S., Spritz, N., Blum, M., Terz, J. and Sherlock, P. (1966). *J. clin. Invest.* 45, 956.

King, R. J. B. (1971). *In* "Some Implications of Steroid Hormones in Cancer" (Eds., Williams, D. C. and Briggs, M. H.). Heinemann, London, p. 62.

Kirkman, H. (1959). *Nat. Cancer Inst. Monogr.* 1, 1.

Kleiner, I. S. and Orten, J. M. (1966)."Biochemistry" 7th Edn. C. V. Mosby and Co., St. Louis, U.S.A.

Klipstein, F. A. (1966). *Ann. intern. Med.* 61, 721.

Klipstein, F. A. (1968). *Gastroenterology* 54, 273.

Klipstein, F. A. (1968b). *Amer. J. clin. Nutr.* 21, 939.

Klipstein, F. A., Schenk, E. A. and Samloff, I. M. (1966). *Gastroenterology* 51, 317.

Klipstein, F. A. and Lipton, S. D. (1970). *Amer. J. clin. Nutr.* 23, 132.

Klipstein, F. A., Samloff, I. M., Smarth, G. and Schenk, E. (1968). *Amer. J. clin. Nutr.* 21, 1042.

Kluyver, A. J. and van Niel, C. B. (1936). *Zbl. Bakt. II Abt. Orig.* 94, 369.

Knott, F. A. (1923).Guy's Hospital Reports 73, 429.

Knott, F. A. (1927). Guy's Hospital Reports 77, 1.

Kojima, S. and Ichibagase, H. (1966). *Chem. Pharm. Bull.* 14, 971.

Korn, E. D., Ulsamer, A. G., Weihing, R. R., Wetzel, M. G. and Wright, P. L. (1969). *Biochim. Biophys. Acta* 187, 555.

Kubota, Y. and Lin, P. V. (1971). *J. inf. Dis.* 123, 97.

Krikler, D. M and Schrive, V. (1958). *Lancet i*, 510.

Krone, C. C., Theodor, E., Sleisenger, M. H. and Jeffries, G. H. (1968). *Medicine* 47, 89.

Krumwiede, E. (1954). *J. exp. Med.* 100, 629.

Kuznezova, L. E. (1969). *Nature, Lond.* 222, 484.

Labrec, E. H., Schneider, H., Magnains, T. J. and Formol, S. P. (1964). *J. Bact.* 88, 1503.

Lacassagne, A. C. (1932). *C. R. Acad. Sci. (Paris)* 195, 630.

Lacassagne, A. C. (1939). *C. R. Soc. Biol. (Paris)* 132, 365.

Lacassagne, A. C., Buu-Hoi, N. P. and Zajdela, F. (1961). *Nature, Lond.* 190, 1007.

Lacassagne, A. C., Buu-Hoi, N. P. and Zajdela, F. (1966). *Nature, Lond.* 209, 1026.

Lack, L. and Weiner, I. M. (1961). *Amer. J. Physiol.* 200, 313.

Laqueur, G. L. (1964). *Fed. Proc.* 23, 1386.

Laqueur, G. L., McDaniel, E. G. and Matsumoto, H. (1967). *J. nat. Cancer Inst.* 39, 355.

Laqueur, G. L. and Spatz, M. (1968). *Cancer Res.* 28, 2262.

Latham, M. J. and Sharpe, E. (1971). *In* "The Isolation of Anaerobes". The Soc. for Applied Bacteriology. Technical series No. 5 (Eds., Shapton, D. A. and Board, R. G.).

Lautemann, E. (1863). *Ann. Chem.* 125, 9.

Lauterbach, F. and Repke, K. (1960). *Arch. exp. Path. Pharmacol.* 240, 45.

Lee, A., Gordon, J. and Dubos, R. (1968). *Nature, Lond.* **220**, 1137.

Lee, C., Anderson, R. C., Henderson, F. G., Worth, H. M. and Harris, P. N. (1959). *Antibiot. An.*

Legler, F. and Zeitler, G. (1964). *Dtsch. med. Wschr.* **89**, 1506.

Leifson, E. (1935). *J. Pathol. Bacteriol.* **40**, 581.

Lesher, S., Walburg, H. E. and Sacher, G. A. (1964). *Nature, Lond.* **202**, 884.

Lester, R. and Schmid, R. (1963a). *J. clin. Invest.* **42**, 736.

Lester, R. and Schmid, R. (1963b). *New Engl. J. Med.* **269**, 178.

Lester, R. and Schmid, R. (1965). *J. clin. Invest.* **44**, 722.

Lester, R. and Klein, P. D. (1966). *J. clin. Invest.* 1839.

Lethco, E. J. and Webb, J. M. (1966). *J. Pharmacol. exp. Ther.* **154**, 384.

Levenson, S. M., Croley, L. V., Horowitz, R. E. and Malm, O. J. (1959). *J. biol. Chem.* **234**, 2061.

Levine, S. Z., Marples, E. and Gordon, H. H. (1941). *J. clin. Invest.* **20**, 199.

Levy, H. R. and Talalay, P. (1959a). *J. biol Chem.* **234**, 2009.

Levy, H. R. and Talalay, P. (1959b). *J. biol. Chem.* **234**, 2014.

Lindenbaum, J. (1965). *Brit. med. J. ii*, 326.

Lindenbaum, J. (1968). *Amer. J. clin. Nutr.* **21**, 1023.

Lindenbaum, J., Gerson, C. D. and Kent, T. H. (1971). *Ann. intern. Med.* **74**, 218.

Linecar, D. (1972). Unpublished results.

Ling, V. and Morin, C. L. (1971). *Biochim. biophys. Acta (Amst.)* **249**, 252.

Linstedt, S. (1957). *Arkiv. Kemi.* **11**, 145.

Linstedt, G., Linstedt, S. and Gustafsson, B. E. (1965). *J. exp. Med.* **121**, 201.

Loesche, W. L. (1969). *Proc. Soc. exp. Biol. (N.Y.)* **131**, 387.

Lower, G. M. and Bryan, G. T. (1969). *J. biol. Chem.* **244**, 2567.

Luckey, T. D. (1963). "Germfree Life and Gnotobiology". Academic Press, N.Y. and London.

Macbeth, W. A. A. G., Kass, E. H. and McDermatt, W. V. (1965). *Lancet i*, 399.

MacFarlane, M. G. and Knight, B. C. J. G. (1941). *Biochem. J.* **35**, 884.

MacFarlane, M. G., Oakley, C. L. and Anderson, G. G. (1941). *J. Path. Bact.* **52**, 99.

Magee, P. N. and Barnes, J. M. (1967). *Advanc. Cancer Res.* **10**, 163.

Maldonado, N., Horta, E., Guerra, R. and Pérez-Santiago, E. (1969). *Gastroenterology (B. Aires)* **57**, 559.

Mallinson, C. N. and Drasar, B. S. (1970). *Gut* **11**, 371.

Mandel, A. D. and Ellison, R. C. (1963). *J. Am. med. Ass.* **185**, 536.

Mandell, A. J. and Rubin, R. T. (1965). *Life Sciences* **4**, 1657.

Marsh, C. A., Alexander, F. and Levvy, G. A. (1952). *Nature, Lond.* **170**, 163.

Martini, G. A., Phear, E. A., Ruebner, B. and Sherlock, S. (1957). *Clin. Sci.* **16**, 35.

Martin, G. C. (1942). *Arch. Biochem.* **1**, 397.

Mason, M. M. and Whiting, M. G. (1966). *Fed. Proc.* **25**, 533.

Mata, L. J., Mejicanos, M. L. and Jiménez, F. (1972). *Amer. J. clin. Nutr.* **25**, 1380.

Mathan, V. I. and Baker, S. J. (1968). *Amer. J. clin. Nutr.* **21**, 1077.

Mawdesley-Thomas, L. E. (1971). *In* "Metabolic Aspects of Food Safety" (Ed., Roe, F. J. C.). Blackwell, Oxford, p. 486.

McCracken. R. D. (1970). *J. Am. Med. Ass.* **213**, 2257.

McMahon, B. and Cole, P. (1969). *Cancer* **24**, 1146.

McMichael, H. B., Webb, J. and Dawson, A. M. (1966). *Brit. med. J. ii*, 1037.

Melnykowycz, J. and Johansson, K. R. (1955). *J. exp. Med.* **101**, 507.

Metchnikoff, E. (1903). "The Nature of Man". Translated by P. Chalmers Mitchell. Heinemann, London.

Metchnikoff, E. (1907). "The Prolongation of Life". Translated by P. Chalmers Mitchell. Heinemann, London.

Meynell, G. G. (1963). *Brit. J. exp. Path.* **XLIV**, 209.

Michel, M. C. (1962). *Amino acids, peptides, proteins, Cahier* No. 5, 157.

Midtvedt, T. (1967). *Acta path. microbiol. scand.* 71, 147.

Midtvedt, T. and Norman, A. (1967). *Acta path. microbiol. scand.* 71, 629.

Midvedt, T. and Norman, A. (1968). *Acta path. microbiol. scand.* 72, 313.

Milburn, P. Personal communication.

Miller, C. P. and Bohnhoff, M. (1962). *J. infect. Dis.* 111, 107.

Mills, S. C., Scott, T. W., Russell, G. R. and Smith, R. M. (1970). *Aust. J. biol. Sci.* 23, 1109.

Minder, R., Schnetzer, F. and Bickel, M. H. (1971). *Naunyn-Schmiedeberg's Arch. exp. Path. Pharmak.* **268**, 334.

Mitchell, D. N. and Rees, R. J. W. (1970). *Lancet ii*, 168.

Mitchell, W. D. and Diver, M. J. (1967). *Lipids* 2, 467.

Moench, L. M., Kahn, M. C. and Torry, J. C. (1925). *J. infect. Dis.* 37, 161.

Monteiro, E., Fossey, J., Shiner, M., Drasar, B. S. and Allison, A. C. (1971). *Lancet i*, 249.

Montgomery, R. D. (1969). *In* "Toxic Constituents of Plant Foodstuffs" (Ed., Liener, I. E.). Academic Press, London and N.Y.

Moon, H. W. and Whipp, S. C. (1971). *Ann. N.Y. Acad. Sci.* 176, 197.

Moore, W. B. (1968). *J. gen. Microbiol.* 53, 415.

Moore, W. E. C. (1965). *Int. J. systematic Bact.* 16, 173.

Moore, W. E. C., Cato, E. P. and Holdeman, L. V. (1969). *J. infect. Dis.* 119, 641.

Morris, C. R. and Bryan, G. T. (1966). *Invest. Urol.* 3, 577.

Mulder, E., Van Den Berg, J. W. O. and Van Deenen, L. I.. M. (1965). *Biochim. Biophys. Acta* 106, 118.

Muller, F. von (1892). *Schlesiche Gesell, Vaterland Cultur.* 70, 1.

Murrell, T. G. C., Egerton, J. R., Rampling, A., Samels, J. and Walker, P. D. (1966). (a) *Lancet i*, 217. (b) J. Hyg. Camb. 64, 375.

Nagler, F. P. O. (1939). *Brit. J. exp. Path.* 20, 473.

Nair, P. P. (1969). *In* "Bile Salt Metabolism" (Eds., Schiff, L., Carey, J. B. and Dietschy, J. M.). Thomas, Springfield, p. 172.

Nair, P. P., Gordon, M. and Reback, J. (1967). *J. biol Chem.*, 242, 7.

Naish, J. and Capper, W. M. (1953). *Lancet ii*, 597.

Najjar, V. A. (1944). *J. Amer. med. Ass.* 126, 357.

Najjar, V. A. and Holt, L. E. (1943). *J. Amer. med. Ass.* 123, 683.

Neale, G. (1968). *Proc. roy. Soc.Med.*, 60, 1069.

Neale, G. (1971). *J. clin. Path.* 24, Suppl.5, 22.

Nelson, D. P. and Mata, L. J. (1970). *Gastroenterology* 58, 56.

Neufeld, F. (1900). *Z. Hyg. Infect.* 34, 454.

Newton, W. L., Pennington, R. M. and Lieberman, J. E. (1960). *Proc. Soc. exp. Biol. (N.Y.)* 104, 486.

Nichols, A. C. and Glenn, P. M. (1940). *J. Lab. clin. Med.* 25, 388.

Nielsen, E. and Evenhin, C. A. (1942). *J. Biol. Chem.* 145, 713.

Noda Institute for Scientific Research, (1966). *Chem. Abstr.* 65, 6262g.

Norman, A. and Grubb, R. (1955). *Acta path. microbiol. scand.* 36, 537.

Norman, A. and Sjovall, J. (1958). *J. biol. Chem.* 233, 872.

Norman, A. and Bergman, S. (1960). *Acta chem. scand.* 14, 1781.

Norman, A. and Palmer, R. H. (1964). *J. Lab. clin. Med.* 63, 986.

Norman, A. and Widstrom, O. A. (1964). *Proc. Soc. exp. Biol. (N.Y.)* 117, 442.

O'Brien, W. and England, N. W. J. (1966). *Brit. med. J. ii*, 1157.

Ogawa, H., Honjo, S., Takasaka, M., Fujiwara, T. and Tmaizumi, K. (1966). *Jap. J. med. Sci. Biol.* 21, 259.

O'Gorman, L. P., Borud, O., Khan, I. A. and Gjessing, L. R. (1970). *Clin. chim. Acta.* 29, 111.

Okamoto, S. and Suzuki, Y. (1965). *Nature, Lond.* 208, 1301.

Okita, G. T., Kelsey, F. E., Walaszek, E. J. and Geiling, E. M. (1954). *J. Pharmacol.* 110, 244.

Olson, G. B. and Wostman, B. S. (1966). *J. Immunol.* 97, 267.

Ozanne, B., Benvenister, R., Tipper, D. and Davies, J. (1969). *J. Bact.* 100, 1044.

Ozawa, A. and Freter, R. (1964). *J. infect. Dis.* 114, 235.

Pala, G., Goppi, G. and Crescenzi, E. (1966). *Arch. Int. Pharmacodyn.* 164, 356.

Palmer, R. H. (1970). *In* "Bile Salt Metabolism" (Eds., Schiff, L., Carey, J. B. and Dietschy, J. M.). Thomas, Springfield, p. 184.

Palmer, R. H. and Hruban, Z. (1966). *J. clin. Invest.* 45, 1255.

Parke, D. V. (1968). "The Biochemistry of Foreign Compounds". Pergamon Press, Oxford.

Parke, D. V., Pollock, S. and Williams, R. T. (1963). *J. Pharm. Pharmacol.* 15, 500.

Pakti, V. M. and Shirsat, M. V. (1961). *J. Sic. Ind. Res. (India)* 20c, 181.

Parkin, D. M., McLelland, D. B. L., O'Moore, R. R., Percy-Robb, I. W., Grant, I. W. B. and Shearman, D. J. C. (1972). *Gut* 13, 182.

Peach, S. L., Fernandez, F., Johnson, K. and Drasar, B. S. (1972). *J. med. Microbiol.* 5, xivP

Pearson, J. (1970). *M. Phil. Thesis, (London).*

Peppercorn, M. A. and Goldman, P. (1971). *J. Bact.* 108, 996.

Perleman, P. and Broberger, O. (1969). *In* "Text-book of Immunopathology" Vol. II (Eds., Muescher, P. A. and Muller-Eberhard, H. J.). Grune and Stratton.

Perry, T. L., Hestrin, M., MacDougall, L. and Hansen, S. (1966). *Clin. chim. Acta* 14, 116.

Phear, E. A. and Ruebner, B. (1956). *Brit. J. exp. Path.* 37, 253.

Phillips, B. P. and Wolfe, P. A. (1959). *Ann. N.Y. Acad. Sci.* 78, 308.

Phillips, G. B., Schwartz, R., Gabuzda, G. J. and Davidson, C. S. (1952). *New Engl. J. Med.* 247, 239.

Phillips, M. J. and Finlay, J. M. (1967). *J. Path. Bact.* 94, 131.

Platt, B. S., Heard, C. R. C. and Stewart, R. J. C. (1964). *In* "The Role of the Gastrointestinal Tract in Protein Metabolism" (Ed., Munro, H. N.). Blackwell, Oxford.

Plaut, A. G., Gorbach, S. L., Nahas, L., Weinstein, L., Spanknebel, G. and Levetan, R. (1967). *Gastroenterology* 53, 868.

Pope, J. L. and Todwell, H. C. (1964). *Fed. Proc.* 23, 426.

Polachek, A. A., Pyanowski, W. J. and Miller, J. M. (1961). *Ann. intern. Med.* 54, 636.

Polter, D. E., Boyle, J. D., Miller., J. G. and Finegold, S. M. (1968). *Gastroenterology* 54, 1148.

Porter, J. R. and Rettger, L. (1940). *J. infect. Dis.* 66, 104.

Powell, D. W., Plotkin, G. R., Maenza, R. M., Solberg, L. I., Catlin, D. H. and Formol, S. B. (1971). *Gastroenterology* 60, 1053.

Price, J. M. (1966). *Can. Cancer Conf.* 6, 224.

Price, J. M. and Brown, R. R. (1962). *Acta Unio. Intern. Contra Cancrum* 18, 684.

Prizont, D. E., Hersch, T. and Floch, M. H. (1970). *Amer. J. clin. Nutr.* 23, 1602.

Proulx, P. and VanDeenen, L. L. M. (1966). *Biochim. Biophys. Acta* 125, 591.

Proulx, P. and VanDeenen, L. L. M. (1967). *Biochim. Biophys. Acta* 144, 171.

Quagliariello, E., Tancredi, F., Fedele, L. and Saccone, C. (1961). *Brit. J. Cancer,* 15, 367.

Quick, A. J. (1932). *J. Biol. Chem.* 97, 403.

Radomski, J. L. and Mellinger, T. J. (1962). *J. Pharmacol. exp. Ther.* 136, 259.

Raven, H. A., Rowley, D., Jenkins, C. and Fine, J. (1960). *J. exp. Med.* 177, 783.

Reis, van der, V. (1925). *Ergebn. inn. Med. Kinderheilk* 27, 78.

Renwick, A. G. and Williams, R. T. (1969). *Biochem. J.* 114, 78p.

Rettger, L. F. and Cheplin, H. A. (1921). "A Treatise on the Transformation of the Intestinal Flora etc." Yale University Press, New Haven.

Rettger, L. F., Levey, M. N., Weinstein, L. and Weis, J. E. (1935). "*Lactobacillus acidophilus* and its Therapeutic Applications". Yale University Press, New Haven.

Richards, P, Metcalfe-Gibson, A., Ward, E. E., Wrong, O. M. and Houghton, B. J. (1967). *Lancet ii*, 845.

Richardson, R. L. and Jones, M. (1958). *J. dent. Res.* 37, 697.

Ridwell, A. G. (1955). *Ann. roy. Coll. Surg. Engl.* 17, 319.

Ringold, H. J., Hayano, M. and Stefanovic, V.(1963). *J. biol. Chem.* 238, 1960.

Robinet, H. G. (1962). *J. Bact.* 84, 896.

Rogers, W. F., Burdick, M. P. and Burnett, G. R. (1955). *J. Lab. Clin. Med.* 45, 87.

Rose, D. P. (1967). *Clin. chim. Acta* 18, 221.

Rose, D. P., Randall, Z. and Cramp, D. G. (1971). *Clin chim. Acta* 40, 276.

Rosebury, T. (1962). "Micro-organisms Indigenous to Man". McGraw-Hill Book Co.

Rosenfeldt, R. S. and Gallagher, T. F. (1964). *Steroids* 4, 515.

Rosenheim, O. and Starling, W. W. (1933). *Chem. Ind. (Lond.)* 48, 238.

Rosenheim, O. and Webster, T. A. (1941). *Biochem. J.* 35, 920.

Rosenheim, O. and Webster, T. A. (1943). *Biochem. J.* 37, 580.

Ross, C. A. C. and Dawes, E. A. (1954). *Lancet i*, 994.

Ross, C. A., Frazer, A. C., French, J. M., Gerrard, J. W., Sammons, H. G. and Smellie, J. M. (1955). *Lancet i*, 1087.

Rowan, R. and Martin, J. (1963). *Biochem. Biophys. Acta* 70, 396.

Rowe, B., Taylor, J. and Bettelheim, K. A. (1970). *Lancet i*, 1.

Roxon, J. J., Ryan, A. J. and Wright, S. E. (1967). *Food Cosmet. Toxicol.* 5, 367.

Russel, P. K., Aziz, M. A., Ahmad, N., Kent, T. H. and Gangorosa, E. J. (1966). *Amer. J. dig. Dis.* 11, 296.

Sabbaj, J., Sutter, V. L., and Finegold, S. M. (1970). *Antimicrob. Ag. Chemother.* 181.

Salen, G., Goldstein, F. and Wirts, C. W. (1966). *Ann. intern. Med.* 64, 834.

Samuel, P., Saypol, G. M., Meilman, E., Mosbach, E. H. and Chaftzadeh, M. (1968). *J. clin. Invest.* 47, 2070.

Samuelsson, B. (1960). *J. Biol. Chem.* 235, 361.

Sanborn, A. G. (1931a). *J. infect. Dis.* 48, 541.

Sanborn, A. G. (1931b). *J. infect. Dis.* 49, 37.

Sander, J. (1968). *Hoppe. Seylers Z. Physiol. Chem.* 349, 429.

Sandler, M., Karoum, F., Ruthven, C. R. J. and Calne, D. B. (1969). *Science, N.Y.* 166, 1417.

Saunders, D. R. and Dawson, A. M. (1963). *Gut* 4, 254.

Savage, D. C. (1970). *Amer. J. clin. Nutr.* 23, 1495.

Savage, D. C. (1972). *Soc. Gen. Microbiol. Symposium Series* 22, 25.

Savage, D. C., Dubos, R. and Schaedler, R. W. (1968). *J. exp. Med.* 127, 67.

Savage, W. E., Hajj, S. N. and Kass, E. H. (1967). *Medicine (Baltimore)* 46, 385.

Saz, A. K. and Marmer, J. (1953). *Proc. Soc. exp. Biol. (N.Y.)* 82, 783.

Saz, A. K. and Slie, R. B. (1954a). *Arch. Biochem.* 51, 5.

Saz, A. K. and Slie, R. B. (1954b). *J. Biol. Chem.* 210, 407.

Scheline, R. R. (1966). *Acta Pharm. Toxicol.* 24, 275.

Scheline, R. R. (1967). *Experientia (Basel)* 23, 493.

Scheline, R. R. (1968a). *J. pharm. Sci.* 57, 2021.

Scheline, R. R. (1968b). *Acta Pharm. Toxicol.* **26**, 332.

Scheline, R. R., Williams, R. T. and Wit, J. G. (1960). *Nature, Lond.* **188**, 849.

Scheline, R. R. and Longberg, B. (1965). *Acta Pharm. Toxicol.* **23**, 1.

Schenk, E. A., Samloff, I. M. and Klipstein, F. A. (1968). *Amer. J. clin. Nutr.* **21**, 944.

Schenkers, S., McCandless, D. W., Brophy, E., and Lewis, M. S. (1967). *J. clin. Invest.* **46**, 838.

Schjonsby, H., Peters, T. J., Hoffbrand, A. V. and Tabaqchali, S. (1970). *Gut* **11**, 371.

Schoenheimer, R. and Sperry, W. M. (1934). *J. Biol. Chem.* **107**, 1.

Scott, T. W., Ward, P. F. V. and Dawson, R. M. C. (1964). *Biochem. J.* **90**, 12.

Scrimshaw, N. S., Taylor, C. E. and Gordon, J. E. (1968). WHO Monograph No. 57.

Sears, H. J., James, H., Saloum, R., Brownlee, I. and Lamoreaux, L. F. (1957). *J. Bact.* **71**, 370.

Seeliger, H. and Werner, H. (1963). *Ann. Inst. Pasteur* **105**, 911.

Seneca, H. and Henderson, E. (1950). *Gastroenterology* **15**, 34.

Senior, J. R. (1964). *J. Lipid Res.* **5**, 495.

Shaw, W. V. (1967). *J. biol. Chem.* **242**, 687.

Shaw, W. V. and Brodsky, R. F. (1968). *J. Bact.* **95**, 28.

Shaw, W. V., Bentley, D. W. and Sands, L. (1970). *J. Bact.* **104**, 1095.

Shearman, D. J. C., Parkin, D. M. and McClelland, D. B. L. (1972). *Gut* **13**, 483.

Sheehy, T. W. and Perez-Santiago, E. (1961). *Gastroenterology* **41**, 208.

Sheehy, T. W., Legters, L. J. and Wallace, D. K. (1968). *Amer. J. clin. Nutr.* **21**, 1013.

Sherlock, S. (1958). *Amer. J. Med.* **24**, 805.

Sherlock, S., Summerskill, W. H. J. and Dawson, A. M. (1956). *Lancet ii*, 689.

Sherris, J. C., Roberts, C. E. and Porus, R. L. (1965). *Gastroenterology* **48**, 708.

Sherwood, W. C., Goldstein, F., Haurani, F. I. and Wirts, C. W. (1964). *Amer. J. dig. Dis.* **9**, 416.

Shimida, S. S., Bricknell, K. and Finegold, S. (1969). *J. infect. dis.* **119**, 273.

Shiner, M. (1963). *Lancet i*, 532.

Shiner, M. (1970). *In* "Bile Salt Metabolism" (Eds., Schiff, L., Carey, J. B. and Dietschy, L.). Thomas, Springfield, p. 41.

Shiner, M., Waters, T. E. and Gray, J. D. A. (1963). *Gastroenterology* **43**, 625.

Shooter, R. A., Cooke, M. E., Rousseau, S. A. and Braden, A. L. (1970). *Lancet ii*, 226.

Sih, C. J., Wang, K. C. and Tai, H. H. (1968a). *Biochemistry* **7**, 796.

Sih, C. J., Tai, H. H., Tsong, Y. Y., Lee, S. S. and Coombe, R. G. (1968b). *Biochemistry* **7**, 808.

Sinclair, T, and Tuxford, A. F. (1971). The Paractitioner **207**, 81.

Siurala, M. and Kaipainen, W. J. (1953). *Acta med. scand.* **147**, 197.

Small, D. M. (1969). *In* "Bile Salt Metabolism" (Eds., Schiff, L., Carey, J. B. and Dietschy, L.). Thomas, Springfield, p. 223.

Smith, G. M. and Worrell, C. S. (1949). *Arch. Biochem.* **24**, 219.

Smith, G. M. and Worrell, C. S. (1950). *Arch. Biochem.* **28**, 232.

Smith, H. W. (1965). *J. Path. Bact.* **89**, 95.

Smith, H. W. (1966). *J. Path. Bact.* **91**, 1.

Smith, H. W. (1971). *Ann. N.Y. Acad. Sci.* **176**, 110.

Smith, H. W. (1972). "Microbial Pathogenicity in Man and Animals". The 22nd Symposium of the Society for General Microbiology. University Press, Cambridge.

Smith, H. W. and Halls, S. (1967). *J. Path. Bact.* **93**, 499.

Smith, H. W. and Halls, S. (1968). *J. gen. Microbiol.* **52**, 319.

Smith, H. W. and Gyles, C. L. (1970). *J. med. Microbiol.* **3**, 287.

Smith, L. D. S. and Holdeman, L. V. (1968). "The Pathogenic Anaerobic Bacteria". Thomas, Springfield.

Smith, R. L. (1966). *Progress in Drug Research* 9, 300.

Snell, S. (1964). *J. Immunol.* 92, 559.

Snog-Kjaer, A., Prange, I. and Dam, H. (1956). *J. gen. Microbiol.* 14, 256.

Solimano, G., Burgess, A. E. and Levin, B. (1967). *Brit. J. Nutr.* 21, 55.

Sompolinsky, D., Ziegler-Schlomowitz, R. and Herczog, D. (1968). *Canad. J. Microbiol.* 14, 891.

Spatz, M., McDaniel, E. G. and Laqueur, G. L. (1966). *Proc. Soc. exp. Biol. (N.Y.)* 121, 417.

Spatz, M., Smith, D. W. E., McDaniel, E. G. and Laqueur, G. L. (1967). *Proc. Soc. exp. Biol. (N.Y.)* 124, 691.

Spink, W. W., Hurd, F. W. and Jermsta, J. (1940). *Proc. Soc. exp. Biol. (N.Y.)* 43, 172.

Spira, W. M. and Goepfert, J. M. (1972). *Appl. Microbiol.* 24, 341.

Springer, G. F., Williamson, P. and Readler, B. L. (1962). *Ann. N.Y. Acad. Sci.* 97, 104.

Sprinz, H. (1969). *Arch. Path. (Chicago)* 87, 556.

Sprinz, H., Sribhibhadh, R., Gangarosa, E. J., Benyajati, C., Kundel, D. and Halstead, S. (1962). *Amer. J. clin. Path.* 38, 43.

Sprinz, H., Gangarosa, E. J., Williams, M., Hornich, R. B. and Woodward, T. E. (1966). *Amer. J. dig. Dis.* 11, 615.

Stahlsberg, H. and Taksdal, S. (1971). *Lancet ii*, 1175.

Stacey, M. and Webb, B. (1947). *Proc. roy. Soc. B.* 134, 523.

Staley, T. E., Corley, L. D. and Jones, E. W. (1970). *Amer. J. dig. Dis.* 15, 923.

Stammers, F. A. R. and Williams, J. A. (1963). "Partial Gastrectomy". Butterworths, London.

Starzl, T. E., Butz, G. W. and Hartman, C. F. (1961). *Surgery* 50, 849.

Sternberg, G. M. (1896). "A Text-book of Bacteriology". J. and A. Churchill, London.

Stewart, G. T. (1966). *In* "Antibiotics, Advances in Research, Production and Clinical Use" (Eds., Herold, M. and Gabriel, Z.). Butterworths, London, p 25.

Sutton, R. G. A. and Hobbs, B. C., (1965). *J. Hyg. Camb.* 66, 135.

Stimmel, B. F. (1954). *Fed. Proc.* 13, 305.

Stocks, P. (1963). *Cancer Progress* 236.

Stokstad, E. L. R. (1954). *Physiol. Rev.* 34, 25.

Stollerman, G. H. and Ekstedt, R. (1957). *J. exp. Med.* 106, 345.

Stoudt, T. H., McAleer, W. J., Kozlowski, M. A. and Marlatt, V. (1958). *Arch. Biochem. Biophys.* 74, 280.

Stoudt, T. H., McAleer, W. J., Chemerda, J. M., Kozlowski, M. A., Hirschmann, R. F., Marlett, V. and Miller, R. (1955). *Arch. Biochem. Biophys.* 59, 304.

Suda, M., Hayaishi, O. and Oda, Y. (1950). *Med. J. Osaka Univ.* 2, 21.

Summerskill, W. H. J. (1969). *Prog. Gastroenterology* 2, 276.

Summers, R. W. and Kent, T. H. (1970). *Gastroenterology* 59, 740.

Sussman, S. (1961). *Pediatrics* 27, 308.

Suzuki, Y., Okamoto, S. and Kono, M. (1966). *J. Bact.* 92, 798.

Suzuki, Y. and Okamoto, S. (1967). *J. biol. Chem.* 242, 4722.

Tabaqchali, S. and Booth, C. C. (1966). *Lancet ii*, 12.

Tabaqchali, S., Okubadejo, O. A., Neale, G. and Booth, C. C. (1966a). *Proc. roy. Soc. Med.* 59, 1244.

Tabaqchali, S. and Booth, C. C. (1967). *Gut* 7, 712.

Tabaqchali, S. and Booth, C. C. (1970). *Mod. Trends Gastroenterology* 4, 143.

Tabaqchali, S., Hatzioannou, J. and Gorbach, S. (1970). *In* "Bile Salt Metabolism" (Eds., Schiff, L., Carey, J. B. and Dietschy, J. M.). Thomas, Springfield, p. 76.

Takahashi, H., Kaihara, M. and Price, J. M. (1956). *J. biol. Chem.* 223, 705.

Takahashi, H., Kaihara, M. and Price, J. M. (1958). *J. biol. Chem.* 233, 150.

Takeuchi, A. (1967). *Am. J. Pathol.* 50, 109.

Takeuchi, A., Sprinz, H., LaBrec, E. H. and Formol, S. B. (1965). *Amer. J. Path.* 47, 1011.

Takeuchi, A. and Sprinz, H. (1967). *Amer. J. Path.* 51, 137.

Takeuchi, A., Formol, S. B. and Sprinz, H. (1968). *Amer. J. Path.* 52, 503.

Tannenbaum, A. and Silverstone, H. (1949). *Cancer Res.* 9, 162.

Taylor, J. Maltby, M. P. and Payne, J. M. (1958). *J. Path. Bact.* 76, 491.

Taylor, K. B. (1972). *In* "Recent Advances in Gastroenterology" 2nd. Edn. (Eds., Badenoch, J. and Brooke, B. N.). Churchill-Livingstone, Edinburgh and London, p 1.

Thannhauser, S. J. and Dorfmuller, G. (1918). *J. chem. Soc.* 144, 1, 513.

Thomas, P. J. (1972). *Gastroenterology* 62, 430.

Thompson, G. R. (1967). *Brit. med. J. i*, 219.

Thompson, R. Q., Sturtevant, M., Bird, O. D. and Glazko, A. J. (1954). *Endocrinology* 55, 665.

Thompson, D., Thompson, R. and Morrison, J. T. (1948). "Oral Vaccines". Livingstone, Edinburgh.

Thompson, S. (1955). *J. Hyg. (Camb.)* 53, 217.

Thorebecke, G. J. and Benacerraf, B. (1959). *Ann. N.Y. Acad. Sci.* 78, 247.

Tomasi, T. B. (1972). *New Engl. J. Med.* 287, 500.

Tomasi, T. B. and Bienestock, J. (1968). *Adv. Immunol.* 9, 1.

Topley, W. W. C. and Wilson, G. S. (1936). "The Principles of Bacteriology and Immunity" 2nd Edn. Arnold, London.

Torrey, J. C. and Montu, E. (1931). *J. Inf. Dis.* 49, 141.

Trexler, R. J., Dawber, N. H. and Lester, R. (1968). *Gastroenterology* 54, 568.

Twort, F. W. (1907). *Proc. roy. Soc.* 79B, 329.

Uno, T. and Kono, M. (1961). *J. Pharm. Soc. (Japan)* 81, 1432.

Urbach, K. F. (1949). *Proc. Soc. exp. Biol. (N.Y.)* 70, 146.

Varela, G., Kean, B. H., Barrett, E. and Keegan, C. J. (1959). *Amer. J. trop. Med.* 8, 353.

Vezina, C., Singh, K. and Sehgal, S. N. (1969). *Appl. Microbiol.* 18, 270.

Vince, A. J. V. (1971). Intestinal Bacteria in Health and Disease. *Ph.D. Thesis*, University of London.

Vlahcevic, Z. R., Buhac, I., Farrer, J. T., Bell, C. C. and Swell, L. (1971). *Gastroenterology*, 11, 420.

Vlahcevic, Z. R., Bell, C. C., Gregory, D. H., Buker, G., Juttijudata, P. and Swell, L. (1972). *Gastroenterology* 62, 73.

Walker, A. R. (1961). *S. Afr. med. J.* 35, 114.

Walker, A. R., Walker, B. F. and Richardson, B. D. (1970). *Brit. med. J. iii*, 48.

Walker, J. G., Emlyn-Williams, A., Craigie, A., Rosenoer, V. M., Agnew, J. and Sherlock, S. (1965). *Lancet ii*, 861.

Wallace, W. C., Lethco, E. J. and Brouwer, E. A. (1970). *J. Pharmacol. exp. Ther.*, 175, 325.

Walser, M. and Bodenlos, L. J. (1959). *J. clin. Invest.* 38, 1617.

Watkinson, G., Feather, D. B., Marson, F. G. W. and Dossett, J. A. (1959). *Brit. med. J. iii*, 58.

Watson, C. J. (1963). *J. clin. Path.* 16, 1.

Watson, E. J., Campbell, M. and Lowry, P. T. (1958). *Proc. Soc. exp. Biol. N.Y.* 98, 701.

Watson, W. C. (1965). *Clin. chim. Acta* 12, 340.

Webb, J. P. W., James, A. T. and Kellock, T. D. (1963). *Gut* 4, 37.

Weijers, H. A., Van de Kamer, J. H., Mossel, D. A. A. and Dicks, W. K. (1960). *Lancet ii*, 296.

Weissenbach, R. J. (1918). *C. R. Soc. Biol. (Paris)* 81, 559.

Welch, A. D., Mattis, P. A. and Latven, A. R. (1942). *J. Pharmacol. exp. Ther.* 75, 231.

Wellcome Trust. (1972). "Tropical Sprue : The Wellcome Trust Study Group". Churchill, London.

Wesselius-De-Casparis, H., Braadbaht, S., Bergh-Bohlken, G. E. and Mimica, M. (1968). *Gut* 9, 84.

West, E. S., Todd, W. R., Mason, H. S. and van Bruggen, J. T. (1966). "Text-Book of Biochemistry" 4th Edn Macmillan, New York.

Wheater, D. W. F. and Hurst, E. W. (1962). *J. Path. Bact.* 82, 117.

Wheatley, D. W. F. (1968). *Arch. Dis. Childh.* 43, 53.

White, L. P., Phear, E. A., Summerskill, W. H. J. and Sherlock, S. (1955). *J. clin. Invest.* 34, 158.

White, F. R. and White, J. (1954). *J. nat. Cancer Inst.* 5, 41.

Whiting, M. G. (1963). *Econom. Bot.* 17, 271.

Wichels, P. (1924). *Z. clin. Med.* 100, 535.

Wiggins, H. S., Bramwell Cook, H. and McLeod, G. M. (1967). *Overdruk. mit. Tijdschrift. voor Gastro-Enterologie* 10, 64.

Wiggins, H. S., Howell, K. E., Kellock, T. D. and Stalder, J. (1969). *Gut* 10, 400.

Williams, R. E. O., Hill, M. J. and Drasar, B. S. (1971). *J. clin. Path.* 24, (Suppl. 5), 125.

Williams, R. E. O. and Drasar, B. S. (1972). *In* "Recent Advances in Gastroenterology" 2nd Edn. (Eds., Badenoch, J. and Brooke, B. N.). Churchill-Livingstone, London.

Williams, R. T. (1959). "Detoxification Mechanisms" 2nd Edn. Chapman and Hall, London.

Williams, R. T. (1970a) (1970b). "Metabolic Aspects Food Safety" (Ed., Roe, F. J. C.) Blackwell, Oxford, pp. 215, 256.

Williams, R. T., Milburn, P. and Smith, R. L. (1965). *Ann. N.Y. Acad. Sci.* 123, 110.

Willis, A. T. (1969). "Clostridial Wound Infections". Butterworths, London.

Wilson, C. W. M. (1954). *J. Physiol. (London)* 125, 534.

Wilson, G. S. and Miles, A. A. (1964). Topley and Wilson's "Principles of Bacteriology and Immunity" 2 Vols. Arnold, London.

Windmeuller, H. G., McDaniel, E. G. and Spaeth, A. (1965). *Arch. Biochem.* 109, 13.

Winitz, M., Adams, R. F., Seedman, D. A., Davis, P. N., Jayko, L. G. and Hamilton, J. A. (1970). *Amer. J. clin. Nutr.* 23, 546.

Wirts, C. W., Goldstein, F. and Wise, R. I. (1959). *Amer. J. Gastroent.* 31, 250.

Wirts, C. W., Templeton, J. Y., Fineberg, C. and Goldstein, F. (1965). *Gastroenterology* 49, 141.

Wiseman, G. (1964). "Absorption from the Intestine". Academic Press, London and N.Y.

Wix, G., Albrecht, K., Ambrus, G. and Szabo, A. (1968). *Acta Micro. Hung.* 15, 239.

Wold, J. K., Khan, R. and Midtvedt, T. (1971). *Acta path. microbiol. scand.* 79, 525.

Wolpert, E., Phillips, S. F. and Summerskill, W. H. J. (1969). *Gastroenterology* 56, 1208.

Wolpert, E., Phillips, S. F. and Summerskill, W. H. J. (1971). *Lancet ii,* 1387.

Woods, D. D. (1953). *J. gen. Microbiol.* 9, 151.

Woods, L. A. (1954). *J. Pharmacol.* 112, 158.

Wostmann, B. S. (1961). *Ann. N.Y. Acad. Sci.* 94, 272.

Wostmann, B. S. (1968). *In* "The Germ-free Animal in Research" (Ed., Coates, M. E.). Academic Press, London and N.Y., p. 197.

Wostmann, B. S. and Wiech, N. L. (1961). *Amer. J. Physiol.* 201, 1027.

Wostmann, B. S. and Olsen, G. B. (1964). *J. Immunol.* 92, 41.

Wostmann, B. S. and Bruckner-Kardoss, E. (1965). *Fed. Proc.* 24, 202.

Wynder, E. L. (1968). *In* "Prognostic Factors in Breast Cancer" (Eds., Forrest, A. P. M. and Kunkler, P. B.). Livingstone, London, p. 32.

Wynder, E. L. and Shigematsu, T. (1967). *Cancer* 20, 1520.

Wynder, E. L. and Hoffmann, D. (1968). *Science* 162, 862.

Wynder, E. L., Kajitani, T., Ushikawa, S., Dodo, H. and Takano, A. (1969). *Cancer* 23, 1210.

Yamada, T., Tipper, D. and Davies, J. (1968). *Nature, Lond.* 219, 288.

Yesair, D. W. and Himmelfarb, P. (1970). *Appl. Microbiol.* 19, 295.

Yoshida, O., Brown, R. R. and Bryan, G. T. (1971). *Amer. J. clin. Nutr.* 24, 848.

Zaki, F. G., Carey, J. B. Jr., Hoffbauer, F. W. and Nwokolo, C. (1967). *J. Lab. clin. Med.* 69, 737.

Zubrzycki, L. and Spaulding, E. H. (1962). *J. Bact.* 83, 968.

Subject Index

A

Abnormal small intestine, 48
Aesculin hydrolysis, 57, 63
Ageing, 233
Amines, 96
    pharmacologically active, 93, 229-230
Amine deaminases, 72, 75, 83, 85
Amino acid deaminases, 72-74
Amino acid decarboxylase, 91-94
Aminoglycosides, 155-158
Amygdalin,
    hydrolysis, 61, 63
    in cassava, 62
Antibiotics (see also under individual
        headings), 150-158
    gut bacteria and 20-22
Arginine dihydrolase, 95
Aromatization, 162, 163
Arylsulphatase, 159-161
Azoreductase, 85-88, 153,154

B

Bacillus
    characteristics, 28
Bacterial flora (see also Microbial flora),
    after surgery, 46-50
    antibiotics and, 21
    bacterial interactions, 23-24
    body defence mechanisms and,
        235-237
    Cancer and, 193-225
    distribution, 36-43
    factors controlling, 9-24
    gastric achlorhydria, 44-47
    hepatic disease and, 226-232
    large intestine, 43
    malabsorption and, 173-181
    mouth, of the 35-38
    normal people, 234-237
    preservation, 5
    small intestine, 38-43
    stability of, 22-23
    stomach of the, 38
    transport systems, 5

Bacterial glycosidases 54-71
    disaccharide metabolism, 65-68
    glucuronide metabolism, 54-57
    glucoside metabolism, 57-65
Bacterial interactions, 22-24
Bacteroides
    achlorhydric stomach, in, 45
    antibiotics, 21
    blind loop syndrome, 175-178
    characteristics, 26
    deamination, 72, 75
    diet and 16-20
    faeces, in, 42
    fatty acids and, 24
    β galactosidase, 67
    α and β glucosidase, 58, 59, 68
    β glucuronidase, 56
    large intestine in, 42
    mouth in, 37
    small intestine, in, 39
Bacteroides fragilis,
    characteristics, 34
Bifidobacterium
    blind loop syndrome, 14
    characteristics, 27
    deamination, 72, 75
    β galactosidase, 67
    α and β glucosidase, 58, 59, 68
    β glucuronidase, 56
    large intestine and, 42
    small intestine and, 39
Bifidobacterium adolescentis
    characteristics, 34
Bile acids, 103-123
    antibacterial action, 10, 11
    cancer and, 212-225
    deconjugation, 104-109
    degradation in gut, 122-123
    dehydroxylase, 116-122
    hydroxido reductase, 109-116
Bile composition, 144
    component metabolism, 144-149
Bile pigments, 145-146
Biliary excretion, 57, 144-149
Blind loop syndrome, 174-178
Bowel sterilization, 21

C

Cancer, 193-225
  bacterial flora, 217
  bacterial production of carcinogens, 193-201
  breast, 222-225
  colon, 212-222
  nitrosamines, 201-203
  steroids, 212-223
  stomach, 210-212
Carbenoxalone, 161
Cardiac glycosides, 58
Cascara sagrada, 54, 58, 60
Chloramphenicol, 22, 71, 79, 90, 152-153
  enterohepatic circulation of, 153
Cholesterol, 124-133
  cholesterol Δ-4-5 reductase, 125-131, 233
  enterococci and, 128
  reduction, 125-131
  side chain cleavage, 132-133
Cholanoyl glycine hydrolase, 104-109
Cirrhosis,
  amines and, 93
  urease in, 78
Clostridium
  bile acid deconjugation, 106-109
  characteristics, 28
  deamination, 72, 75
  diet and, 16-20
  β galactosidase, 67
  α and β glucosidase, 58, 59, 68
  β glucuronidase, 56
  nuclear dehydrogenation, 137-143
  phospholipase, 148
Clostridium perfringens (welchii), 28, 31, 185
  characteristics, 34
Corynebacterium,
  characteristics, 28
Cycasin
  hydrolysis of, 62-65
Cyclamate, 19, 20, 159-161

D

N-deacylase, 79
N-dealkylation, 79-80, 82, 83-85
Deamination, 72-78

Decarboxylation, 166, 167
Dehydroxylation, 164-166
Diarrhoea (see also Food poisoning), 183-192
  agents of disease, 173, 184-188
  alterations in flora, 190-191
  protective function of flora, 184
  travellers diarrhoea, 190
  weanling diarrhoea, 189, 190
Diazo reductase, 85-88
Diet
  gut bacteria and, 16-20
  and cancer, 202-4, 213-14, 223-225
Dissacharidase deficiency, 66
  β galactosidase and diarrhoea, 67
L-dopa, 74, 98-100

E

Enterobacteriaceae
  achlorhydric stomach, in, 45
  blind loop syndrome, 175-178
  characteristics, 26
  colicines, 24
  diet and, 16-20
  faeces, in, 42
  mouth in, 37
  resident strains, 22
  small intestine in 39
Enterohepatic circulation, 68-71, 152, 153
  bacteria and, 68, 71
  bile acids, 103
  bile pigments, 145
  cholesterol, 125
  detoxication, 70
  drugs, 70, 71
  β glucuronidase, 70
Enterococci
  diet and, 16-20
Environment
  antibacterial drugs, 20-22
  bacterial contamination, 15
  diet, 16-20
  Eh, pH, 7
Enzymes (see also under individual enzymes)
  limitations to study, 8
  study of micro-organisms in 3-7

Escherichia coli
  characteristics, 34
  deamination, 72, 75
  α and β galactosidase, 67
  α and β glucosidase, 58, 59, 68
  β glucuronidase, 55, 56
  in diarrhoea, 185-186
  N-esterase, 79, 152, 161
  N-ester synthetase, 78, 150, 151, 157
Eubacterium
  characteristics, 28
Eubacterium aerofaciens
  characteristics, 34

F

Faeces
  normal flora, 42, 43
Fatty acid reduction, 163
Fibre and cancer, 215-216
Folic acid, 9
Food poisoning,
  Bacillus cereus, 184-185
  Clostridium perfringens (welchii), 185
  Salmonella typhimurium, 186
  Staphylococcus aureus 187
  Vibrio parahaemolyticas, 187-188
Fusobacterium
  characteristics, 26

G

α and β galactosidase, 65-68
Gastric acid, 9, 10
Gastric achlorhydria
  bacterial flora in, 44-45
  following surgery, 46
Gastric flora, 38
  pernicious anaemia and gastric achlor-
    hydria, 44-45
Germ free animals, 13-14, 173, 233
  ageing, 233-234
  immunity, 235-237
  limitations to study, 8
  nutrition, 234-235
Glucosides, 57-65
α and β glucosidase, 57-60, 65
Glucuronides, 54-57
β-glucuronidase, 54-57
Glycoside cathartics, 58-60

Gram positive anaerobes,
  diet and, 16-20

H

Hepatic disease, 226-232
  amines and, 93, 229
  gallstones and, 230, 232
  hyperammonemia, 226-229
  phenols and, 229
  steatorrhoea and, 230
Hydroxycholanoyl dehydrogenase, 109-
    116
  7α hydroxycholanoyl dehydrogenase,
    111-114
  12α hydroxycholanoyl dehydrogenase,
    114-115
  3α hydroxycholanoyl dehydrogenase,
    115-116
Hydroxycholanoyl dehydroxylase, 116-
    122, 136-138
Hydroxysteroid oxidoreductase, 109-116

I

Ileostomy, 49
Indole production, 95, 101, 181
Intestinal absorption, 172
Intestinal bacteria,
  cultivation, 5-7
  examination, 7, 8
  growth rate, 23
  identity, 25-35
  isolation, 5-7
  specimens, 4, 5
Intestinal immunity, 12-15, 235-237
Intestinal motility, 14-15
Intestinal mucosa, 11-12
Intestinal secretions, 10-11
Intestinal structure,
  bacteria and, 235
  mucosa, 11
Immunology,
  intestinal, 12-14, 236

K

Kanamycin, 20, 21

L

Lactobacillus
  achlorhydric stomach, in, 45
  characteristics, 27
  diet and, 16-20
  faeces in, 42
  β galactosidase, 67
  α and β glucosidase, 58, 59, 68
  β glucuronidase, 56
  implantation of, 22, 23
  large intestine, 42
  mouth, in, 37
  small intestine, in, 39
Large intestine
  normal flora, 42, 43
Lactulose, 226
Lincomycin, 20
Lysozyme, 11, 13

M

Malabsorption, 172-182
  blind loop syndrome, 174-178
  normal flora, 181-182
  post pathogen, 173
  tropical, 178-181
  Whipples disease, 181
Methyl amphetamine, 79-80
Microbial flora (see also Bacterial flora)
  bacterial species comprising, 29-31
  environment, 15
  gastric juice and, 10
  host physiology and, 9
  immune mechanisms and, 12
  intestinal motility and, 14
  intestinal mucosa and, 11
  intestinal secretions and, 10
  limitations to study, 3
  metabolic activity, 28, 54-167
Morphine
  enterohepatic circulation, 71
Mouth
  bacterial flora, 36-38
Mucin, 167-168

N

Neomycin, 20
Neoprontosil, 85, 154

Neisseria,
  characteristics, 27
Nitrate reductase, 88-90, 152
Nitrite reductase, 88-90
Nitro reductase, 88-90, 152
N-nitrosation, 80-83, 201-202
  and cancer, 201-212
Nuclear dehydrogenation of steroids, 134-143
  dehydration reactions, 136-138
  double bond conjugation, 135-141

O

Oral flora, 35-38

P

Penicillin, 154-155, 156
Peptococcus
  characteristics, 27
Peptostreptococcus,
  characteristics, 27
Phenolphthalein glucuronide,
  enterohepatic circulation, 71
  hydrolysis, 55
Phenols, 96-98, 181, 197-198, 229-230
Phospholipase, 82, 147
Phospholipids, 146-149
Phosphatase, 82
Propionobacterium
  characteristics, 27
Pseudomonas
  characteristics, 26
  implantation, 26
Prontosil, 69, 85, 154

Q

Quinic acid, 163

S

Salazopyrin, 87, 154
Salmonella,
  antibiotics, 21, 22
  in diarrhoea, 186
Sarcina,
  characteristics, 27
  in faeces, 18

Senna, 54, 58, 60
Small intestine
  diverticulosis, 47
  flora and intestinal abnormalities,
    47-48, 175
  flora and surgery, 45-47
  gastric achlorhydria and, 44
  gastric surgery, 45-47
  normal flora, 38-41
  in tropical residents, 40-43, 178-179
Staphylococcus,
  characteristics, 26
  enterocolitis, 21
  in diarrhoea, 187
Specimen collection, 4, 5
Steatorrhoea, 175-177, 230
Streptomycin, 21, 155-158
Steroids, 134-143
  and cancer, 194, 212-223
  excretion, 124
Steroid nuclear dehydrogenase, 134
Stilboestrol
  enterohepatic circulation, 69
Stomach
  achlorhydria, 44
  normal flora, 38
Streptococcus,
  achlorhydric stomach, in 45
  characteristics, 27
  mouth in, 37
  small intestine, in, 39
  faeces, in, 42
Streptococcus faecalis,
  characteristics, 34
  deamination, 72, 75
  β galactosidase, 67
  α and β glucosidase, 58, 59, 68
  β glucuronidase, 56
Stickland reaction, 72, 76

Sulphatase, 159
Sulphonamides, 153, 154
Surgery,
  colonic transplant, 47
  gastric, 46
  ileostomy, 50
  ileostomy effluent, 49
  specimen collection, 4

T

Tetracycline, 20, 21
  tropical sprue and, 180
Tropical sprue, 179-181
Tryptophan, 94, 100-102, 198-201
Tryptophanase, 100-101
Tyrosine, 94, 96-98

U

Ulcerative colitis,
  salazopyrin, 154
  bacterial flora and, 237, 238
Ureamia,
  urease in, 77
Urease, 76-78, 226-229

V

Vibrio cholerae 187
Vitamin B$_{12}$, 175
Vitamins,
  bacterial production of, 234
  blind loop syndrome, 175-177

W

Weanling diarrhoea, 189-190